MEDICINE IN THE REMOTE AND RURAL NORTH, 1800–2000

STUDIES FOR THE SOCIETY FOR THE SOCIAL HISTORY OF MEDICINE

Series Editors: *David Cantor*
   Keir Waddington

TITLES IN THIS SERIES

1 Meat, Medicine and Human Health in the Twentieth Century
David Cantor, Christian Bonah and Matthias Dörries (eds)

2 Locating Health: Historical and Anthropological Investigations
of Place and Health
Erika Dyck and Christopher Fletcher (eds)

FORTHCOMING TITLES

A Modern History of the Stomach: Gastric Illness, Medicine and British
Society, 1800–1945
Ian Miller

War and the Militarization of British Army Medicine, 1793–1830
Catherine Kelly

MEDICINE IN THE REMOTE AND RURAL NORTH, 1800–2000

EDITED BY

J. T. H. Connor and Stephan Curtis

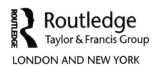

Routledge
Taylor & Francis Group

LONDON AND NEW YORK

First published 2011 by Pickering & Chatto (Publishers) Limited

Published 2016 by Routledge
2 Park Square, Milton Park, Abingdon, Oxfordshire OX14 4RN
711 Third Avenue, New York, NY 10017, USA

First issued in paperback 2015

Routledge is an imprint of the Taylor & Francis Group, an informa business

BRITISH LIBRARY CATALOGUING IN PUBLICATION DATA

Medicine in the remote and rural north, 1800–2000. – (Studies for the Society for the Social History of Medicine)
1. Medical care – Europe, Northern – History – 19th century. 2. Medical care – Europe, Northern – History – 20th century. 3. Medical care – North America – History – 19th century. 4. Medical care – North America – History – 20th century.
I. Series II. Connor, James Thomas Hamilton, 1952– III. Curtis, Stephan Michael.
362.1'094'09034-dc22

ISBN-13: 978-1-138-66154-7 (pbk)
ISBN-13: 978-1-8489-3157-2 (hbk)

Typeset by Pickering & Chatto (Publishers) Limited

CONTENTS

ACKNOWLEDGEMENTS

This collection of essays began as a series of conference papers delivered at Memorial University, St John's, Newfoundland and Labrador, Canada. Those who were invited to participate in this event hailed from Scotland, England, Norway, Sweden, Denmark, Iceland, Finland, as well as Atlantic, central and western Canada. Most of the papers presented at the conference appear in this volume.

Many who attended the conference commented that it was *worthwhile*. If so, then we have the Hannah Institute conference funding programme to thank. This programme, sponsored by Associated Medical Services, Inc. of Toronto, Canada, generously supported travel and accommodation costs for all visiting participants. We are grateful to Drs Bill Seidelman and Bill Shragge, presidents of this philanthropic agency during the time of the conference and subsequent publication of this collection of essays. Additional thanks are extended to Bill Shragge for approving the publication subvention.

Many attendees also commented that it was an *enjoyable* conference. If so, then additional funding allowed us all to savour the many sights, sounds and flavours of Newfoundland – at the most north-eastern edge of the North American continent. Accordingly we wish to express our thanks to: Dr Axel Meissen (former president, Memorial University), Dr James Rourke (Dean of Medicine), Dr Reeta Tremblay (former Dean of Arts), Mr Andy Wells (former mayor, City of St John's), colleagues in the Department of History Memorial University, and the Newfoundland and Labrador Centre for Applied Health Research.

Others also helped in many material ways in making this conference worthwhile and enjoyable, or assisted in the production of this book: Terry Bishop-Stirling, Dr Anders Brändström, Anne Budgell, Dr Jennifer Connor, Dr Catherine Donovan, Dr Nancy Earle, Dr Ólöf Garðarsdóttir, Dr Paul Hackett, Stephanie Harlick, Carol Hedd, Dr Monica Kidd, Dennis O'Keefe, Dr Marie Clark Nelson, Rosalind Nichols, Nigel Markham, June McGuire, Sinikka Okkola, Dr John Rogers, Dr Peter Sköld, Christopher Smith, and Claire Wilcox. We also would like to acknowledge the advice and encouragement of Dr David Cantor (Deputy Director, Office of History, National Institutes of Health) in his capacity as the Society of the Social History of Medicine series editor along with the external reader of these essays; their comments greatly strengthened this book.

J. T. H. Connor and Stephan Curtis

CONTRIBUTORS

Astri Andresen PhD is Professor in History in the Department of Archaeology, History, Cultural Studies and Religion at the University of Bergen. She is researching Sami History, the History of Children and Childhood and the History of Health and Medicine. She has published books and articles within the three fields, including works on rural health.

Steven Cherry PhD is Reader in the History of Medicine at the University of East Anglia, Norwich UK. He has published work on the organization of medical and hospital services from eighteen to the late twentieth centuries; mental health care in Britain; and aspects of health care in rural Europe.

J. T. H. Connor PhD is John Clinch Professor of Medical Humanities and History of Medicine, Faculty of Medicine, Memorial University of Newfoundland, St John's, Canada; he also holds an appointment in the Department of History, Faculty of Arts. He has published widely on science, technology and medicine in nineteenth- and twentieth-century North America, as well as aspects of medical museums.

Stephan Curtis is Associate Professor, in the Department of History, Memorial University of Newfoundland, St John's, NL, Canada. His interests include infant and maternal mortality, childhood diseases and the dissemination of medical knowledge in nineteenth-century Sweden.

Megan Davies is an Associate Professor in the Health & Society Programme, York University, Toronto. Current projects include: a history of home and community health in the British Columbia Peace River region; a study of health and poor law practices in the Shetland Islands; an oral history project on home birth and lay midwifery in British Columbia, 1970–90; and collaborative educational and research website projects on the history of mental health and deinstitutionalization in Canada (www.historyofmadness.ca).

Marguerite Dupree is Professor of Social and Medical History at the University of Glasgow in Scotland and a Fellow of Wolfson College, Cambridge. She is co-author, with Anne Crowther, of *Medical Lives in the Age of Surgical Revolu-*

tion (Cambridge University Press, 2007), and of articles on the history of the medical profession, on the history of hydropathic establishments, on medical practitioners and the business of life assurance and on issues of integration in the National Health Service 1948–74. She is also the author of books and articles on family history and on the history of government–industry relations in Britain in the nineteenth and twentieth centuries.

Sören Edvinsson is Associate Professor and senior lecturer at the Centre for Population Studies, Umeå University, Sweden. He is also employed at the Demographic Data Base at the same university. His research has mainly been within the fields of historical demography, and particularly health and mortality patterns of historical epidemiology and the history of public health. He has also been very strongly involved in the development of the Demographic Data Base.

Dr Francis King is a Research Fellow in the School of History, University of East Anglia, and has published on aspects of political and economic history of Russia/the USSR.

Marianne Junila holds a PhD and is University Lecturer in the Department of History, University of Oulu, Finland. Her areas of expertise include the social history of the twentieth century, war and the home front, migration, sickness and health, childhood, power and gender and Northern Finland.

Linda Kealey PhD has been a faculty member at the University of New Brunswick since 2002 and was previously a faculty member at Memorial University of Newfoundland. Her recent research and publications have focused on health care history in Canada and particularly the role of women as nurses and midwives. This research builds on her previous studies of Canadian women at work and women's involvement in labour and socialist policies in the twentieth century.

Øivind Larsen, Professor of Medical History (ret.), Institute of Health and Society, University of Oslo, Norway, studies the history of diseases, especially infectious ones, and of the development of the medical profession.

Sasha Mullally PhD is Assistant Professor of History at the University of New Brunswick in Fredericton, New Brunswick, Canada. Her research investigates the social transformation of rural medical practices in the first half of the twentieth century, focusing on the eastern borderlands between Canada and the United States.

Mette Rønsager, previously a nurse from 1987–95, obtained her PhD (2006) and has been Associate Professor at Copenhagen University 2002–3 and 2006–7, and archivist 2007. She is currently a Postdoctoral Research Fellow at Copenhagen University. Her fields of research are Greenlandic health service

1800–1955, Greenlandic women's education, and the role of women as go-betweens between Danes and Greenlanders in colonial Greenland.

Dr Art Teemu Ryymin is senior researcher at Stein Rokkan Centre for Social Studies, Uni Research, in Bergen, Norway. He wrote his doctoral thesis in history at the University of Tromsø (2003). Ryymin works with nineteenth- and twentieth-century history of health and medicine and minority history, chiefly in a northern European context.

LISTS OF FIGURES AND TABLES

INTRODUCTION:
CORES/PERIPHERIES – RURAL/REMOTE:
MEDICINE, HEALTH-CARE DELIVERY AND
THE NORTH

Stephan Curtis

This collection of essays emerged from a conference held at Memorial University in St John's, Newfoundland, in 2007 in recognition of the Fourth International Polar Year (IPY). One theme of the IPY was the investigation of the 'cultural, historical and social processes that shape the resilience and sustainability of circumpolar human societies, and to identify their unique contributions to global cultural diversity and citizenship'.[1] The maintenance of health and treatment of illness and accidents in locations such as northern Scotland, Scandinavia, Finland, Russia and northern Canada, and coastal regions such as Newfoundland and Labrador can certainly be easily linked to notions of human 'resilience and sustainability' (even if some of these northern locales are not circumpolar).

Of course climate, topography, cultural animosies or at least suspicions between providers and recipients of health care, and the financial capacity of various governments in other remote areas of the world, all shaped what could be done just as they do today. The essays in this volume focus on northern, polar societies but the strength of this collection is best demonstrated by envisioning 'the North' not solely as a unique geographical part of the world. Of course it is that but it also kindles in us images of numbing cold, and constant hardship and isolation on the one hand, and of opportunity, excitement and welcome solitude on the other. Thinking about what the 'North' means or, better still, the images it evokes enables us to see the many similarities between the societies studied in these papers and other parts of the world that were and are best understood as frontier regions characterized by the obstacles, challenges and opportunities they present.

Historians and others have modified Frederick Jackson Turner's concept of frontier and used it to frame studies in far-flung regions of the world. Many early works argued that frontiers were pushed back either because of the demands of domestic and/or export markets, or because of the initiative of adventurous people eager to carve out a livelihood for themselves. Neither case involved any great concern for people already living in these areas. More recently, Magnus Mörner demonstrates that this 'policy of exclusion' did not characterize all attempts to move into new territories. Instead, he argues that Swedes who moved northward during the nineteenth century generally pursued a 'policy of inclusion' that involved taking into account the needs and concerns of the local Sami. This is not to say that there were no sources of contention or that the relationship between the Sami and the new settlers was free of conflict and suspicion.[2]

The point here is that there are considerable advantages to envisioning 'the North' in a variety of ways that has little to do with its geographical location. The most useful of these encourage us to focus our attention on the way government officials, new arrivals and local inhabitants perceived this area. It is also worthwhile to view this area as a fluid frontier best characterized as a region of compromise and negotiation but also one where underlying sources of conflict were often aroused.[3] Both approaches offer the opportunity to discover many regions in the world that were and are, in some way, similar to the northern societies studied here.

Numerous themes and topics are raised in these essays that are relevant not only to a discussion of how medicine was practised in rural and remote areas of the recent past, but also to current attempts to improve medical care in more isolated regions of the world in the twenty-first century. For example, it is no secret that many governments and NGOs are engaged in an ongoing struggle to improve maternal and infant health throughout much of the world. These organizations and individual practitioners are confronting many of the same logistical and cultural obstacles as did their counterparts in northern Europe and North America who are the subject of this volume. How can these governments of today rationalize access to medicine and entice trained medical practitioners to work in remote areas? There has been a long history of opposition to outsiders attempting to impose new medical practices on local populations.[4] How did those doctors and midwives earn the trust and respect of their patients? What role is there for traditional and unlicensed practitioners with the encroachment of more modern medical practices?

There is obviously an argument for extending the geographical and temporal scope of any collection of essays that addresses such questions but those presented here focus on the various challenges and rewards of practising medicine in northern latitudes from the second half of the nineteenth century to the late twentieth century. It would be impossible to overstate the hardships that doctors, nurses, midwives, folk healers and patients confronted in their pursuit of good health or, at the very least, a little less discomfort in their daily lives. Similarly, it would be unfair to belittle the efforts various governments have undertaken in the past to improve the provision of health care for small and widely dispersed populations while being simultaneously constrained by very limited financial resources. However, instead of dwelling solely on these formidable obstacles that confronted practitioners and government officials, these contributions also make a compelling case for highlighting the sense of duty, of responsibility, and of genuine care for the sick shared by all those charged with bringing medical care to those who needed it.

In addition to providing a window on the development of medical practice and health care delivery in remote areas and harsh environments, these papers also augment our understanding of illness and health by complementing the numerous historical studies dealing with more densely populated environments. People who lived and worked in remote northern settlements were subject to illness and injury just as were their southern or urban counterparts but perhaps even more so. Yet our understanding of the history of medicine and health care in these pockets of population remains spotty owing in part to a lack of interest by professional historians and in part to the logistical difficulty of accessing and retrieving archival evidence from such areas. The few existing studies that touch upon medicine in isolated areas are generally focused on the United States of America and particularly the rural South. Many of these can be more accurately described as histories of rural medicine and small-town doctoring and are not particularly germane to our northern project.[5] Nonetheless, their concern with 'everyday medicine', race, class, gender and the role of the state in nation building and other related bureaucratic activities in under-populated and under-funded rural and remote areas provides additional context in which to ground this collection of essays.

If it is wise to consider 'the North' in a way that downplays its geographical characteristics, a similar case can be made in reassessing what we mean by 'rural'. There are many reasons for defining 'rural medicine' within larger social, cultural, political and even medical frameworks than simply using the geographical location in which that medical care occurred. One can, albeit unwisely, conjure up dichotomous images of rural, generally healthful environments with inhabitants engaged in all manner of quaint folk cultures on the one hand, and the disease infested urban centres with their more cosmopolitan and allegedly more scientifically advanced populations on the other. Using simplistic spatial or demographic definitions to define rural and urban areas in the regions of the world examined in this volume is bound to fail. One would be hard pressed to consider the locales and regions examined here as being even remotely 'urban' but they were all rural and remote in many different ways.[6]

These essays can certainly stand individually on their own merits or, as has been done here, be organized into groups centring on various themes such as gender, professionalization and the increasing role of the state in the provision of medical services. They also make contributions to studies investigating how innovations – whether administrative or cultural – gain support among local populations, particularly those living in rural parts of the world.[7] One way to frame such a discussion is to explore the nature of relationships between core and peripheral regions while remaining constantly aware of the limitations of such terms and particularly the potentially negative associations often made with the latter.

A recent conference held in Heidleberg entitled, 'Global Developments and Local Specificities in the History of Medicine and Health' attempted to move us away from core/periphery models because of the inferior characteristics often and mistakenly attached to the periphery *vis à vis* the core.[8] While the objective to provide more 'value neutral' terms is a noble one, a designation of 'local' or 'global' can easily evoke the same sense of struggle, domination, compliance, weakness etc. often attached to cores and peripheries. More important than perceiving our areas of study as being divided into two distinct and largely antagonistic entities engaged in a constant struggle to either impose or resist a particular practice or relationship, it is far more useful to explore the mechanisms that enabled these relationships to serve the interests of both parties. This is neither an attempt to suggest that conflict did not exist, nor is it the intention to offer a rose-coloured interpretation of the past in which everyone was prepared to sacrifice their own wishes and wants for the common good. The essays presented here make it abundantly clear that suspicion if not outright loathing often coloured the relationship between the providers and receivers of medical care. However, these essays also demonstrate that the form of care that finally emerged was the product of negotiation rather than declaration, and of compromise rather than intransigence.

Immanuel Wallerstein's seminal work of the early 1970s examined the economic relationships and mechanisms by which core regions of the world were able to exploit those at the periphery.[9] Historians and other academics quickly adopted this model of exploitation and dominance and applied it to their own studies. For example, Heikki Vuorinen's examination of infant mortality patterns dating from the late 1980s identifies core regions as those that exert 'economical, social, cultural and political dominance over [the] periphery at the hierarchial [*sic*] level under investigation'.[10]

In recent years two major challenges to the assumptions underlying Wallerstein's work have emerged and this collection of essays adds support to these new interpretations. The first questions the ability of the core to exert hegemonic control over areas outside of it, and the second recognizes the multiplicity and fluidity of core and peripheral regions within single countries.[11] Historians, especially those engaged in anti-colonial studies, are increasingly challenging the assumption of an inherently passive periphery and the result has led to the not surprising discovery that peripheries have not always been as acquiescent as politicians and central bureaucrats may have wished.[12] To some degree this opposition was possible because of the logistical difficulties central governments faced when trying to introduce and enforce new reforms in remote areas. However, ascribing the delayed acceptance of new innovations solely to the inefficiency of past bureaucracies is only a partial explanation and increasing attention is being placed on the fortitude of local populations to influence decisions and practices. Nonetheless, the importance of local providers of health care and regional administrations who brought improvements to distant communities continues to be frequently overlooked and this is especially so when discussing underdeveloped regions of the world.[13] Instead the focus of attention tends to fall most heavily upon the efforts of leading bureaucrats and medical officials who more often than not lived in far distant capital cities.

We have also become more aware that countries typically consist of multiple domestic cores and peripheries. This is an important development for two reasons. First and foremost, it highlights that research ought to focus on exploring the mechanisms by which these different areas form relationships rather than looking at them in isolation. Secondly, it demonstrates more clearly than examining international connections the fluid nature of relationships. That is to say, one region might be considered a 'core' *vis à vis* some other territory but it may well find itself to be peripheral to developments occurring elsewhere.

Certainly the articles in this volume examine the relationship between core regions of political and medical authority and the peripheral, distant outposts in which many of the doctors and other medical practitioners found themselves. However, while many of these locales certainly shared the geographical and demographic characteristics we associate with designations of 'rural', they were also defined by their social and cultural distance from the nearest administrative centres. City-trained doctors, nurses and midwives frequently complained about the relative isolation of the communities and regions in which they worked but many also found it difficult to understand and adapt to local cultures that were as alien to them as the remote locales in which they lived. Simply stated, these articles examine medical practice in rural settings but these environs were more than just physically distant from the centres of administrative influence. Those charged with the responsibility of bringing medical innovations to these areas also had to consider the unique environments consisting of unfamiliar cultures and social structures, and the local concerns of the people they encountered. These challenges were as daunting as were the logistical obstacles to delivering medical care to a sparse population in largely isolated communities.

This collection of essays also adds to the recent literature that employs notions of core and peripheral areas to help understand the process by which ideas are spread through a community and the circumstances under which innovations are either accepted or rejected by local populations?[14] There has been a large shift away from Torsten Hägerstrand's works of the mid-twentieth century that explained geographical patterns of innovation diffusion largely as a result of 'distance decay'.[15] Researchers have more recently included in their analyses many more social, demographic and cultural variables into their calculations to understand the forces that determine receptivity to innovations.[16] By so doing they are challenging the largely top-down model of diffusion and emphasizing instead a process of dissemination that takes into account the role played by those who are encountering new methods and ideas for the first time.[17] In short, emphasis has shifted somewhat away from exploring the way in which innovations are spread through a society, to examining why they are either accepted or rejected. This requires a thorough understanding of the environment in which those new methods and ideas were introduced.[18]

The work of Thomas Valente and others who explore the importance of social networks in determining an individual's decision to either accept or reject a new innovation is particularly relevant to the works in this volume.[19] While none of the articles presented in this volume specifically examine processes of diffusion and dissemination, many of them do demonstrate the importance of local networks to the acceptance of new innovations. These networks came in many forms: the numerous lay women Megan J. Davies studies who incorporated various medical theories in the Peace River region of British Columbia, Canada; the distant networks of patients in northern Newfoundland and the local physicians who kept in contact with their colleagues in the United States of America that are the subject of J. T. H. Connor's research, or the Greenlandic midwives with their ties to Danish and indigenous societies that Mette Rønsager examines. In each case the creation of networks between practitioners and their patients contributed to the gradual acceptance of new medical techniques and forms of organization.

It is within these larger debates about the characteristics of cores and peripheries and the relationship between them that these papers make significant contributions. These authors are not simply examining rural medicine as a wholly autonomous entity produced and delivered in parts of the countries far from central authorities. Instead, they all illuminate the interaction of medical practitioners and the people they encountered, and how the medical care that emerged was the result of cultural negotiation, administrative limitations, political agendas and the initiatives of local doctors, midwives and nurses.

What did medical care entail for those charged with providing it in the nineteenth century and onwards? For many of the practitioners studied here it meant much more than simply attending to the physical needs of the sick. Sören Edvinsson demonstrates that for Dr Ellmin in nineteenth-century northern Sweden, providing medical services to the people in his region was both a consequence and an expression of a political radicalism that demanded he provide the best care possible to all who needed it regardless of their social status. At the same time, there is no denying that he very much wanted to 'improve' and 'civilize' many of those he encountered in much the same way as colonial powers wanted to do the same to the people they encountered in far distant colonies. Teemu Ryymin shows that early twentieth-century physicians in northern Norway who were responsible for bringing medicine to the Sami, and the state officials who sent them there, expressed similar goals as did Ellmin almost a century earlier. Norwegian voluntary groups also saw the medical care they provided as a means to introduce modern ideas to what they perceived as a largely 'backward' population. Mette Rønsager's contribution to this volume reveals that Danish authorities tried to use midwives to bring more advanced medical practices to the people in Greenland throughout the nineteenth and into the twentieth century.

There is no doubt that many practitioners were attracted to their profession and the remote parts of their countries by a sense of adventure. Dr Ellmin certainly felt it as he set off to tend to those in distant villages. The nurses in New Brunswick, Canada, who are the focus of Linda Kealey's contribution, and their counterparts in twentieth-century northern Finland who are the subject of Marianne Junila's study, also saw their work as an adventure and enjoyed the professional autonomy of working without the close supervision of a physician.

We should not forget that medical care also had a political function. It could be used to try and create a sense of unity among the people as was attempted in nineteenth- and twentieth-century Norway. By the late 1900s numerous countries sought ways to safeguard the cultures and rights of indigenous peoples. The Norwegian Government, for example, recognized that native medical practices were integral to preserving Sami identity and therefore introduced measures to ensure that they survived. In Scotland, the Highlands and Islands Medical Service attempted to bring medical care to a region that quite simply could not otherwise afford it. As it turned out, this experiment was so successful that its influence can still be seen in how the National Health Service (NHS) is organized today.

This collection does not specifically try to interpret the wishes, fears, concerns and frustration of those who needed medical care, but their voices are not entirely absent. Of course we are limited by the sources available to us. Very few people indeed kept personal diaries of their innermost thoughts or their usually infrequent encounters with medical practitioners. If such sources did, at one time exist, it is highly improbable that they are still extant. It is sometimes possible, as Davies does so brilliantly in her contribution to this volume, to conduct interviews or rely on oral histories to inform our knowledge of relatively recent times. Unfortunately, the range of sources available when seeking a more comprehensive understanding of earlier times is much more limited. In most cases we only have the records of those responsible for bringing medicine to those people who either needed it or, in some cases at least, had it imposed upon them; the patients themselves are seldom clearly heard.[20] Despite the emphasis of the essays presented here and the limitations of the authors' sources, one can discern the constant murmur of patients' voices in the background. Whether we are relying on official documents, physicians' reports, diaries, interviews or the multitude of other sources used in this collection of essays, there is no mistaking patients' suspicions regarding new methods and practitioners, their concerns about the possible consequences of those innovations for their culture and their fears when confronted with childbirth, debilitating diseases or severe accidents. Finally, we are constantly made aware of their demands to be included in decisions regarding their health and the medical care they would receive. These sentiments were as present in the nineteenth century as they were in the twentieth and were heard throughout the regions studied here. Nonetheless, even today governments and other agencies continue to ignore the wishes and concerns of those living in remote regions upon whom new innovations are to be practised.

The first group of papers by Steven Cherry and Francis King, Marguerite Dupree, Teemu Ryymin and Astri Andresen provide a thorough examination of the attempts by the Russian, Scottish and Norwegian governments to exert greater control over the medical services in the distant parts of their respective countries. In 'Medical Services in a Northern Russian Province', Cherry and King explore the cultural and logistical obstacles to providing improved medical care in the period of *zemstvo* government between 1864 and 1917. On the one hand, local officials faced a well-entrenched hostility directed towards outside authority, a peasantry that was loathe to accept new medical innovations and a constant shortage of funds. Bureaucrats worked diligently to address these problems but there was nothing that they could do about the region's isolated location, extreme poverty or harsh environment. For all of these reasons it is not surprising that they found it difficult to recruit medical practitioners. Russia's defeat in the Crimean War highlighted the need to rationalize the administrative districts and the provision of medicine. The various levels of administration quickly learned that the number of trained medical practitioners was far short of the number needed; but a lack of funds made it impossible to hire additional doctors or even the less-skilled *feldshers*. One option was to find ways to entice those few physicians already present to take on additional duties. Unfortunately, this met with only very limited success and the state found it necessary to improve the training of *feldshers* who could attend to the medical needs of the rural population. Such measures proved fairly successful but the cultural distance between the trained practitioners and the people they tried to help was not so easily overcome. Local traditions were difficult to change, and efforts to impose new public health measures were often met with suspicion.

Dupree's contribution demonstrates the ability of a remote, relatively poor and scarcely populated area, in this case the Highlands and Islands of Scotland, to influence the reorganization of the NHS in 1974. After the creation of the national insurance legislation in 1911, the Highlands and Islands Medical Service (HIMS) was devised to respond to the very poor health of the population, and the poverty and lack of medical care that characterized the region. Trained medical practitioners were in especially short supply and hospitals were few and far between. The goal of the HIMS Fund was to provide finances that could be used to entice practitioners to the area and to improve communications and hospitals. As part of the plan, in return for providing medical services regardless of where the patient lived, a doctor was able to charge a fee collected from the patients themselves or, if they were too poor to pay, the doctor received compensation from the HIMS Fund. In this way doctors received state funding administered directly by the Scottish Office in Edinburgh, but remained 'independent contractors', neither entirely dependent upon the state for their livelihood nor on the patients they treated. The HIMS received glowing recommendations in the Cathcart Report of 1936 and again a decade later when the NHS (Scotland) Bill was introduced. The question emerged how best to administer a healthcare system to which everyone had access, and in 1948 in the Highlands and Islands the NHS replaced the HIMS with the same tripartite mixture of agencies as in the country as a whole. It consisted of regional hospital boards, executive councils overseeing local general practitioners, and local authorities employing medical officers of health responsible for enforcing public health measures. Another examination of the provision of health care in the Highlands and Islands occurred between 1964 and 1967 and, although some measures were recommended similar to those found in rural Norway, there was little sense that anything substantial had to be changed. This is not to say that no problems existed; many of those that had prompted the creation of the HIMS still remained. The high costs, difficult transportation and the large distances between physicians and widely dispersed patients could not easily be overcome. The major problem, however, was with the way in which the different types of medical care were provided. Few people in the Highlands and Islands felt that the tripartite division of administration was particularly efficient and welcomed the proposal that all health services be brought under one central authority. This structure was to serve as the basis for the reorganization of the NHS in 1974.

Teemu Ryymin's article examines the Norwegian Government's campaign against tuberculosis among the Sami during the first half of the twentieth century. There had been a long history of 'Norwegianization' which sought to eliminate or certainly minimize differences within the population and this policy survived until the mid-1940s. Underlying this official policy was the assumption that the Sami people were a backward people who needed to cast aside their culture and language if they were to survive. Government appointed medical officials and voluntary organizations were responsible for providing care to the inhabitants of the northern County of Finnmark where extreme poverty contributed to very high rates of tuberculosis. Early missionaries to the region in the late 1800s flouted official policies and preached to the population in the local language in an effort to spread the word of God which they assumed would help the Sami avoid poverty and disease. Various religious associations were responsible for providing much of the care the Sami received and, despite some opposition, they found that the people were grateful for it. The problem was that these missionaries were caught trying to preserve Sami culture and identity on the one hand, while simultaneously trying to 'improve' the Sami on the other in what Ryymin calls a 'paternalistic civilizing project'. It was in this context that the state and various voluntary organizations launched their campaigns against tuberculosis which included the construction and staffing of nursing homes, sanatoria and hospitals. In addition to these physical improvements to the medical landscape, it was also decided that there should be a comprehensive health education programme put into place. What is crucial here is that tuberculosis was no longer blamed primarily on the alleged backwardness of the Sami but rather on the effects of industrialization and the introduction of modern society. This did not mean that the Sami were seen as being as culturally advanced as the Norwegians but rather that economic and social change was now considered to have contributed to their plight. The state began providing funds to improve housing and education – most often in Norwegian – all in the hope of 'improving' the Sami. The agenda shifted in the 1920s and 1930s when the state began screening children throughout the country for signs of tuberculosis. Part of the reason for this shift was new medical knowledge that no longer saw tuberculosis as one of the inevitable consequences of economic growth and civilization, but as an infectious disease that could be combated by purely medical rather than cultural means. Nonetheless, efforts to create a homogenous, Norwegian-speaking population persisted until the early 1950s when the government agreed to print public health information in the Sami language at the same time as its screening campaigns became ever more comprehensive. The period from the late nineteenth century to the mid-twentieth century had witnessed a major change in the status of the Sami. From being perceived as a backward people who needed to be Norwegianized for their own benefit, state officials in the 1950s became more attuned to the needs of the Sami and to providing medical care on their own terms.

Astri Andresen examines the provision of health care to the Sami in northern Norway during the second half of the twentieth century. Immediately after the Second World War, the state committed to providing a uniform standard of medical care across all of Norway. During these early years there was little attention paid to the possibility that the Sami ought to be recognized as a distinct population: this only occurred in 1989. Language was one of the major obstacles to providing health care to the Sami and recognizing them in their own right. Initially they were simply expected and required to learn Norwegian but in 1959 Sami became an official language in the area where they lived. This was partly seen as a way for the state to disseminate public health information to those whose command of Norwegian prevented them from discussing such things with local, Norwegian-speaking physicians. By the 1950s there was no doubting that levels of health among the Sami were much lower than among those living in the rest of the country and medical authorities, and the Sami Committee (the group charged with making recommendations to the government) in particular, saw this not only as unacceptable but contrary to the government's alleged goal of ensuring the health of everyone living in Norway. By this time it was no longer accepted that the poor health of the Sami was due to some alleged racial or biological inferiority. The only agreed upon remedy was greater state intervention but the question then arose about what form that involvement should take. While it may have been advantageous to provide physicians who spoke the local language, this was not seen as practical especially as the number of patients who spoke Sami seemed to be declining. Nonetheless, the government did begin to encourage Sami students to attend medical schools with the hope that they would be able to take what they learned back to their communities. The problem of language was only one of those faced by government officials. There also remained those of large distances, poor transportation and a harsh climate which made it difficult to recruit physicians and other health practitioners. One solution was to create a northern university that could recruit students from the Sami-speaking population and train doctors who could tend to the needs of those living in the north.

The 1980s and 1990s saw the question of how to provide adequate health care to the Sami take on an international perspective with the ratification of ILO Convention 169 in 1990 concerning Indigenous and Tribal Peoples in Independent Countries. Matters of health were now framed within the larger context of legal rights and, as such, now demanded not just equal access to medical care but also the preservation of Sami identity. However, as Andresen demonstrates, this did not result in the Sami assuming sole control over the social services provided to them. Instead, the Norwegian government now addresses the specific needs of this population but as part of the national policies it offers. An example of this can be seen in the government's willingness to promote knowledge of traditional medicine as a way to preserve Sami culture while simultaneously providing doctors with all the skills and knowledge one might expect them to receive from a medical school. This contribution demonstrates the process by which the 'marginal' or 'peripheral' Sami was assimilated into the larger Norwegian discourse of medical care and how they were able, despite this assimilation, to maintain their distinct culture and to at least partially dictate the pace and form of their inclusion into Norwegian society.

The second group of papers in this volume explores how physicians attempted to establish identities for themselves and the strategies they employed when interacting with local populations and central authorities in their struggle to combat a plethora of medical problems. Here cores and peripheries are not solely administrative or geographical constructs but rather suggest a cultural distance between those who are bringing new methods to remote communities and those who are exposed to them. Sören Edvinsson locates Dr Ellmin, a physician who found himself under suspicion because of his alleged radical activities in Stockholm, firmly within the various cultural ideas and medical debates that characterized nineteenth-century Europe. Ellmin found himself stationed in a remote part of the country and his annual reports to state authorities not only fulfilled his professional obligations, but also reflected a desire to discover, record and enlighten a people about whom he felt much of Swedish society knew nothing. His topographies also illuminate debates within the medical field about the direction that state medicine should take. Should it be primarily concerned with improving the environment in which people lived, or modifying the behaviour of those people to ensure they adopted more suitable and healthy habits? Here then is a doctor who had considerable experience working in the Swedish capital thrust into an economically, socially and culturally peripheral society. One sees in his annual medical topographies the nineteenth-century obsession with the discovery of new lands and new peoples. Ellmin certainly believed that he and the state had a moral obligation to civilize the people he encountered but he was no mere government lackey. There is no doubt that he was a hard-working doctor who took his duties seriously but his reports also reveal his genuine concern for the local population and his sincere attempts to exert pressure on the government to improve their living conditions and access to health.

Øivind Larsen uses a combination of several physicians' medical topographies from much of the nineteenth century and modern statistics to reveal the tremendous obstacles that Norwegian physicians encountered in their efforts to ensure a healthy population. More importantly, these sources reveal what these doctors *thought* were the most pressing areas of concern and how legislation was often the product of perception rather than quantitative data. The Sanitation Act of 1860 represents one of the key pieces of legislation as it marked the state's commitment to preventing outbreaks of cholera. As a result of this legislation the powers of district physicians expanded and, as representatives of the state, they worked closely with local officials. The doctors' annual reports thus record a variety of voices representing different levels of administration particularly during the last third of the nineteenth century. Larsen's work demonstrates that there was not always a clear correlation between the doctors' perception of the general state of the public's health and levels of mortality or morbidity. For example, doctors in the capital of Christiania (Oslo) appear to have paid little notice to the high level of mortality in the city. Larsen suggests this may have been due to the fact that they had become somewhat accustomed or perhaps immune to it. Whatever the case, it appears that simply exploring quantitative mortality data will not always explain the introduction of legislation aimed at improving the public's health. If we are to make sense of the actions of bureaucrats and physicians we must recognize the importance of what they perceived to be the causes of concern and at what point those concerns demanded action. As Larsen suggests in his work, although urban centres may have been characterized by their lack of sanitation and their unhealthy populations, this did not necessarily mean that physicians were more active in the towns and cities than in rural areas. In fact, it is entirely possible that outbreaks of disease among formerly healthy people living in pristine and wholesome countryside may well have been more likely to gain the attention of health officials.

J. T. H. Connor's study of Dr Robert Ecke, who came from the United States to work in the small, isolated town of Twillingate, Newfoundland, during the 1930s illustrates the importance of personal networks for the diffusion of ideas – in this case from Europe via Baltimore in the United States of America, to this distant island community in the North Atlantic. The provision of medicine in and around the town had a relatively long history and Ecke certainly continued many of the local traditions. However, this study illuminates the importance of Henry Sigerist, Director of the Johns Hopkins Institute of the History of Medicine, for the type of medical care that the people of Twillingate received. His 'fervent advocacy of socialized medicine' was to influence those who later moved to this isolated town to deliver health care. However, the local population also had a tradition of helping one another and this practice of mutual assistance in times of need served as the foundation upon which Ecke and others were to build their medical careers. Although Ecke certainly came from an urban environment and possessed considerable formal medical training, Connor shows that he was forced to adapt quickly to local customs and the limitations imposed upon him by the harsh environs in which he worked. Twillingate was indeed far removed from the life and intellectual climate of Johns Hopkins University. Nonetheless, this geographically peripheral town was very much the centre of the medical and cultural world of north-eastern Newfoundland.

Sasha Mullally examines the creation of a medical profession in the Canadian maritime and bilingual province of New Brunswick during the early twentieth century. Using the case of an American trained physician who may or may not have completed his studies, Mullally demonstrates that the New Brunswick College of Physicians and Surgeons took its gate-keeping function very seriously indeed. However, despite the provincial College's efforts to marginalize and eliminate unlicensed medical practitioners, the geographical and cultural distances between the trained, primarily urban physicians and the rural population divided between anglophones and francophones were not easily overcome. It is in New Brunswick, Mullally argues, that we see tensions emerge between different economic, political, social and cultural regions. One common feature of all these areas was a population determined to receive good medical care. This demand enabled unlicensed doctors and midwives to practise despite the best efforts of the College to prosecute them and remove them from the medical landscape. What we see is not the emergence of a clear-cut division between professional physicians united against unlicensed and 'unorthodox' practitioners, or between urban and rural. Instead, the medical landscape of New Brunswick during the 1920s and 1930s allowed for compromise, accommodation and shifting alliances and agendas.

The final group of contributions examines the role of women as medical practitioners in the past two centuries as they negotiated the fuzzy boundaries between orthodox and unorthodox, core and peripheral medicine. There is no doubt that women have a long history of being the main providers of care although their role has often been marginalized in the historical record partially because of their presumed lack of formal training. Of course recent research has done much to restore both traditional and formally trained female practitioners to the medical landscape. The contributions of Mette Rønsager, Linda Kealey, Megan Davies and Marianne Junila represent important additions to this literature and illuminate the importance of midwives, nurses and unlicensed healers in bridging the gap between administrative and cultural cores and peripheries. Moreover, in all four works we see women challenging the constraints that society imposed upon them. While it might be argued that here were women still confined to the more traditional roles of midwives and nurses, they fulfilled these roles in very untraditional ways. They often undertook lengthy and dangerous journeys by themselves during which they demonstrated that they were very well skilled and could act independently of male supervision. Their activities, devotion to duty and the proficiency with which they carried out their responsibilities frequently earned them the respect of all their patients.

Rønsager explores how Greenlandic midwives in the nineteenth century not only mediated between Danish authorities and the native population, but also how they brought ideas and methods from Europe into the periphery of Greenland. In this case we see the coming together of two disparate cultures aided by the ability to overcome the problem of distance between two widely separated geographical regions. It is not surprising that early Danish doctors seldom treated native Greenlanders. First, the distances they would have needed to travel were enormous. Second, the language barrier made it almost impossible for patients and doctors to converse with one another. High infant and maternal mortality was of primary importance to local authorities and physicians and all agreed that well-trained midwives could do much to improve the likelihood of mothers and infants surviving childbirth. Greenlandic women were initially trained in Greenland but increasingly were sent to Copenhagen to receive their training. However, those who travelled to Denmark usually belonged to the Greenlandic elite and this introduces a class dimension, in addition to those of gender and culture, to the analysis of medical care in Greenland. As does Edvinsson, Rønsager shows the cultural distance that existed between the urban administrators and trained male practitioners on the one hand, and the native population that they perceived as childlike and primitive on the other. Although intrinsically important to the introduction of modern medicine to the people of Greenland, the midwives educated in Denmark fulfilled an additional role that was no less important. This was to bring European culture to the people. Some did so quite eagerly but the majority did so only reluctantly thereby enabling them to maintain their native identity at times that suited them.

The contributions by Kealey and Davies also examine the essential role that nurses and unlicensed female medical practitioners played in providing care to people living in rural parts of Canada during the 1920s when the government and other organizations first began to focus more attention on the state of rural medicine. As Kealey demonstrates, those living in non-urban parts of New Brunswick were particularly dependent upon the public health nurses of the Canadian Red Cross Society (CRCS) who remained a main source of medical care into the 1970s. These women often worked far from urban centres and found that they were very much on their own during times of medical emergency. While this autonomy provided tremendous opportunity for improving one's skills and certainly appealed to many of the nurses, many also found it intimidating to be forced to engage in practices for which they were not trained. Moreover, there was always the possibility, if not the likelihood, that physicians would perceive them as encroaching upon their areas of alleged expertise. While these women initially responded primarily to the medical needs of the local populations, by mid-century they were also taking on the responsibility of introducing public health measures as dictated by the provincial government. What we see throughout the whole period from the 1920s through to the 1970s was the close relationship between the voluntary CRCS and the provincial government as they pursued the common goal of improving the health of the population in New Brunswick.

Davies shifts our attention away from the formally trained female nurses and focuses instead on the importance of lay women as healthcare providers in a remote interior region of northern British Columbia during the 1920s. The case of Emily Tompkins reveals this woman's resourcefulness in dealing with a serious emergency and the plethora of lay and scientific medical practices that she and others employed when dealing with common ailments and diseases. By using a variety of different oral and local histories, Davies is able to conclude that women used their capacity as primary caregivers to create an identity for themselves which they used to enhance their social position in the 'belated frontier' of the Peace River region. This contribution clearly illuminates the intersection of lay, folk medical practices and the more 'scientific' ones to which the sick were exposed. During the 1930s the Peace River region was increasingly integrated in the provincial economy and roads linked it to other centres. In this environment doctors, nurses and midwives provided medical care but so, too, did women with no formal training whatsoever. 'Home medicine' competed equally with 'scientific medicine' and the experienced (or most resourceful) women of the communities were afforded the same respect as their more formally trained female and male counterparts.

Junila also examines the challenges that distance can bring to the provision of medical care in her study of northern Finland during the two decades after the Second World War. It continues to be the case in the countries examined in the volume that it is in the most remote areas that medical practitioners are least likely to be found. Various strategies to entice trained physicians, midwives and nurses to these regions have seldom proven entirely successful. However, Junila is less concerned with illuminating how these difficulties hampered efforts to bring medicine to Lapland and instead focuses her attention on the allure of such harsh conditions on the women who became public health nurses. For some it was the sense of duty that enticed them to head north; for others it was a sense of adventure, while others welcomed the opportunity to enjoy much more autonomy than was available elsewhere. Whatever the case, there was no doubt that they were embarking on an often dangerous journey that would put tremendous geographical and cultural distance between them and all that had been familiar. Far from urban centres and the supervision of doctors, these women performed diverse tasks that they otherwise would have been prohibited from undertaking. In many cases public health nurses had to adapt to local customs while simultaneously trying to introduce new medical techniques to a sceptical or fatalistic population. In other cases, these women were welcomed by enthusiastic and grateful people who had long sought access to a skilled medical practitioner.

These essays deal with nineteenth- and early twentieth-century societies found in the northern latitudes that shared similar topographies and similarly harsh northern climates. They were, then, in what we commonly call 'the North'. While some of the characteristics of this region were unique to it, there were and still remain other frontiers and peripheries of the world that present many of the same challenges and opportunities. The medical practitioners found in these essays were responsible for providing health care to local populations. They endured the daily hardships of surviving in such an inhospitable environment and had the added burden of negotiating between different cultures. They represented the state and outside authority, and brought new innovations to previously isolated communities. It is no wonder that their arrival often caused the sick to view them with no small amount of suspicion. Nonetheless, in relatively short order these practitioners became integral members of community life. This was no small feat and can be attributed only to the perseverance of these men and women, their resourcefulness, and their willingness to find areas of common ground between them and their patients. Government officials similarly struggled to provide the best level of care possible within often strained financial circumstances. It would be a gross exaggeration to suggest that these bureaucrats were able to divorce themselves entirely from their own prejudices and beliefs about those living in the rural, distant lands. These people were seldom seen as social and cultural equals but it would be difficult to see in these essays anything but a sincere effort to improve their health and well-being.

PART I: REMOTE MEDICINE AND THE STATE

Introduction

The authors of this section illuminate some of the major challenges states confronted in their efforts to provide medical care in remote areas. One problem was to attract and retain skilled medical practitioners willing to work in such isolated and physically demanding surroundings. Government officials also found it difficult to maximize the medical benefits they could offer while keeping costs firmly under control. This certainly was no easy feat when a small population was dispersed widely over a hostile environment. A sense of suspicion, both on the part of the medical practitioners and the intended recipients of medical innovations further complicated the efforts to introduce a more uniform level of medical care. Those living in the northern-western province of Russia that Steven Cherry and Francis King discuss were particularly reluctant to accept medical 'outsiders' and this was a major obstacle to the spread of academic medicine. Taken together, the contributions by Teemu Ryymin and Astri Andresen reveal a long history of state involvement in the provision of medicine to the Sami. During the course of the twentieth century the Norwegian government gradually abandoned its efforts to impose its perception of medical 'improvements' upon those living in the far north. Instead, it launched a comprehensive medical initiative particularly during the second half of the century that consisted of large financial expenditures and a new-found respect for Sami culture. This coincided with international movements whose mandates were to preserve and acknowledge the importance of indigenous cultures. To that end, newly trained Sami doctors are now able to provide their patients with modern and traditional medicines. The major challenge facing government health officials in twentieth-century Scotland was largely logistical rather than cultural, but tensions existed even within this homogeneous population. Marguerite Dupree's analysis demonstrates that although the Scottish government introduced a much more rational and streamlined form of medical care than had ever existed, local residents frequently questioned whether the organization of the HIMS provided the best possible solution to their medical needs. Their input helped inform the legislation that finally emerged.

The contributions to this section reveal that attempts to introduce cost-effective medical systems was as much a challenge to the Russian authorities of the late nineteenth to early twentieth century as they were to Scottish and Norwegian authorities even in the late 1990s. In each case the success of central governments depended upon their ability to adopt policies that would enable them to overcome logistical problems while simultaneously minimizing sources of cultural tension. Some of these movements were motivated and directed entirely by domestic concerns but Ryymin and Andresen show that international forces eventually influenced medical legislation that emerged in Norway during the second half of the twentieth century.

1 MEDICAL SERVICES IN A NORTHERN RUSSIAN PROVINCE, 1864–1917

Steven Cherry and Francis King[1]

Russian zemstvo medicine is a purely social matter. Treatment by a doctor in the zem-stvo is not a personal service to the patient at his expense, nor is it an act of charity. It is a social service.

M. Ia. Kapustin[2]

This paper investigates the organization of medical services under extreme con-ditions, in some northerly parts of European Russia during the era of *zemstvo* reform: the period of rural self-government that existed between 1864 and 1917. It concentrates on the north-western *guberniya* (province) of Olonets, now largely part of the Republic of Karelia.[3] An area characterized by its remote-ness, relatively harsh geographic and climatic conditions and meagre economic resources from which to finance medical services, Olonets was also perceived as 'culturally backward'. Its inhabitants were often suspicious of or antagonistic towards outside influences, whether in the form of governmental authorities or would-be improvers in health, hygiene and medicine. Arguably, the reluctance of health-care professionals to work in such an environment aggravated mat-ters, although there were also distinct attractions in practising *zemstvo* medicine. Given such contexts, the study has relevance to suggested 'core and periphery' and 'distance decay' issues (see the introduction to this volume) affecting health care provision in remote areas.

The wretchedness of Russian peasant life in the late nineteenth century, readily apparent to contemporary observers, has also been a reoccurring theme for modern historians.[4] Russia's northern provinces posed particular difficulties, as each contained *uezds* or districts,' that were remote and barren, lying on or within the Arctic Circle. The northernmost province of Arkhangel included the strategically important ports of Murmansk and Arkhangel'sk but was otherwise very sparsely populated. With much of economic activity featuring the sea-sonal migration of reindeer and the nomadic Sami herders, the *zemstvo* reform of 1864, whose system of local government depended on settled communities, was not extended to Arkhangel *guberniya*. The provinces of Vologda and Perm' also had very sparsely populated northern *uezds*, though their southern districts were considerably more developed. Olonets was thus the most northernmost province included within the *zemstvo* reform. A wholly rural and sparsely populated area, it featured a harsh climate with average temperatures hovering around freezing point.[5] The local provision of rudimentary – but largely free – health care therefore occurred under extreme conditions, yet shared the characteristics of the emergent *zemstvo* medical system as it was implemented throughout European Russia.[6]

Early Health Measures and the *Zemstvo* System

During the eighteenth century, Russia's size, poverty and alleged 'backwardness' constituted formidable barriers to the erratic and top-downwards modernization of the body politic. Measures to promote commerce, business and the professions using controlled electoral procedures and the granting of charters to towns and nobility also produced local leaderships concerned with public health, morality and limited philanthropic effort.[7] By the early nineteenth century, the Ministry of the Interior assumed some responsibility for public health, conventionally depicted as 'hampered by extreme shortage of medical personnel and medical stores, both of which were still further reduced by the demands of the army ... the hostility of the peasants and the indifference of the educated classes'.[8]

Medical qualification, licensing and regulation were state controlled. Amongst the 8,000 physicians practising in 1845, the degree-qualified and licensed *vrach* were outnumbered by *lekar* with their basic, five years' training.[9] Physicians might harbour professional and even political reform agendas but their official status and functions in sanitary policing, dissection, hospitalization and the supervision or monitoring of local healers led district populations to identify them with state authority.

Although health measures, private practice and medical personnel were concentrated on St Petersburg and Moscow, several agencies offered patchy and rudimentary provincial services. *Prikaz* (Office of Public Welfare) provision, largely uncoordinated and urban, included some 500 provincial hospitals with almost 19,000 beds by the early 1860s. Provincial and district public health committees, established from 1845 onwards, monitored epidemics to little immediate effect and, like the provincial hospitals, had a poor reputation with the peasantry. Since the 1820s the Ministry of Appanages had provided physicians and *feldshers* (semi-trained health workers) for 'court' peasants in the service of the imperial family, and the Ministry of State Domains made similar arrangements for peasants on state lands. During the 1850s this constituted a rural system of sorts, and by 1867 some 350 physicians provided training and supervision for roughly 5,500 *feldshers* who were mainly responsible for outpatient clinics and domiciliary visits.[10] Meanwhile, the number of village pharmacies had tripled between 1827 and 1852, by which time there were 1,200 in operation, along with some 250 *lechebnitsy* (local clinics) reportedly attracting increased peasant attendances.[11]

Defeat in the Crimean War in 1856 emphasized Russia's need of modernization and reform, seen in the emancipation of the peasantry from 1861 and the establishment of the *zemstvo* system in 1864. This system, consisting of locally elected assemblies based on a restricted, property-owning franchise, offered a degree of self-government in thirty-four *guberniyas* of European Russia. In addition to the provincial assemblies, *zemstvos* were simultaneously created for district subdivisions. The Ministry of Internal Affairs retained its own 'reach' into the countryside but the *zemstvos* were granted powers of local taxation and greater responsibilities, notably for education and public health. 'Improvement' in these areas had no specific form or agency, however, and the position of the *zemstvo* was ambiguous: conceived as part of state power and a source of expertise, they were potentially also a forum for opposition and professional interest, as seen in the development of health care.[12]

The *zemstvos* inherited limited *guberniya*-level health facilities and hospitals, although those at the *uezd* level barely existed and more remote areas were completely devoid of trained medical practitioners. With no template to shape its emergence, the '*zemstvo* system' of health care was piecemeal but innovatory and acclaimed by its supporters. Thus A. A. Sinitsyn, an early *zemstvo* physician recalled, 'nowhere in the West did we have any precedents for this, and in Russia up to that time nothing had been done in this direction: therefore, we had to start from scratch, not having any models for guidance'.[13] The system was characterized by its devolved organizational forms, an emphasis upon public hygiene and preventive medicine as well as treatments, and the promotion of modern medical care not conditional upon the payment of fees to physicians.[14] Another strongly influential but sometimes constraining feature was the emphasis on 'fairness'; the ambition that medical service provision should be equally accessible to all inhabitants, wherever they lived. In 1894, the *Entsiklopedicheskii slovar* described *zemstvo* medicine as 'the pride and glory of the *zemstvos*, Russia's unique contribution to public health, developed without previous example in the West and adapted especially to Russian needs'.[15] However, the historian and leading contemporary authority Boris Veselovsky also noted uneven or delayed developments in many areas, particularly in the deployment of public health measures and the organization of *guberniya*-level doctors' congresses.[16]

Veselovsky's observations are relevant to the situation in the province of Olonets *guberniya*, where the delivery of medical services to a scattered, poverty-stricken population provided a daunting challenge. Three-quarters of the province's 150,000 km² – an area the size of England and Wales – were covered by forests and lakes, the latter aiding communications during the short summer. A limited growing season vulnerable to unreliable weather and poor quality soils in all but the southernmost districts meant that agriculture was underdeveloped. Serf-owning landlordism had hardly featured in most areas prior to emancipation, and peasants on former state lands practised subsistence farming, often using slash-and-burn methods because there was insufficient open ground or livestock to manure the soil.[17] Agricultural productivity remained low, and although hunting, logging and fishing were vital supplementary activities, the province was still a net importer of foodstuffs in the twentieth century.[18]

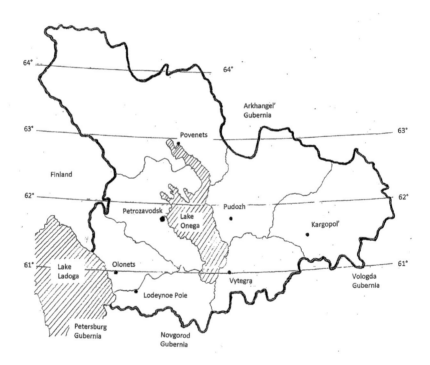

Figure 1.1: Map of Olonets *guberniya* and *uezd* towns, Russia.

The Olonets *guberniya* was divided into seven *uezds*: Petrozavodsk, Olonets, Vytegra, Kargopol', Lodeynoe Pole, Povenets and Pudozh. Each of these were named after principal towns which were mainly marketing or administrative centres but essentially agglomerated village settlements. Rural peasants still comprised 92 per cent of the provincial population in 1913, with just 4 per cent regarded as 'townsfolk'. One half of the latter lived in Petrozavodsk, from 1781 the *guberniya* 'capital' and easily the largest town with 10,961 people in 1868 and 18,878 by 1913. Olonets town was more typical of the remainder of the villages; its 1913 population was just 2,095.[19] Generally the provincial inhabitants were dispersed, numbering barely 300,000 in 1867, 368,000 at the 1897 census and over 425,000 in 1913, when 78 per cent were Russian, 16 per cent Karelian and 4 per cent Estonian.[20] Logging, which employed roughly 3,000 people, and iron-working, developed from mining and works begun under Peter the Great before 1714, were the principal industries. There was no railway link between major cities until 1914 and, in 1916, Petrozavodsk was the last Russian *guberniya* capital to be connected to St Petersburg. Steamship and inland navigation was confined to the summer months which meant that settlements were linked to one another only by tracks, paths and a few seasonal roads for most of the year. Further industrial development, particularly after 1861, produced more wage and migratory labour but also brought associated health problems as discussed below.

Zemstvo medical services in Olonets *guberniya* broadly developed according to a pattern seen elsewhere in Russia. In a flush of reforming zeal, delegates at the first *guberniya* assembly in 1867 resolved:

> To instruct the guberniya uprava [executive board] to act immediately to put an end to the population's lack of medical assistance. It should establish how many feldshers will be needed in the volosts [rural subdistricts], what medicines are needed, whether village midwives are required and how many. It is to report on all this to a future assembly.[21]

The gulf between the assembly's potential as an improving agency and its likely attainments was exposed within months when the second assembly was informed that seven doctors (one per *uezd*) and fifty-five *feldshers* (one per *volost*) were needed to bring health care up to standard. Yet there were currently no *uezd* *zemstvo* doctors and only thirteen *feldshers*; to recruit and pay such personnel would cost almost 20,000 roubles annually – double the entire first health care budget.[22] In 1868 this cost increased to 21,500 roubles, with state-funded hospital treatments for sick soldiers, prisoners and certain state employees providing limited forms of subsidy, notably for doctors' salaries.[23] Meanwhile the provincial *nachal'nik*, the state official overseeing local administration, complained that the *uezd zemstvos* had neither produced proper annual budgets nor allocated funds for medical services. Optimistically attempting to square this circle, the second *guberniya* assembly resolved 'to find ways in which medical work can be improved without spending significant sums on it'.[24] One short-term expedient was to pay supplements to state-employed town doctors undertaking *zemstvo* duties additional to their usual work of examining army recruits, conducting autopsies and so forth.[25] Even then, the town of Pudozh had no doctor and four other towns each relied upon medically qualified political exiles.[26]

The *guberniya* hospital in Petrozavodsk had just one doctor, whose salary, along with those of the town doctors, was 'paid from the money received from the Office of Public Welfare for keeping sick servicemen in hospital'.[27] Initial assessments of existing hospitals, services and equipment and of obligations inherited from the Office of Public Welfare were not encouraging. Ninety-one general hospital beds were available, including fifty-four at Petrozavodsk hospital, which also had a six-bed psychiatric wing, plus twelve or so at district hospitals in Lodeynoe Pole, Olonets and Pudozh. These were poorly equipped and, according to Dr I. A. Shif, 'were exclusively in the hands of the fel'dshers ... the degree of trust shown by the population corresponded with the overall state of these hospitals'.[28] As for the provision of other medical services in the *guberniya*, he concluded, 'in the first ten to twelve years of the *zemstvo*'s existence it retained the same insignificant organization ... bequeathed by the Prikaz and the Chamber of State Property'.[29]

Prior to any improvements much of the existing infrastructure required making fit for purpose. Thus Vytegra *uezd zemstvo* took over the town hospital in 1867, finding this institution 'extremely run down, without money, without linen, without the necessary medical equipment ... its first task was to ensure the hospital was properly run'.[30] The *guberniya nachal'nik* complained in 1870 that district health care provision remained 'unsatisfactory' but did not offer any obvious remedies so the *zemstvos* canvassed their doctors for suggestions.[31] Dr Krashevsky of Lodeynoe Pole suggested the subdivision of each *uezd* into six medical districts, each with a resident *feldsher* who would be visited and supervised by a *zemstvo* physician. A modified version of this plan using four sub-districts was adopted, 'until ways of increasing the *zemstvo*'s funds can be found which are more reliable and less burdensome for the population'.[32] However, Dr Lit (Pudozh) was already emphasizing preventative medicine, implementing better health education in schools and homes, and hygiene improvements. These public health measures were to be 'achieved partly by spreading correct views among the population about health ... and partly by removing those factors which continually act to cause disease'.[33]

Feldshers, Doctors and Hospitals

Feldshers comprised the majority of front-line medical personnel in areas such as Olonets with some rural stations previously established by the Ministry of State Domains passing into *zemstvo* control after 1864. Most *feldshers* were then untrained or semi-trained male nurses, either ex-army medical orderlies (*rotnye fel'dshera*) or former children's home residents who had been apprenticed to hospitals. For example, in 1867 the Ministry of Internal Affairs sent Moscow orphanage boys to Olonets province as newly-trained *feldshers*, although they were fit only for hospital work under the supervision of a doctor.[34] With each physician responsible for an area larger than an English county, such supervision was notional although, with the developing *raz"ezd* or circuit system, physicians undertook month long tours of their districts two or three times each year, holding clinics and monitoring local *feldshers*. These arrangements also reflected the goal of 'fairness', providing people with the opportunity to access qualified doctors. One-time Moscow *zemstvo* doctor Evgraf Osipov recalled how initially '*uezd* zemstvos tried to organize physicians' services in such a way as to be equally accessible to all zemstvo ratepayers'. In the eyes of this physician, 'they were too concerned with the idea of "zemstvo equality"'.[35] Yet other *zemstvo* representatives approved this extension of medical services into the countryside that did not necessitate finding, appointing and funding too many scarce and expensive physicians: according to contemporary historian Veselovsky, 'the dominant view was that cheap feldsher services were adequate for the peasants'. They were seen as 'necessary as an intermediary between the doctor and the population', and, with the *feldshers*' salaries lower than those of doctors, 'the zemstvo can only afford the former'.[36]

Doctors bemoaned their time lost in travelling and doubted the clinical capabilities of *feldshers*, criticizing their 'scattering' of medicines and emphasizing instead the need for preventive measures.[37] Most eventually favoured Dr Osipov's system of 'rational medical help', that is, seeking to combine Western sanitary models with fixed facilities within smaller medical districts (*uchastki*), with the prospect of sustained treatments and greater medical influence over proximate populations.[38] The *uchastok* model combined public health measures with medical care in smaller subdistricts that ideally included a physician, a small hospital, a pharmacy, outpatient clinics, a midwife and *feldshers*. Just nineteen *uezds* in *zemstvo* Russia (eight within Moscow *guberniya* itself) had adopted the stationary system by 1878, but forty-seven had done so by 1890 and 138 by 1900. In the same period, *uezds* solely employing the circuit system fell from 134 in 1880 to just two by 1900, leaving perhaps 200 *uezds* using hybrid systems.[39]

Diagnoses and treatments made by *feldshers* remained the norm for most of the population of Olonets *guberniya*, particularly in remote areas, despite *zemstvo* doctors' reservations and insistence that 'the right to treat illnesses independently is the exclusive preserve of the doctor'.[40] There were 1,350 *feldsher* medical stations across Russia in 1870 and this number rose to 2,800 by 1890 when numbers stabilized partly in response to the increasing presence of physicians.[41] Given prevailing conditions, no *uezd* in the province of Olonets fully adopted the system of fixed surgeries in manageable medical districts, and local *zemstvo* doctors still spent at least some time on tours. Yet the establishment of a comprehensive network of *feldsher* stations represented considerable progress: the thirteen *feldshers* in *zemstvo* service in 1867 rose to seventy-five by 1891, even if fifty of them were under-trained and required replacement according to the 1896 Olonets doctors' congress.[42] Replacements remained difficult to attract to the region: Dr Isserson of Lodeynoe Pole acknowledged that he 'had on more than one occasion approached the *feldsher* schools in Moscow and St Petersburg and had always received the same reply: nobody wants to come to work for you.'[43]

Rather than dispense with the *feldshers*, Olonets *guberniya* involved doctors in the development and qualification of these practitioners. The training school, opened in Petrozavodsk in 1899, aimed to overcome shortages and deficiencies by offering *uezd* grants to suitable students. In return they were obligated to provide eighteen months of qualified paid service as a district *feldsher* for each year of financial assistance.[44] By 1906 a network of over ninety *feldsher* stations with roughly 100 personnel, sixty-five suitably trained, boosted popular access to basic levels of treatment.[45] The level of general education, capabilities and medical knowledge of these practitioners also improved and, reflecting their new-found pride and status, seventy-five Olonets *feldshers* established their own professional and mutual aid association in 1913.[46]

By 1881 every *zemstvo* district had at least one doctor, although geographical areas and potential patient numbers varied enormously, the 1905 ratios of doctors to inhabitants ranging from 1:4,900 in Petersburg *uezd* to 1:65,200 in Nikol'sky *uezd*, Vologda *guberniya*. The average *zemstvo* doctor's area varied between 130 km^2 in Moscow *uezd* and 24,202 km^2 in the *uezd* of Ust'sysol'sky, again in Vologda *guberniya*.[47] Veselovsky heroically concluded from such diversity 'that the typical *uezd* at this time is one with a radius of sixteen to seventeen versts per doctor's district and one doctor per 25,000 inhabitants'.[48]

Although Olonets *guberniya* was not the worst provisioned for qualified doctors, the situation there was extremely challenging for practitioners. Five doctors in the north-eastern district of Povenets were each responsible for about 6,000 people scattered over 8,000 km^2 and limitations aggravated by climate and terrain were only partly offset by the work done by *feldshers*.[49] With just 3,500 roubles available for doctors' salaries in 1868, the *zemstvos* initially sought to contract existing government doctors for their medical work. Thus Dr Lyubichankovsky, appointed as Olonets *uezd zemstvo* doctor, was already the state-employed district and town doctor for Olonets and 'also held the same three positions in Lodeynoe Pole *uezd*. He lived in Lodeynoe Pole and visited patients if he was in Olonets'.[50] These unfeasible arrangements were exposed by the 1871 cholera outbreak, which affected 518 people and killed 293. During this period the Ministry of Internal Affairs had to provide three additional epidemic doctors, since local practitioners, 'obliged to be in two different places at the same time, one on government service, and another as a *zemstvo* doctor', were unable to cope.[51]

Advancements occurred all the same. Fifteen *uezd zemstvo* doctors attended the first Olonets doctors' congress in 1887, suggesting limited improvement, although *feldshers* still provided most medical treatments. Dr Isserson of Lodeynoe Pole reported that he undertook monthly circuits around six *feldsher* stations under his supervision and personally saw 22 per cent of their 6,212 outpatients in 1886. He also visited some larger settlements lacking any medical personnel, but found that emergencies or epidemic outbreaks disrupted methodical work:

> [I]t would be useful for the doctor to visit more often, and it is highly undesirable to leave patients entirely to the care of the feldshers. But we have to accept this as a necessary evil ... given the size of the uezd and the appalling state of the roads ... Even with monthly visits, the doctor spends almost two-thirds of the time travelling about the uezd [52]

At the 1896 doctors' congress, Isserson described the appearance of an additional *feldsher* station and the medical subdivision of his district into three *uchastki*. This meant that the doctors required less travelling time and were able to hold extra clinics for patients.[53] Since 1892 over 14,000 patients had been treated annually, possibly suggesting greater confidence in medical treatments and their improved efficacy and availability.[54] Yet some villages and settlements remained over 50 km from the nearest surgery in 1907 when Dr Shif estimated that just 15 per cent of the provincial population had access to *zemstvo* doctors in cases of serious illness.[55] Similarly, Dr Libov of Lodeynoe Pole hospital reported in 1912 that, because of isolation, workloads and travelling, 'doctors' posts in our *uezd* remain unfilled for a long time and doctors often leave after a short period of service'.[56]

Nevertheless, there were more qualified personnel like Dr Libov on the scene by the early 1900s. *Zemstvo* hospital services expanded in European Russia from the 11,400 beds inherited from *prikaz* arrangements in 1864 and was able to provide roughly 26,600 beds in 1890 and 30,100 by 1898.[57] Although the initial focus upon provincial-level hospitals consumed limited resources, later developments featured better rural hospital services, often in conjunction with moves towards the stationary system and the abolition of fees in most district hospitals. During the 1890s the number of *zemstvo* village hospitals rose by almost 50 per cent to provide roughly 12,900 beds compared with 11,700 and 5,500 beds available in the town and provincial hospitals, respectively.[58] This suggests that there was greater accessibility, although the ratios of population to hospital beds still varied enormously: at least 11,900:1 in Tula, an industrializing province south of Moscow, compared with 300:1 around St Petersburg.[59]

Hospital development in Olonets *guberniya* was slow before the mid-1880s while existing facilities were upgraded, but thereafter each *uezd* had its own hospital offering between twenty and twenty-six beds. In 1887 Petrozavodsk *guberniya* hospital still officially had fifty-four beds, with just five for women patients, although Dr Andrusevich reported up to eighty-five inpatients in the hospital at any one time.[60] Kargopol' hospital, which also had facilities for six-teen prisoners, was 'old, and could not withstand criticism from the hygienic point of view'.[61] Povenets hospital had been 'built without regard for the lat-est requirements of hygiene', while amenities were poor at Lodeynoe Pole.[62] However, the Olonets and Pudozh hospitals were better and construction of a new district hospital was underway in Vytegra, a town of 2,800 inhabitants.[63] Subsequent developments included a degree of medical specialization, some rebuilding or renovation and the addition of outlying facilities. Thus by 1903 Petrozavodsk hospital had 202 beds with an additional surgeon, psychiatrist and ophthalmologist, appointed respectively in 1890, 1900 and 1903. District-level facilities were complemented by the addition of nine village hospitals, the smallest in Arkhangely with five beds, and in more remote areas some thirteen self-contained 'casualty wards', each with a few beds served by the local district doctor.[64] Concerns over fairness and accessibility shaped hospital provision to the extent that in 1890 the *guberniya zemstvo* assembly rejected a request from Kargopol' for funds to build a cottage hospital in Konevo village since 'it should not be built in Konevo, but in a more distant and remote location'.[65]

Public Health Measures

Most *zemstvo* doctors adopted a 'root causes' approach to sickness, regarding their public health work as critical. The development of bacteriology aided diagnoses and preventive measures thereby reinvigorating the 'medical enlightenment' of the uncivilized which involved hygiene and health education.[66] Antisepsis, asep-sis and specific treatments for diphtheria and syphilis, successively building upon the success of the earlier smallpox vaccination, also bolstered the claims and sta-tus of scientific medicine. Yet genuine progress remained patchy and uneven, not least because the underlying social conditions associated with ill-health went unimproved. Grinding poverty accompanied by insufficient diet and clothing, appalling domestic conditions, little appreciation of hygiene and extensive disease levels, accompanied by the worst infant and child mortality in Europe, were identifiable in Russia long before they were quantified.[67]

In practice, many doctors merely condemned the peasantry or bemoaned their own isolation. Thus Dr V. Smidovitch, formerly an unpaid hospital assistant in St Petersburg *guberniya* and *zemstvo* doctor, felt that 'anyone who is but slightly acquainted with the conditions of our rural life will agree that its poverty and lack of culture entirely shut off the ordinary practitioner.'[68] Veselovsky quoted a woman doctor D. I-va: 'you and the inhabitants speak entirely different languages and neither understands the other. There is nobody with whom to exchange a few words, with whom to share impressions, to ask for advice or instructions.'[69] Frieden's broader study of Russian physicians similarly suggested that 'the most serious defect was Russia's cultural backwardness. Illiteracy, compounded by ignorance, fatalism, distorted religiosity, and centuries of tradition reigned in the countryside.'[70]

Peasants might link illnesses with spirits, winds, words or glances and, in addition to prayer for protection or assistance, their traditional healers 'to some degree accompanied their treatment with chants, invocation and suggestion and ... surrounded the procedure with mystery'.[71] Midwives *(povitukhi, babki)* had a wider healing role and used herbal remedies, as did shamans *(znakhari)* and witches *(kolduny)*.[72] O. Tian-Shanskaia, an 1890s eye-witness, was highly critical of untrained midwives, citing their usage of sacramental wine for malnourished babies; of chewed-up food in rag pacifiers and their shaking or turning of infants suffering from diarrhoea.[73] Others joined with mothers in leaving it to God to decide the fate of sick or emaciated 'old' babies not expected to survive.[74] Stoic practicality matched grim realities, for example in the practice of making gifts of dead children's clothes.[75] Moreover, peasants who identified doctors and isolation procedures with intrusive authority might hide their sick children or deny the presence of infection.[76] As Dr Smidovitch noted, 'doctors in the employ of our *zemstvos* constantly draw attention to the reluctance displayed by peasant women, and especially girls, in availing themselves of medical aid'.[77]

Zemstvo medicine battled against these customs and attitudes with variable success and gave them serious consideration in the planning of particular campaigns and general organizational arrangements. In 1872 the Perm' *guberniya zemstvo* appointed Dr I. I. Molleson as Russia's first public health doctor *(sanitarnyy vrach)*. He and other *zemstvo* doctors were initially limited to gathering information, without clear guidelines as to subsequent procedures, let alone tangible results.[78] Responses to the 1865 legislation and central directives to combat smallpox outbreaks, for example, were variable rather than uncooperative. Such directives frequently relied upon minimally trained clergy or school teacher vaccinators *(ospenniki)*. During the early 1870s these pandemic personnel were demonstrably ineffective; vaccine supplies were inadequate or spoiled and few follow-up checks or revaccinations occurred. Simeon Leskov, a priest and *zem-stvo* deputy in Petrozavodsk, had expected improvement but complained in 1874 that

> the feldsher of Sholtozerskaya was paying no attention to ... smallpox, for which a reli-able method of controlling its spread had been discovered long ago ... we have seen no help either from the doctor, or from the feldsher, not to speak of the other diseases.[79]

Subsequent developments included better vaccine supplies and administra-tion by trained *feldshers*, midwives and medical students, particularly under the stationary *uchastok* model.[80] In Olonets, Dr Isserson advocated compulsory vaccination to overcome peasant resistance, but acknowledged that supply prob-lems led to hazardous child-to-child vaccination:

> [W]hen vaccinating using human lymph, it is very easy to inject some constitutional disease, primarily syphilis, as there are many syphilitic children in the villages and it is impossible to ensure that cowpox is taken only from healthy children[81]

Such difficulties were only overcome after the *guberniya* hospital established its own calf shed, and by 1901 almost 8,500 vaccinations were undertaken annually with an almost 97 per cent success rate.[82]

Cholera was less destructive in Olonets *guberniya* than elsewhere and occa-sional outbreaks, as in Lodeynoe Pole in 1892, were associated with river traffic. Counter-measures included isolation procedures with 'strict supervision of all steamers arriving and departing ... and barracks for those infected were set up in Lodeynoe Pole, Sermaks and Voznesen'e'.[83] These barracks aroused considerable peasant suspicion and during the 1908 typhus outbreak in Kondushi village no one would enter them. Overcrowded dwellings were an accepted fact of peas-ant life, as were traditions of visiting those affected by disease, 'sometimes not because of need, but out of curiosity'.[84] The steam cleaning or disinfection of clothes was also resisted, partly because the chemicals involved were associated with some 'trace of the infectious spirit', and conflicts arose over 'the custom of the better-off population giving away the deceased's clothing'.[85] Nevertheless, doctors claimed that, 'by strictly carrying out disinfection measures, we were able to limit the spread of scarlet fever and cholera'.[86]

Efforts to combat syphilis, which was in rural areas initially associated with increasing trade and communications and spread largely by non-sexual means, faced particular difficulties.[87] Experimental measures, such as seasonal syphilis hospitals at Voznesen'e village (1872) and Vodlitsa (1876) for migrant workers on the inland waterways, failed to attract patients.[88] Because communications and transport relied heavily upon local, state or police authorities, confiden-tiality in relation to syphilis cases requiring hospital treatments was always threatened, further compounding peasant suspicions of surveillance and authority.[89] Most Olonets doctors thus opted for educative and persuasive methods, arguing that coercion would merely produce evasion. Meanwhile, the number of registered syphilis cases steadily increased from 2,410 in 1899 to 6,146 in 1910. It is significant that in this year, even in remote Olonets, physicians knew of the introduction of Salvarsan – no evidence of distance decay here. Kargopol' *uezd* sanitary council requested the drug for trials as early as November 1910 and arranged for medical training in its administration by February 1912.[90]

Midwifery

Olonets *guberniya*'s infant mortality rate, averaging 344 per 1,000 births from 1867 to 1881, considerably exceeded European Russia's rate of 276 per 1,000.[91] Seeking to establish one trained midwife *(akusherka)* in each *volost*, the provincial medical administration initially substituted peasant girls with one-year's training under medical direction.[92] Unimpressed, Dr Isserson argued that in his district, 'most of the *zemstvo* midwives are women who can hardly sign their own name' and were ill-equipped for the 'almost missionary activity' needed to overcome peasant suspicion.[93] Despite claimed affinities with local women, trained midwives attended only about 6 per cent of births in the province by the early 1890s, with *uezd* doctor Shepilevsky attributing continued high infant mortality to peasant customs, notably 'a firmly rooted view that the act of birth, to have a successful outcome, should take place in strict secrecy, so that nobody could cast the "evil eye"'.[94]

Unless the midwife herself was known and trusted, *zemstvo* midwifery services were used only by less superstitious peasants or those seeking medical help in the event of complications. Midwife Kropacheva attended just three births in Kargopol' *uezd* in her first year, 1882, compared with sixty-six in her final year, 1893. A year later her successor attended only twenty-four deliveries, leading Dr Ol'gsky to conclude that 'in general peasants do not get used to "the midwife" but to "Praskov'ya Mikhaylovna", "Appolinar'ya Alekseevna" and so on'.[95] The *guberniya* medical authorities persisted with attempts to use trained midwives or *feldsher*-midwives to win over peasant women on the basis of personal familiarity, since such personnel might then also act as vaccinators, health visitors or advisers on gynaecological problems and sexually transmitted diseases. Yet the forty-two midwives and *feldsher*-midwives in *zemstvo* service in 1896 still attended under 7 per cent of births – a problem not unique to Olonets province.[96] Some twenty Russian midwifery schools offered peasant girls one or two years of hospital training in exchange for a period of rural practice in the late 1870s. By 1905 a similar number of rural *zemstvo* schools contributed to the 10,000 or more trained midwives. However, at least 6,000 of these women ended up in urban or private practice compared with the less than 2,500 midwives who remained in rural areas. Obviously these women were not particularly attracted to such remote locations and rural populations.[97]

Partly in response to Russian government medical departmental guidelines, Olonets *guberniya* appointed Dr Nikolaevsky to undertake a broad 'topographical-medical and statistical-sanitary survey' in 1885.[98] Government officials then met northern *guberniya* representatives to discuss the establishment of sanitary bureaux and councils; notification procedures for infectious diseases; morbidity and mortality data; and public health budgets, which duly became agenda items at the inaugural Olonets doctors' congress in 1887.[99] Dr Chuvaev, head of Kargopol *uezd* hospital also proposed 'common measures for stopping, as far as possible, the further spread of syphilis'.[100] Yet he was required to allay fears among unsympathetic *zemstvo* deputies that such congresses wasted public money and doctors' time, arguing that 'the congress, even with all the travelling to it from the most remote points, would not take a doctor away from his district for more than twenty days'.[101] The assembled doctors duly pronounced there were insufficient resources, personnel and time for effective sanitary bureaux to develop, arrangements restated as 'unmanageable' at their 1896 congress, because doctors were still 'spending massive amounts of time travelling about, owing to the particular geographical conditions of Olonets *guberniya*'.[102] Although Dr A. A. Tsvetaev was eventually appointed to develop a *guberniya* sanitary bureau in 1912, there were no signs of assisting personnel before 1914.[103]

Conclusions

Improving health care in Olonets *guberniya* was not simply a matter of inputs from core to periphery being affected by distance, though remoteness was a seasonally compounded underlying problem. Medical appointments, better hospital facilities, smaller medical districts and greater attention to public health issues suggested progress in terms of professional, medical 'supply side' criteria, by inference of benefit to rural populations, even in more remote and inhospitable areas. Yet central initiatives were rare and 'improvement' was interpreted by provincial and district assembly representatives who, even when sympathetic, had to consider differing medical and lay views concerning how to proceed alongside financial constraints. Problems were compounded by the need to convince a pragmatic and sometimes suspicious peasantry, resentful of any coercion.

Local doctors regarded increasing usage of medical facilities as evidence that 'the population's trust in medical personnel has grown'.[104] Yet the latter were not necessarily physicians since, in poor or remote areas like Olonets, the training and supervision of auxiliary health workers rather than their displacement was the feasible option for medical and lay authorities. Even as the stationary *uchastok* system extended, *zemstvo* doctors needed to compromise, acknowledging economic realities and also mediating scientific knowledge, perhaps in recognition of their peasant clientele and political paymasters, or because their outlook was shaped by broader forms of social medicine. For many 'the socio-logical approach to disease, couched as it was in socio-economic terminology, perhaps appeared as *a more recognizable* medical theory than others of a more purely laboratory nature'.[105] If such approaches shaped *zemstvo* medical practice, they were also not unknown in France, Germany or Britain before specific and bacteriological measures became predominant in preventive medicine.[106]

Doctors aiming to shape health services and assert professional dominance had to acknowledge the influence of *zemstvo* deputies over limited health budgets. In 1905, most of Russia's 23,500 qualified medical practitioners were actually urban-based directors of hospitals, with more than 4,500 in private practice and 6,800 in military service.[107] For the minority seeking alternatives, not least to 'serve the people' in rural areas, *zemstvo* medicine offered health care arrangements more independent of state or commercial controls. Yet in 1910 the 3,082 *zemstvo* doctors were still outnumbered by government non-military medical personnel (3,940 in 1907), although Table 1.1 illustrates their improv-ing district-level profiles.[108]

Table 1.1: *Uezd*-based *zemstvo* doctors, 1865–1904.[109]

Year	Number of *zemstvo* doctors in *uezds*	Doctors per *uezd*	Total *uezd* doctors in Olonets *guberniya*
1865	48	0.087	6 (1866)
1875	904	2.30	8
1885	1,347	3.76	14
1895	1,840	5.41	21
1904	2,608	7.08	26

Health auxiliaries possibly acted as a bridge between initially suspicious local populations and practitioners of modern medicine, although in Olonets this appears to have been more true of *feldshers* than trained midwives. Peasants' familiarity with medical personnel was critical in shaping attitudes towards health care services and their endorsement of prescribed measures was shaped by their experiences and subjective attitudes as well as by distance, terrain and physical communications. Effective measures, such as vaccination or cataract procedures, were met with peasant pragmatism rather than overt hostility but ineffectual practices, notably the inability to arrest the process of infection once underway, did little to abate older customs.[110] In many respects modern medicine had yet to demonstrate its claimed superiority, particularly concerning surveillance, isola-tion or seemingly invasive measures and, meanwhile, untrained but experienced midwives and other healers were valued.[111] Coercive measures and bureaucratic complexities or inflexibility aggravated these problems: in Pudozh *uezd* the organization of patient transport and arrangement of inevitable documentation alone could take a whole month before the process of hospitalization began.[112]

Veselovsky's early twentieth century comparison of *zemstvo* with non-*zemstvo* areas in European Russia, broadly demonstrated that greater proportions of the sick, whether as hospital patients or outpatients in domiciliary settings, were seen by qualified doctors under *zemstvo* medicine.[113] *Zemstvo* medical spending per capita was also higher than elsewhere in Russia, barring the Baltic provinces.[114] However, John F. Hutchinson suggests there was a retrenchment in *zemstvo* medicine after the 1905 Revolution. He criticizes its lack of sanitary engineering and underdevelopment of bacteriological measures, although his conclusion that 'the administration of public health at the local level was such a shambles that it almost defies description' seems harsh.[115]

Whether as exception or rule, experiences in Olonets commend cautious interpretation of the more fulsome claims made for *zemstvo* health care. Veselovsky cited the Olonets *guberniya* as 'the worst provided with medical services, while at the same time taxation is higher here than anywhere else', attributing this to the conservatism of leading provincial *zemstvo* figures.[116] Vadim Badanov's recent comparative survey noted medical services spending by 1903 of 1.05 roubles per capita in Olonets, compared with 0.97 and 0.64 roubles respectively in the 'model' Moscow and St Petersburg *guberniyas*.[117] This situation might reflect the extremities surrounding health services provision: unlike many *guberniyas*, Olonets did not charge outpatients for treatments or medicines, presumably because few were able to pay.[118] Dr Shif, a direct participant, attributed limitations before 1880 to 'a shortage of funds, a low population density and a low cultural level', making unfavourable comparisons with those provinces quicker to establish smaller medical districts headed by doctors.[119]

Apparent medical spending inefficiencies might thus reflect extra costs imposed by free treatments, huge distances, rudimentary infrastructure and harsh climatic conditions. Health spending actually increased in absolute and proportional terms within district budgets, noticeably in Olonets *uezd*, from 13.5 to 35.0 per cent between 1877 and 1901. The Povenets *uezd* allocation had the least expansion, but still grew from 18.6 to 25.2 per cent in the same period.[120] With responsibilities also for education and other services it is difficult to see how significantly higher proportions of district budgets could be allocated to health care: this was not a case of an 'improving' centre and unresponsive peripheral agencies. Provision still varied: there were 6,000 people per doctor in Povenets *uezd* but an average of 23,200 in Kargopol' *uezd* in 1905, although such ratios were less than in most parts of *zemstvo* Russia.[121] Neighbouring Arkhangel *guberniya* lacked *zemstvo* institutions but had a population of comparable size, just exceeding 400,000, albeit scattered over a still wider area where features such as distance decay might loom larger. Here in 1909 there were just sixteen doctors, only half of whom were engaged with the rural population, compared to the thirty in Olonets *guberniya*.[122]

Allowing for the suggested conservatism and bureaucratization of some leading *zemstvo* personnel, there were considerable efforts in Olonets *guberniya* to develop medical services and their more equitable distribution. Initial consolidation of existing facilities was followed by additions to *feldsher*, midwife and medical personnel, as with district and village hospitals or outlying casualty wards, with greater emphasis also upon public health measures. Central prompting was not the key feature and extreme conditions largely determined that the province retained hybrid arrangements featuring *feldshers*, the *raz"ezd* (circuit) system and *uchastki* (medical stations), but which were still very much part of the *zemstvo* medical system. Olonets *guberniya* was not unique or stubbornly 'backward' in the persistence of some older forms of healing or in its underdevelopment of sanitary engineering and health education measures in comparison with metropolitan standards. Its continuing medical shortcomings need to be contextualized, not within the limits of the *zemstvo* system but within the more general inequities and unevenness of Tsarist Russia.

2 CHANGING MINORITY CULTURE: HEALTH SERVICES AND HEALTH PROMOTION IN NORTHERN NORWAY, 1900–50s

Teemu Ryymin

A fundamental feature of Norwegian public health work since the 1860s has been the conviction that reforming popular culture could prevent disease and promote health. The aim of many medical doctors and state public health officials in late nineteenth- and early twentieth-century Norway was to inculcate a healthy 'culture' where it was deemed absent. The culture promoted was one defined as healthy by mostly middle-class medical doctors and representatives of the state medical establishment; the lifestyles and 'bad habits' that were to be changed or discarded altogether could vary depending on factors relating to gender, class, or spatial dimensions – for example, rural and remote regions.

Ethnic minorities have historically represented a challenge for public health work. The habits and ways of living among such minorities could be – and often were – deemed as 'foreign' and condemnable by the medical establishment, which subjected these populations to vigorous campaigns of cultural change. This was, of course, also the case with the Norwegian rural population after the 1860s and the urban working class from the turn of the twentieth century. Ethnic minorities posed an additional challenge because of language: both the straightforward issue of how to convey a health message to a population that did not always understand the Norwegian language, but also more complex issues pertaining to the relationship between language, culture and health.

In this article, I will analyse the work of the Norwegian Sami mission to build social and health institutions for the indigenous Sami population in Finnmark, as well as the fight against tuberculosis in this county in the first half of the twentieth century, in order to elucidate the changing role that language and culture played in the shaping of public health work in a multi-ethnic context.

Multi-Ethnic Finnmark *c.* 1900

Finnmark is the northernmost county of Norway, extending over approximately 46,400 km² north of the Arctic Circle. It borders with Russia to the east, Finland to the south, and the county of Troms to the south-west.[1] In 1900, the county's population numbered approximately 32,800, making it the most sparsely populated county in Norway.[2] The Norwegian-speaking population, chiefly fishermen and small farmers, constituted 55 per cent of the county's population, with the rest divided among the indigenous Sami (28 per cent) and Finnish-speaking immigrants and their descendants, known in Norway as Kvens (17 per cent).[3] Along the fjords, coastal Sami, Kven and Norwegian fishermen and farmers were settled in partly segregated communities, while the interior of the county formed the heartlands of the nomadic reindeer-herding Sami. Among the minorities, knowledge of Norwegian was often scant or non-existent, despite official efforts to teach them the language of the national majority.

Since the mid-nineteenth century, the Norwegian state authorities were concerned that the minorities could pose a threat to national security by acting as a 'fifth column' for Russian (and from 1918, Finnish) interests.[4] Accordingly, the minorities were subjected to a state policy of linguistic assimilation; school teachers and priests were instructed to use Norwegian instead of minority languages in their services. This 'Norwegianization' policy was also informed by the dominant nationalist ideology, which stressed the need to build a homogenous Norwegian nation-state.

The assimilation policy was accompanied by social evolutionist thought emphasizing the hierarchical relation between Norwegian, Sami and Kven cultures. The Sami, and to a lesser extent the Kvens, were seen as primitive and underdeveloped compared to the Norwegian majority. The Sami (particularly the coastal Sami) were placed on the lowest rung of the cultural ladder in terms of development and the potential for 'culture'.[5] Some Norwegian commentators even described the Sami as a 'doomed people', thus sharing a common metaphor used for indigenous groups in the throes of modernization and assimilation around the globe at this time.[6] This hierarchy legitimized attempts to 'civilize' or 'uplight' the minorities by representatives of the putative 'higher culture' in many fields and also affected the provision of health services and health promotion in Finnmark.[7]

Provision of Health Services and Health Problems in Finnmark

The provision of health services in Norway as a whole in the first half of the twentieth century was based on a cooperative effort between official and voluntary agencies. The state and the county and municipal authorities supplied public health officers (district medical officers in Finnmark) and midwives, and financed and supported some key medical institutions. In 1900, Finnmark had ten medical districts served by district medical officers; in addition, an ambulatory district medical officer and two other practising doctors brought the total to thirteen medical doctors.[8] The county of Finnmark supported three hospitals, one in each of the largest urban settlements (Hammerfest, Vardø and Vadsø); a few small provisional hospitals were also established during the seasonal fisheries, which attracted great numbers of fishermen from all over the Norwegian coast.[9] The scope of public health services gradually expanded in the following decades, despite economic depression and the constantly crisis-ridden county finances, so that in 1942 there were twenty-six medical doctors (fifteen of them district medical officers) and a network of health and social institutions in Finnmark. In 1940, the county had 636 hospital beds in all, tuberculosis institutions included.[10] In addition, a number of social institutions (mainly children's homes and homes for the elderly), diagnosis stations for detection of pulmonary tuberculosis and other health institutions had been established in the previous decades, many by voluntary associations.

After 1900, voluntary associations became an important provider of health services to the population in Finnmark as elsewhere in Norway. In Finnmark, their role was particularly evident in the two largest health-related problems in the county: poverty and tuberculosis.[11] Poverty was widespread in Finnmark, where incomes were largely dependent on seasonal fisheries. When the fisheries failed, poverty quickly asserted itself. International economic difficulties of the 1920s and 1930s were also felt in the north.[12] The precarious economic situation of income-earners resulted in inconsistent and often low tax revenues for local and county government. The housing conditions and sanitary arrangements in the county reflected this private and public poverty and were deemed very unsatisfactory by medical observers in the early years of the century. Many Sami families, particularly in coastal areas, resided in turf huts, sometimes sharing their dwellings with domestic animals. These circumstances supported the doctors' view of Sami primitiveness: one physician dubbed such shared dwellings and the life in them as 'the rock bottom of human existence in Europe'.[13] Although many Norwegian and Kven families lived in small, overcrowded wooden houses, medical doctors considered the housing and the bathing habits (particularly among the Kvens, who used traditional saunas) of these groups to be superior to those of the Sami.

The main cause of death in Finnmark in 1900 was tuberculosis – a common companion of poor social conditions. This was also true of Norway as a whole but the tuberculosis mortality rate in Finnmark considerably exceeded that in the rest of the country. In Finnmark, tuberculosis mortality peaked at around 51 per 10,000 inhabitants in 1906–10, roughly double the national average.[14] Tuberculosis took a heavy toll among Finnmark's Sami, and contemporary observers agreed on that the group's character as an uncivilized 'people of nature' contributed to the wastage (see Table 2.1).[15]

Table 2.1: Deaths from tuberculosis per 10,000 inhabitants 1901–40.[16]

	1901–5	1906–10	1911–15	1916–20	1921–5	1926–30	1931–5	1936–40
Finnmark	50.6	50.9	49.0	44.2	42.5	29.3	20.1	15.1
National Average	28.2	26.0	23.6	22.6	20.4	16.1	12.4	9.1

The Fight against Poverty: Social Mission among the Sami

Poverty and its associated social problems became an issue among missionaries working among the Sami in Finnmark in the late 1890s. The main missionary organization was the Norsk Finnemission, established in 1888 by the bishop of Tromsø, J. N. Skaar. Skaar was critical of the state minority policy of the time.[17] The Norwegianization policy made the work of the church among the Sami difficult; it was also at odds with the Lutheran ethos of providing the Gospel in the people's vernacular. Thus, Norsk Finnemission chose to utilize Sami language in their evangelization, thereby challenging the official assimilation policy. The Sami mission also combated Læstadianism, a Lutheran pietistic movement which had emerged in northern Sweden in the 1840s and rapidly spread to the northern parts of Norway. Læstadianism won adherents in many Sami communities, as it did among the Kvens and the Norwegians. The movement was critical of the established Church structures and was perceived as a threat by the Norwegian State Church.[18] The main tasks of the Norsk Finnemission, outlined in 1892, were to preach the word of God to Sami who lived in the peripheries of the diocese of Tromsø (which also included Finnmark) or who had not mastered the Norwegian language, to provide the Bible and other religious literature in the Sami language and to make sure that the Church's religious message was promoted.[19]

From the late 1890s the Sami missionary organization engaged in a wide-ranging social mission, prompted by the missionaries' experience of social misery in the region. In 1896, one of the missionaries stated that it was

> unbelievable how many sick and crippled, limp, blind and deaf of all ages one finds among the Finns [Sami]. In certain places one is appalled over their numbers and over the nameless wretchedness they have to live in. I believe I safely dare say that there is no other place in this country with such an abundance of remote places which the priest never has the opportunity to visit, and such a sad profusion of cripples, who never may partake of the table of the Lord, than Finnmark.[20]

The missionaries thus interwove the bodily and material misery among the Sami with their perceived spiritual needs, creating a forceful impetus for the social mission.

The expansion of the Sami mission's field of work also reflected an overall growth of social work within the Norwegian inner mission, as many missionary organizations came to see the alleviation of need among the poor and sick as a central task.[21] Such work was partly conceived as a Christian duty, but also as a way of negotiating the social consequences of modernization and urbanization. The education of deaconesses started in Kristiania in 1868, and deacons followed in 1890. Tellingly, it was a deacon working for the Norsk Finnemission, Bertrand Nilsen, who suggested in 1899 that the organization establish a nursing home for elderly Sami in Kistrand in Finnmark, opening in 1903.

Several health and social institutions in the Sami-dominated areas of northern Norway were built and run by the Norsk Finnemission, Norsk lutersk finnemisjonsforbund, Kvinnelige Misjons Arbeidere (KMA) and other, mainly southern-based, religious associations in the early 1900s. This constituted the first serious effort to provide more than basic health and social services, such as district medical officers and public hospitals, to the Sami population in northern Norway.[22] In Finnmark alone, the two main organizations engaged in the Sami mission, the Norsk Finnemission and the Norsk lutersk finnemisjonsforbund, established the following institutions in the first decades of the twentieth century (see Table 2.2).

Table 2.2: Sami mission social and health institutions in Finnmark, 1903–31.

Year	Name/place	Organization
1903	Kistrand home for the aged	Norsk Finnemission
1914	Leirpollen home for the aged	Norsk lutersk finnemisjonsforbund
1917	Lebesby home for the aged	Norsk Finnemission
1918	Nyborg tuberculosis nursing home, Nesseby	Norsk lutersk finnemisjonsforbund
1919	Karasjok tuberculosis nursing home	Norsk lutersk finnemisjonsforbund
1920	Kolvik children's home	Norsk lutersk finnemisjonsforbund
1921	Bygøyfjord home for the aged	Norsk Finnemission
1923	Kautokeino tuberculosis nursing home/home for the aged	Norsk Finnemission
1928	'Hans Schanckes Minde', children's home, Tana	Norsk Finnemission
1931	'Sollia', home for pretubercular children, Sør-Varanger	Norsk Finnemission

Some of these institutions were established in cooperation with the Norwegian National Association Against Tuberculosis and received state funds. Other religious organizations also built up social and health institutions in Finnmark, so that by 1929 nearly 40 per cent of all medical and social institutions in the county had been established and/or were administered by different religious organizations (fifteen out of thirty-nine institutions, hospitals included).[23] Nine out of ten children's homes in Finnmark in the interwar decades were run by such organizations.[24] The Sami mission also established institutions in Troms and Nordland. Even though the institutions were nominally designated for the Sami, people were cared for regardless of ethnicity.

The second main aspect of the social mission was the engagement of parish nurses (*menighetssøstre*), i.e., voluntary nurses employed by the mission organizations, in local communities.[25] In addition to staffing the social institutions, parish nurses also served the wider communities. The Sami mission engaged nurses from 1911 onwards, and during the interwar years, many municipalities in Finnmark had one or several parish nurses present. During the 1930s, they became increasingly involved in the public health work against tuberculosis, as discussed in detail below.[26] During the economically harsh interwar decades these women undoubtedly strove hard to alleviate social misery in the region, treating not only the body but also the soul.[27]

The missionaries wanted to provide social and health services to the Sami, but also to win souls for the 'proper' variety of Christianity. To accomplish both was not easy. In some areas, such as Tysfjord in Nordland, evangelization proved to be difficult. On the one hand, according to one of the KMA sisters working at a nursing home in Tysfjord, attempts at celebrating Christmas during her first winter in the area – with a 'wonderful Christmas tree' – conflicted with the views of the local, strongly Læstadian, population, who regarded this as 'Norwegian idolatry'.[28] On the other hand, the social and medical work organized at the nursing home was highly regarded and sought after by the local population.[29] This example, among many others, indicates that the local population approached the new institutions and services pragmatically: if the services were conceived as beneficial, they were used and sought after, but those practices, religious or otherwise, that were deemed unpalatable were discarded and resisted.[30] Such a pragmatic approach to medical and social services presented from the outside is well known from other rural areas, and there is no reason to expect that the Sami in northern Norway should have acted significantly differently.[31]

The pro-Sami language policy of the Sami mission organizations probably eased the acceptance of the social and health services provided by the mission. Use of the Sami language was facilitated by Sami emissaries engaged by Norsk Finnemission, who dominated the organizations' field workers to begin with. However, from the 1910s the workers in the Sami mission were increasingly recruited from southern Norway.[32] The extent to which the Sami language was actually used in the social mission is somewhat uncertain, as the children's homes operated by the Sami mission paid little heed to the lingual and cultural background of the Sami children. However, the Sami mission's explicit goal was to use the Sami language 'to the necessary extent, as long as the Sami themselves wish that the Sami language is used'.[33] The children's homes in general in Finnmark did not have an explicit policy of Norwegianizing their residents.[34] Moreover, many emissaries and parish nurses from the south were in fact educated in the Sami language (northern Sami) to enable them to work according to the language policy of the mission and in order to promote the Gospel in their patients' mother tongue; some were even capable of using all three main languages of Finnmark in their work.[35]

The role assigned to cultural change in the health and social work of the Sami mission was ambiguous. On the one hand, the Sami mission wanted to preserve and protect the Sami language and other cultural symbols of Sami-ness, such as traditional costumes and handicrafts. On the other hand, one central aim of the Sami missionaries' social work was to transform aspects of Sami culture that were perceived as 'primitive' and 'backward'. On a collective level, the Sami were to be 'lifted upwards'.[36] This ambition was legitimized in many ways: the state assimilation policy was sometimes emphasized as the reason for the problems the Sami faced, such as poverty, bad housing, inadequate clothing and nutrition.[37] To alleviate the situation, the missionaries had to 'descend' among the Sami.[38] This paternalistic civilizing project could sometimes emphasize the superiority of Norwegian culture, exemplified by the missionary G. Tandberg who wrote in 1911 that the Sami mission had to 'heighten their (the Sami) cultural level by imparting them the advantages of our Norwegian culture'.[39] But 'uplifting' could also be seen as a Christian project, critical to Norwegianization. In 1921, the administrative board of Norsk lutersk finnemisjonsforbund stated that the goal of the mission was to 'lift the whole of this our sister nation up to the light of Christ's love' as

> [The Sami] have for long enough been held in contempt, they have for long enough had to live in earthen holes, they have for long enough been pushed aside from the best places, their mental capacities have for long enough been crippled by Norwegianization, they have for long enough been told that they are no good, but that it would be fine if they could become Norwegians' servants. Little by little, this will change under the merciful sun of God.[40]

This collective 'uplift' was translated to mean that the transformation of the individual Sami by the missionaries, would be achieved for instance through the mission's social and health institutions. In children's homes the Sami children were to be transformed spiritually and culturally: they were to receive Christian

upbringing as well as training in order to become 'good and useful' people.[41]
Training in ordinary domestic chores was taught to encourage the children to
live a 'well-ordered house-life'.[42] In homes for the elderly, the aim was spiritual
transformation, as the aged and ill were to be 'prepared for their final journey to
eternity'.[43] In schools for Sami children established by the mission in Finnmark
(1916, 1936) and Nordland (1910), the children were to receive a practical
education suited to their needs, as defined by the missionaries.[44] The schools
were also to cultivate the children in Christian, civilized values and practices,
as expressed for instance in the 1917–18 annual report of the Sami school in
Håvika in Nordland:

> Also of great importance is to set the child on an even keel while it is so little. One
> may thereby hope to remove the congenital inclinations and edges that are more dis-
> cernible among a people of nature such as the Lapps [Sami] than among people who
> have been under culture for years.[45]

Cleanliness, diligence and industriousness, together with Christian values, were
among the virtues to be inculcated in children. In theory, the pupils in the Sami
mission's schools were to use their traditional costumes and speak their own language, even though in practice the teaching was often done in Norwegian.[46] The
Sami mission also became involved in attempts to improve housing standards
among the Sami, a task that was given a prominent place in the campaign against
tuberculosis in Finnmark.[47]

The 'civilizing' or 'uplifting' of the Sami represented a common aim shared
both by the Norwegian state authorities and the missionaries. However, for the
Sami mission linguistic assimilation was not necessarily a part of the promotion
of cultural change. The work of the mission aimed to change those aspects of Sami
culture and individual ways of life deemed unhealthy, such as housing, cleaning
and eating habits, and to inculcate in children and other residents of their institutions an ethos of Christian and 'civilized' values. The Sami language *per se* was not
seen as a hindrance to adapting the Sami to a more 'healthy' way of living. From
the perspective of the Sami mission, it was evidently possible to conceive of a citi-
zenry acting and living in accordance with values and norms defined as 'healthy',
while at the same time holding on to their Sami heritage and language.

Language, Culture and Tuberculosis in Finnmark

A different view of the relation between language, culture and health dominated
the campaign against tuberculosis in Finnmark, which was organized jointly by
state medical authorities and voluntary associations in the 1910s. The characteri-
zation of the Sami culture, including their language, as primitive, uncivilized and
non-developable contributed to a policy of cultural uplift as the fundamental

solution to the tuberculosis problem in Finnmark. However, differentiating it from the policy of the Sami mission organizations, the state policy also implied linguistic change for the Sami.

The Norwegian public health campaign against tuberculosis was formed as a cooperative effort between public authorities on state, county and municipal levels on the one hand and voluntary associations on the other.[48] The legal basis for the campaign was defined in the Norwegian Tuberculosis Act of 1900, which aimed to isolate disease carriers in advanced stages of the disease. The Act defined the municipal health boards and their leaders, usually the state-appointed district medical officer of health, as the main actors in the struggle against the disease. The building and running of local nursing homes where isolation could be carried out became a local responsibility. In Finnmark, the county authorities established the first such nursing home in 1905, and many more were built towards the early 1920s, largely by voluntary associations. Usually, the state contributed financially to the dietary expenses of patients isolated in such nursing homes, and oversaw these and other tuberculosis institutions through the state Chief Medical Officer for Tuberculosis. The state also built and ran large-scale, expensive curative institutions such as sanatoria and coastal hospitals (*kysthospitaler*) and financially supported voluntary organizations engaged in tuberculosis work. The Norwegian National Association Against Tuberculosis (hereafter National Association), established in 1910 and the Norwegian Women's Public Health Association (NKS), established in 1896, were the two most significant voluntary associations working against tuberculosis in Finnmark in the early twentieth century.

However, the state extended its contribution to the anti-tuberculosis work in Finnmark in an exceptional manner, compared with the rest of the country. Annual state funds for the running of tuberculosis nursing homes and grants to enhance the local medical doctors' competence in tuberculosis diagnosis and treatment were allocated to Finnmark beginning in 1909, and in 1915–16 the state opened a coastal hospital for scrofulous patients in Vadsø in Finnmark and Vensmoen sanatorium in Nordland, catering for tubercular patients from northern Norway. A second coastal hospital was opened in Tromsø in 1924, serving patients from Troms and western Finnmark. This exceptional state activity, particularly pertaining to the nursing homes, was motivated by the difficult economic situation in Finnmark, which hindered local activity against tuberculosis, as well as 'national' considerations. The fears underlying the official Norwegianization policy in the north made the state authorities more willing to contribute public funds to the development of Finnmark, in order to secure the national borders and to integrate the county more firmly into the national state.

In 1914, the National Association published a report discussing the tuberculosis situation in Finnmark. Three specific means to combat the disease were suggested: in order to provide enough isolation sites, new nursing homes should be built; the standard of dwellings in Finnmark should be heightened through state intervention, and a vigorous campaign of public education should be set in motion, in order to heighten the population's knowledge of tuberculosis and how to best avoid it. Moreover, the committee that authored the report emphasized that the state, as well as the voluntary associations, had to support every initiative that would 'develop the province in economic, cultural and hygienic respect'.[49]

The fundamental rationale for these measures provided in the 1914 report lay in an understanding of tuberculosis as a disease of civilization that had been introduced to Finnmark by the general process of integrating the county into the rest of the nation. The connection of tuberculosis with industrialization, urbanization, the growth of modern communications and the establishment of a poor industrial working class living in unsanitary conditions was a widely accepted notion in the late nineteenth century and early twentieth century, in Norway as elsewhere.[50] According to the National Association report, the development of modern communications between Finnmark and southern Norway had led to an increased import of the tubercle bacillus in the last decades of the nineteenth century.[51] Given the lack of natural immunity against the bacillus, the harsh climatic conditions, and not least, the uncivilized character of the county's population, the bacillus found a particularly fertile ground in Finnmark. The 'primitive' and weak Sami, particularly those living on the coast in a state further worsened by their use of turf huts as dwellings, were seen as the most vulnerable to tuberculosis.[52] Such unhygienic dwellings also hindered the public education campaign among their residents.[53] Thus, the population in Finnmark had to be 'developed' in general and the Sami and their dwellings in particular were to be 'civilized', i.e., they were to be re-housed in what was seen as more hygienic wooden houses. Such action was the result of the National Association viewing tuberculosis as a societal disease: infection was not only a function of exposure to the tubercle bacillus itself, but also of the level of a population's susceptibility to disease in general, which was somehow socially and culturally determined. Thus, to civilize the population was to strengthen its resistance to tuberculosis.

The building of new nursing homes in Finnmark was intensified in the wake of the National Association report. Six new homes opened their doors between 1917 and 1923, established by local branches of NKS and the National Association and other voluntary associations, such as the Sami mission organizations. The state opened Norway's only state-driven nursing home in Talvik near Alta in 1923. All of the nursing homes in Finnmark received state funds for their management.[54] In the 1920s the nursing homes were complemented with a number of institutions for pre-tubercular children, in accordance with new emphases in Norwegian tuberculosis control.[55] The proposed housing reform got under way in 1915, when the Parliament decided that state loans for building purposes could be granted at lower interest rates in Finnmark than elsewhere in Norway.[56] National considerations, that is, concerns about the exposed geopolitical situation of Finnmark, played a key part in the legitimization of this special treatment.[57] The state loans were to be spent on new wooden houses. Between 1915 and 1920, the National Association financially supported the destruction of a number of turf huts (and poorly built wooden houses) in Sami-dominated districts in Finnmark, northern Troms and Nordland by burning them with the intent to replace them with more hygienic dwellings.[58] Social measures such as this reform gained a stronger position in Norwegian anti-tuberculosis policy in general in the 1920s.[59] An educational campaign promoted by the National Association report was seen as imperative, given the overall 'low cultural level' of the Finnmark population. Not only was it necessary to educate the population specifically about tuberculosis, it was of importance 'to support everything that aims at increasing the general level of enlightenment among the population' in the county.[60] State boarding schools were ascribed a central role in the education about the disease and, more generally, in the molding of the children of Finnmark to a more hygienic, civilized way of life. Such boarding schools had been built in the county since 1905, in part as a response to the state's anxiety about national security: in these institutions, children of minority backgrounds were to learn – and use – Norwegian.[61] The National Association promoted a forcing of the pace of construction of such boarding schools as a way of civilizing the population and, thus, combating tuberculosis. The significance of these institutions in the combat of the disease was deemed very important:

> With respect to hygiene their [boarding schools] importance cannot be overestimated. Besides teaching the usual school subjects, the children also learn to undress, to lie orderly in the bed instead of lying fully clothed on the floor as they often do at home, to make the bed when they rise and to aerate their bed clothes, to wash themselves, as well as to keep their rooms tidy. Further, they learn to sit properly at the dining table, to eat with knife and fork, and to have their own cups and so on under the meals.[62]

Such molding of individuals to 'civilized' habits was quite similar to the aims of the Sami mission, as we have seen. Crucially, the strengthening of the schools in Finnmark, which was seen as a precondition for the 'civilizing' of the county's population by the National Association, would also further the linguistic assimilation of the minorities.[63] In general, the aim of cultural development or uplift as a part of disease control was expressed as a process of assimilation of the Sami into the 'superior' Norwegian national culture and language. In practice, this meant that the enlightenment campaign was conducted mainly in Norwegian, rather than in Sami or Finnish. Even though the Sami language had been used sporadically in local efforts to inform the population about the contagious nature of tuberculosis, the enlightenment campaign in the schools of Finnmark after 1914 was conducted only in Norwegian, while among adults it was partly carried out also in Sami and Finnish.[64] The prevalent view of minority culture and language, particularly Sami culture and language, as primitive and incapable of development, made it impossible to carry out the task of civilizing school children in any other language than Norwegian.

The adoption of this strategy of cultural uplift by the National Association is in striking contrast to the linguistic policy of the Sami mission. The different strategies may be understood in the light of the differing relations between the state and the voluntary agencies: while the Sami missionaries were from the outset critical to the state policy of linguistic assimilation, several National Association committee members were among the prominent architects of the state minority policy, among them the later Prime Minister Johan Ludwig Mowinckel, the later Finnmark county governor (*fylkesmann*) Hagbart Lund and reindeer inspector Kristian Nissen. Mowinckel and Lund in particular were central figures in the development of the Norwegianization policy in Finnmark, while Nissen was well known for his opinion that the Sami language was not a 'language of culture'.[65]

The primary intention of the anti-tuberculosis campaigners was to combat the disease, but the means they chose also promoted linguistic assimilation; the Sami missionaries wanted to alleviate material and spiritual need, but did not regard the Sami language a hindrance to the 'uplifting' of the Sami. Instead, the opposite was true. The work among the Sami was legitimized with different arguments by the respective voluntary agencies. In the tuberculosis campaign, 'national' considerations played an important role, as expressed by the National Association committee in 1914:

> The location of Finnmark is so exposed, its population so blended with foreign elements, that any effort, even the most minor, to bind this province to the rest of the country, also becomes a national effort of importance. It enhances patriotism and strengthens solidarity and those days may come, when both are put to the test.[66]

The Sami missionaries' imperative to lift the Sami 'sister nation' to the light of God's merciful sun, under which they were fundamentally equal to their Norwegian brethren, ultimately had a religious motivation. However, as we have seen, the goal of cultural change, expressed as 'uplift' or civilizing, was shared between the agencies, who also co-operated closely in the establishment and running of several health institutions. Moreover, the minority languages were not totally absent in the enlightenment campaign designed to combat tuberculosis, but the extent to which Sami missionaries and health workers actually were able to use the Sami language is questionable. Thus, although linguistic assimilation was persistently advocated by many health-care workers in Finnmark at the beginning of the twentieth century, it is reasonable to conclude that the main characteristic of health promotion in the region was the straightforward desire to replace a cultural lifestyle that was perceived as unhealthy by one that was believed to inhibit the spread of disease.

The role assigned to cultural change as a main means of tuberculosis control diminished from the early 1930s, as the Norwegian anti-tuberculosis work shifted emphasis towards more technical measures.[67] A greater emphasis was placed on mass medical examinations of school children, the earliest possible diagnosis of pulmonary tuberculosis with the help of a network of diagnosis stations equipped with X-ray facilities, and active surgical treatment of pulmonary tuberculosis. This development towards a more 'epidemiologic' strategy in tuberculosis control had profound consequences for the role assigned to culture and language, more generally 'civilization', in the understanding of tuberculosis and how to combat it.

In Finnmark, the public health work against tuberculosis became firmly committed to the 'epidemiologist' line during the 1930s.[68] Voluntary screenings of school children were carried out in almost every municipality by 1932. Norway's first county-owned diagnosis station, fitted with X-ray equipment, was established in Talvik near Alta in 1930, and by 1936 four such stations were in operation in Finnmark. New public health nurses, instrumental for mass screenings of school children and families and thus for the rational operation of the diagnosis stations, were employed. Many of them also worked as parish nurses for the Sami mission.[69] In 1939, the Finnmark County Tuberculosis Board that organized the public health campaign in the county described its activities during the thirties as 'direct and active' work against tuberculosis. The Board emphasized that it regarded general improvement of hygienic conditions, work for better housing, more correct nutrition and help to needy school children as important, but that it had deemed it necessary to concentrate its efforts on the most essential activity, that is 'early diagnosis of new cases, tracking down of possible sources of infection, new and old, and treatment and preferably the rendering harmless of every detected case' of tuberculosis.[70]

The medical reorientation in the fight against tuberculosis in Finnmark meant that the older understanding of tuberculosis as a societal disease and as an illness of civilization, was replaced by a modern view of tuberculosis as an infectious disease on a par with other infectious diseases. Since many medical doctors now rejected the previously held connection between tuberculosis and civilization, there was little support for cultural or social concerns, or attempts of social reform, when the anti-tuberculosis measures were redefined during the economic depression of the early 1930s. Even though the language strategy in tuberculosis work in Finnmark schools was not altered, linguistic or minority culture no longer played a significant part in the medical discussions about tuberculosis, the distribution of infection, or the measures to be used against the disease in Finnmark in the 1930s. Presence of an infectious source in homes, not 'race', ethnicity, culture or language, was the all-important factor.[71]

During the Second World War, the national tuberculosis work increasingly followed the epidemiological strategy. In 1940, Norwegian collaborators with the German occupation forces took over the administration of the medical sector. A new State Tuberculosis Inspector, Sophus W. Brochmann, was appointed by the Quisling government in 1940. Brochmann, who had been a relentless advocate of the new tuberculosis control strategy in the 1930s, enforced strict epidemiological measures against tuberculosis in 1942, through an amendment of the Tuberculosis Act of 1900 and a new Act making mass radiography tuberculosis screening mandatory.[72] In Finnmark, the epidemiological policy was implemented as far as was possible under war-time conditions. However, in the last stages of the conflict, the retreating German forces carried out a 'scorched earth' strategy in most of Finnmark (and Northern Troms) and evacuated the county's population by force in the face of the advancing Soviet troops. In consequence, nearly all infrastructure in Finnmark, medical institutions included, was completely destroyed in the autumn of 1944.

Universal Measures, Minority Language – Finnmark after the Second World War

After the country's liberation in May 1945, the reinstated State Director General of Health, Karl Evang, and his State Tuberculosis Inspector, Otto Galtung Hansen, continued the epidemiological tuberculosis policy established during the war. In 1947, Parliament passed new acts regulating tuberculosis work that were essentially copies of those passed earlier by the Quisling government, with the addition that the anti-tuberculosis BCG vaccination was made mandatory. Evang and his staff also emphasized the need for social measures in the combat against the disease, in accordance with their social democratic political outlook, thus combining the measures of tuberculosis work of the 1920s and 1930s in a new post-war state policy on tuberculosis prevention.

The tuberculosis policy was a part of Evang's general public-health policy for liberated Norway.[73] Evang's approach had a firmly universalist point of departure: when it came to provision of health services and health promotion, the only relevant dividing lines in the population were differences in income and geographical location. The budding welfare state was to equalize disparities in access to health services, and the health services themselves were to be universal and free of cost.

This vision of state responsibility to equalize social and, to a certain degree, geographical differences in order to promote health had no place for considerations of cultural differences in the population. Even though Evang was highly conscious of the difficult situation in Finnmark and knew that new medical institutions were desperately needed – not least to curtail the rapidly blossoming tubercular infection among the returning evacuees – he did not pay any heed to the multi-linguistic, multi-ethnic character of the county's population. In fact, Evang explicitly stated in 1947 that Norway had a homogenous population.[74] This indifference to cultural variety in the population was quite common in the social democratic party that dominated political Norway after the liberation: the earlier class-based outlook had been replaced by a wish to represent 'the people', and the 'people' were seen as indivisible.[75]

However, when the new epidemiological means of tuberculosis prevention mandated through the 1947 acts were deployed in Finnmark, the language question so to speak seeped back in, at first in order to make prevention more efficient. During the 1950s, Finnmark became the county in Norway where the mass tuberculosis diagnosis apparatus was deployed most often: the state-organized X-ray teams trawled the county seven times between 1952 and 1966. This unparalleled frequency reflected the county's still rather high tuberculosis morbidity compared with the national average. It also exemplifies the social democratic equalization project: the welfare state directed its resources in public health work to those areas which were perceived as worst off in terms of health and social conditions.

To make tuberculosis prevention as efficient as possible, the National Association responded in 1952 to pleas from Finnmark to produce propaganda materials on tuberculosis prevention in Sami. The first Sami-language brochure promoting the BCG vaccination was printed in 1953.[76] In 1954, the state agreed to pay for brochures in Sami that urged participation in the upcoming X-ray campaign.[77] According to Finnmark County Medical Officer Øyvind Jonassen, who had taken the initiative, such brochures would have a strong impact among the Sami, particularly since so little else was published in their language.[78] New brochures in Sami were produced to promote screenings in 1958 and 1960, and the screenings were also announced in a Finnmark-based Sami newspaper.[79] Thus, the one-language strategy that had dominated tuberculosis work in Finnmark since 1914 was replaced by a bilingual approach.

Meanwhile, the Finnish-speaking Kvens seem to have been ignored by medical doctors in Finnmark and the central health authorities. The pre-war efforts to secure the national borders in Finnmark through public health work were nevertheless in effect abandoned through the mass X-ray and vaccination campaigns, which in the Tana River valley also stretched over to the Finnish side of the border from 1952. The mostly Sami population in the valley had lively interaction across the border, and Jonassen pointed out that it was inexpedient to limit the campaign only to one side of the border: from an epidemiological point of view the population of the valley was a single unit.[80]

Furthermore, the mass X-ray screening campaigns carried out in Finnmark from 1952 were from the start designed to accommodate the seasonal migration pattern of the reindeer-herding nomadic Sami, in accordance with suggestions from the county medical officer.[81] The point was to make the screenings as comprehensive as possible, and to achieve this, the state X-ray teams were deployed to the Inner Finnmark at Easter, when the reindeer-herders were gathered at the church villages of Kautokeino and Karasjok. The X-ray apparatus were transported to the Inner Finnmark from the coast by snowmobiles; the rest of the county was screened during the summer months by boat and bus-based teams. This pattern was repeated throughout the 1950s.

These adjustments to Sami language and way of life in the 1950s were admittedly minor, but they nevertheless signalled that the view of the relation between minority culture, language and health promotion was changing on a more fundamental level. A new attitude was particularly evident in the pages of the *Journal of the Norwegian Medical Association*. In 1956 Professor Johan Torgersen, an anthropologically interested radiography specialist, disputed the long-standing notion of the Sami as a 'doomed people'. He insisted rather that the Sami were a 'vigorous people, culturally adapted to the circumpolar environment' that was by no means threatened by physical extinction; what *was* threatened was the Sami culture, which was 'exposed to a violent pressure connected with the recent years' industrialization and mechanization of rural life'.[82] Even though Torgersen shared an essentialist notion of Sami culture with his colleagues of the 1910s, his view of the relationship between culture and health promotion was the opposite of theirs. According to him, the 'vigour' of a people was dependent on its cultural well-being and vice versa, and physicians could – through their superior knowledge of the population and its plight – contribute to this interaction.[83] One way to accomplish this was to use the Sami language in health promotion. As the Finnmark county medical officer, Øyvind Jonassen, argued in 1959:

> The nomadic Sami have barely been able to participate in the material and cultural progress of the times. So far no Sami doctor, Sami engineer or dentist has ever been educated. The Sami have no opportunity to get basic education in their native tongue. They are referred to obtain such education in Norwegian during a short primary school, where Norwegian has to be learned first ... Medical doctors ought to use the Sami language in the health education where it can be done.[84]

Jonassen was even clearer than Torgersen that the Sami should not be assimilated to enable their participation in 'progress'; on the contrary, assimilation to the majority way of life would withhold material and cultural progress from the

Sami. Jonassen further insisted that public health work in Finnmark should 'as far as possible try to build on the valuable things in the old Sami way of life. Otherwise things may turn from bad to worse'.[85] Thus, the view of the role of cultural and language change in the promotion of health and health services was turned upside down: from the pursuit of cultural and linguistic assimilation of the Sami as a prerequisite for achieving better health to an emphasis on the need to adjust public health work to the Sami language and way of life. Jonassen's redefinition of cultural factors in public health work and his emphasis on the necessity of education in the Sami language also reflect the move of official minority policy in Norway in a more culturally pluralist direction.

Concluding Remarks

The early twentieth-century policy of encouraging cultural change in order to promote health and combat social problems such as poverty was fundamentally similar in Finnmark and elsewhere in Norway: the population was to be educated and 'uplifted' to a way of life that was more in accordance with the norms and values of medical expertise and others providing health and social services. However, multi-ethnic Finnmark presented a special challenge to this approach. The emphasis on the need to Norwegianize the minorities in order to achieve the desired 'cultural uplift' varied over time and also among the different actors involved.

It is possible to discern three phases regarding the role assigned to culture and language in health promotion among the indigenous Sami in the first half of the century. In the first phase early in the century, the need to 'civilize' the population of Finnmark, particularly the 'primitive' Sami, who were seen as an easy victim of the scourge of civilization, tuberculosis, was stressed. Changing the Sami ways of living, cleaning, eating and housing habits was seen as essential to the combat tuberculosis, and the promotion of such cultural change also played an important role in the social work of the Sami mission. The pursuit of cultural 'uplifting' was not restricted to the Sami; rural and working-class people throughout the country were subject to the same kind of policy of advocating cultural change as a means of promoting health, combating disease and alleviating social need. However, as we have seen, the importance assigned to linguistic change, i.e., linguistic assimilation of the Sami, varied among the Sami mission and the medical doctors involved in public health work in Finnmark. As the understanding of tuberculosis changed during the interwar years, the intimate connection between tuberculosis and 'civilization' was dissolved in the eyes of many medical doctors. The concomitant changes in tuberculosis control rendered the earlier emphasis on changing minority culture (and language) in order to promote health obsolete. This second phase was evident in Finnmark from the 1930s to the early 1950s. However, the adoption of an anti-tuberculosis strategy based on mass X-ray screenings and the BCG vaccination, procedures that in theory obviated cultural factors, led in the early 1950s to a reintroduction of language and cultural considerations into public health work. The result was a third phase that saw propaganda materials in Sami produced to make the new measures of tuberculosis control as effective as possible, and the mass campaigns were adjusted to the nomadic reindeer herders' seasonal cycle of migration. The adaptation of tuberculosis work to the Sami language and way of life in the 1950s also signified a more fundamental change in the view of the relations between culture, language and health. Medical doctors started to emphasize the necessity of adapting public health work and health education to the language and culture of the Sami people, instead of the other way around. This course adjustment brought the public health work among the Sami closer to the linguistic strategy adopted by the Sami mission organizations in the previous decades.

3 THE SAMI, SAMI-NESS AND THE STAFFING OF HEALTH SERVICES IN NORTHERN NORWAY, 1960s–2001

Astri Andresen

In 2001, the Norwegian Ministry of Health and Social Affairs established the country's first centre for Sami health research. It is hosted by the University of Tromsø, the northernmost university in Norway, but also based in Karasjok in Finnmark; thus, it is set in a region that for hundreds of years has been ethnically diverse and, in certain areas, predominantly Sami. The centre is an institutionalized manifestation of political and academic will to consider the interrelatedness of Sami-ness, sickness and health. Members of the Sami Medical Association (a physicians' association), founded in the mid-1980s, played no small part in laying down the principles upon which the centre was to be based: first, it was to focus solely upon the Sami population; secondly, it was to produce new knowledge concerning the health and living conditions of the Sami; and, thirdly, it was to educate researchers in Sami medicine and public health.[1]

Such principles indicate that regarding health issues being Sami is conceived of differently from both other minority groups and the Norwegian majority. But why should this be so and what are the practical implications? The question of why Sami-ness matters touches on two different aspects of health: a variable influencing sickness and health, and a variable that is relevant to designing health services. The two aspects are intertwined, and this article will investigate the shifting approaches to Sami-ness as relevant to health services from the 1960s, when a specific quota system for Sami youth entering medical education was implemented, until the establishment of the centre for Sami Health Research in 2001. The first voices proclaiming that Sami patients needed Sami-speaking physicians were, however, heard in the late 1940s and the 1950s, and we will shortly examine the context in which this happened.

Health services comprise a broad range of activities, but ever since the 1950s and until quite recently, particular Sami needs, with a few exceptions, have been defined more in relation to the staffing of health services than to the structure of these services. How to recruit health personnel, whom to recruit, how to educate them and what to require from them have been recurring topics in discourses over health services for the Sami, and the shifting answers contribute to understanding why, or why not, Sami-ness has mattered. This article deals with staffing, broadly speaking, as problematized by the different agents involved in shaping health services: pro-Sami and Sami spokespeople, medical professionals, and state and county authorities.

Overall national health policies form the basis of health services both to minority and majority populations in Norway. In the period following the Second World War Norwegian governments implemented a policy to provide all citizens with equal access to health services regardless of social status or place of residence; this historical context is essential to understanding the development of health services for the Sami. Regional equalization has in fact been described as one of the most characteristic traits of Norwegian welfare state policies after 1945 – and northern Norway figured prominently on the welfare agenda.[2] Thus, also in periods when Sami-ness as such did not matter to the authorities, health services to the Sami population expanded due to an overall desire for equality between urban and rural communities and central and peripheral regions.

Two developments regarding the status of the Sami are of particular relevance when discussing health services. The first concerns minority policies and changes in Sami legal status. During this period Norwegian minority policy underwent two decisive shifts. First, after the Second World War long-standing discriminatory practices were gradually replaced by a policy of recognition and inclusion.[3] From the 1980s onward, minority rights were formally inscribed in law.[4] The second development concerns shifting definitions of what constitutes Sami-ness. In the interwar period, the dominant view was that the Sami constituted a race different from other Nordic peoples, and non-Sami Norwegians generally regarded the Sami as inferior. However, no firm conclusion was ever drawn regarding the interrelatedness of biology, culture and health, even though this topic was discussed on several occasions both in Norway and in neighbouring Sweden.[5] Beginning immediately after the Second World War, but in particular since the 1970s, a new understanding has been established: the Sami has been defined as an ethnic group and ethnicity has come to be understood as culturally, not biologically, constructed. Fredrik Barth's ground-breaking book *Ethnic Groups and Boundaries,* published in 1969, played a major role in shifting attention from what is often conceived of today as essentialism towards constructivism, from biology to culture and, not least, from ethnic boundaries conceived as resulting from an isolated position to a product of interaction between different groups.[6] After the breakthrough of Barth's theory, Sami-ness as essence, be it biological or cultural, was generally not considered relevant, although it should be noted that old definitions of what a people 'is' seldom disappear quickly or completely. A recent doctoral thesis, for example, illustrates that biological and social ethnic characteristics shared by at least some Sami informants were conceived of as being inherited – but, somewhat contradictorily, without ethnicity necessarily being regarded as a biological matter.[7]

In the 1950s, the study of genetic markers was introduced to Sami research.[8] The Sami attracted special attention as constituting 'population isolates'. Since then, the genetic composition of the Sami has been investigated for a number of purposes, including the aim to trace 'genetic origin' and to map likely emigration routes and emigration periods.[9] It has however also been suggested that 'the genetic structure of the Sami population' makes it particularly suitable for the investigation of genetic and environmental factors influencing particular diseases.[10] Medical studies have indicated that certain differences in the prevalence of some diseases between the Sami and neighbouring peoples might be a product of genetic variances.[11] Archaeologists and historians have questioned the methodologies applied, in particular the selection of who is to be considered Sami.[12] Furthermore, concerns have been voiced that genetic research might be used to once more link Sami-ness to 'blood'.[13] Such debates are not restricted to Norway or the Nordic countries; for example, in the United States of America (US) a main issue has been the 'relative merit of the concept of "race" or "ethnicity", especially from the genetic perspective'.[14] This article will demonstrate that some traces of 'blood' re-entering the discussion via genetic research can be discerned, but I have found no indication of genetics actually having influenced health services towards the Sami. The long-standing issue regarding health services is a more pragmatic one, namely language, to various degrees intertwined with cultural understanding.

The 1950s: Language and Respect

In the interwar period, in accordance with official assimilation policy the Sami population had a duty to learn the Norwegian language in order to communicate with members of the medical profession.[15] The Sami language had no official status in Norwegian society; in the 1936 School Act, it was designated an auxiliary language only.[16] In 1948 a parliamentary committee submitted its report on Sami education and enlightenment, and as a result, Sami became an official educational language in some districts in 1959.[17] It was hoped that the official status would enable the Sami to keep their self-respect and to enjoy the benefits of modern society like any other citizen.[18] The so-called Sami Committee that presented its final report the same year urged the government to take steps to recruit Sami-speaking health personnel, and proposed that a quota be established for Sami youth who wanted to study medicine, together with educational grants.[19] The recommendations were grounded in, first, an observation that the health situation was worse among the Sami, who had particularly high infant mortality rates, compared to other populations,[20] and second, that to communicate with the Sami, the Sami language was a must since many Sami neither spoke nor understood Norwegian. This shift in health-care policy was accompanied by a shift in thinking about what constituted Sami-ness. Even if the 1950s were a period of some confusion over this issue, long-standing assumptions about the relation between race, race-mixing and health were being replaced by an understanding that seems inspired by the UNESCO declarations on race (1950, 1951).[21] Medical research, for example, concluded that health differentials in Finnmark were not the consequence of race or racial mixing but were due instead to the health services and general welfare not having reached the Sami, in particular the nomadic communities.[22] The language barrier and dire economic conditions, remote living and/or a nomadic lifestyle all were seen as contributing to health issues. In fact, to the extent that health differences between groups of the population were specifically discussed, they were typically described in terms of where people lived: in central or remote locations. Sometimes residence and livelihood reinforced each other: the nomads were commonly described as a particularly vulnerable group.[23]

The 1960s: Equality and/or Quota Systems?

Progress in fulfilling the Sami Committee's recommendation to recruit Sami-speaking health professionals was slow. The reception of the recommendation in the Ministry of Social Affairs was negative. Rejecting the proposals of both quotas and grants, the Ministry maintained that the more important task was to provide the whole county of Finnmark with health services of equal quality to the rest of the country.[24] It conceded that it would be favourable if physicians in Sami districts understood the local language 'as long as there are still some Norwegians who use the Sami language only or have problems in understanding Norwegian', but insisted that language barriers were probably of little importance for the quality of medical services in Sami districts.[25]

The reception of the recommendations on quotas and grants can be compared to another recommendation, most likely put forward by the chief county medical officer in Finnmark, Øyvind Jonassen. He promoted a wider solution to problems regarding health care in Finnmark: large-scale Nordic co-operation in the north regarding all health services to the border populations regardless of ethnic belonging. This initiative benefited from the experiences of X-ray screenings that had been carried out since 1952 in the Tana River valley, which straddled the Norwegian-Finnish border (see Teemu Ryymin's essay in this collection). Nordic cooperation regarding health services was put into practice very quickly. In 1960 an amendment to the 1927 Act on Physicians' Rights and Duties (Endringer i lov av 29. april 1927 om lægers rettigheter og plikter) allowed Swedish and Finnish physicians to practise in the Norwegian border districts – and vice versa for Norwegian physicians on health missions. The Act also encompassed other health personnel and allowed sick persons to be hospitalized in neighbouring countries without special formalities. In short, Nordic resource allocation could alleviate some of the most pressing difficulties in providing not just the Sami in particular, but the entire population in the sparsely populated border districts of inner Finnmark, with adequate medical services. In the long run the collaborative project did not turn out to be a success, but that is a story of less interest in the context of this article.[26]

The Ministry did not follow principles of equality in only its rejection of quotas. The Ministry could point to an increase in bilingualism in northern Norway and a steady decline in the number of persons using the Sami language – a logical consequence of a century of official policy to suppress it. In the 1930 census the Sami-speaking population officially numbered approximately 20,000 individuals, whereas in the 1950 census only 8,778 persons gave Sami as their first language.[27] Hence it is understandable that the Ministry of Social Affairs, which was responsible for the health of the entire nation, would decide that its limited resources could be better used for other purposes than educating physicians to serve a relatively small – and seemingly diminishing – group. Less understandable, from today's perspective, was the Ministry's view that communication between health professionals and the Sami population was not overly hampered by the lack of a common language. This might be seen as a defensive justification of the unwillingness to educate Sami- or Sami-speaking physicians, but mainly it reflected the widespread belief in the medical community that well-trained physicians were fully able to diagnose and treat ill-health even without patients' verbal explanations of their conditions:

> The Ministry of Social Affairs finds that for a physician with a good medical training who is generally well educated and endowed with human understanding and empathy, the process of adaption [to a different culture] does not create problems that affect the quality of medical services.[28]

This was largely in tune with the expressed confidence of Karl Evang, the Director General of Health in 1938 and from 1945 to 1972, that the medical profession – and the medical sciences – were capable of solving almost any problem.[29] But, furthermore, it was in tune with overall Labour policies in post-war society that placed various expert groups in key positions in the planning and 'running' of the state.[30] The attitude of the Ministry of Social Affairs in these issues furthermore signalled the official position that 'the Sami' were a variant of 'Norwegians', a view-point grounded in the social democratic striving for policies based on the essential equality of all citizens. The interwar socio-political discourse about minorities that assigned an important role to race and culture was overturned without formal debate.

The Ministry of Social Affairs did not have the final word on medical training, however. At the medical faculty at the University of Bergen, Professor Torstein Bertelsen – himself born in northern Norway – took up the Sami Committee's idea of educating Sami physicians. He convinced the faculty council to pass a motion that 'talented, Sami-speaking students' could be admitted to the faculty after a closer scrutiny of their 'circumstances'.[31] Sami youth, Bertelsen argued, had never had the opportunity to compete with others on an equal footing; they had always been hampered by the fact that the teaching language had been Norwegian.[32] Since students were admitted to medical studies on the basis of marks only, it was unsurprising that the country had no Sami physicians.

Moreover, the negative attitude of the Ministry of Social Affairs was not shared by colleagues in the Ministry of Church and Education, which was responsible for minority affairs. When this ministry submitted the Sami Committee's report to Parliament, it supported the recommendation to establish a Sami quota for medical students. It emphasized the crucial importance of the Sami language in bringing health information to the general public in northern Norway. It furthermore recognized that the female population played a key role regarding nutrition, domestic science and health and urged that young Sami women be encouraged to enter the health professions 'to serve among their own'.[33] Parliament supported these views, and in its positive treatment of the Sami Committee report it broke decisively with pre-war assimilation policy by unanimously supporting the idea that it was time for policies that promoted the cultural and economic interests of the Sami themselves.

In 1963 the first two Sami students were admitted into the medical school at the University of Bergen. The first school of nursing in Finnmark, established three years earlier, introduced a quota for students born in the county as well as one for Sami-speaking students.[34] Furthermore, when the 1957 act on community nursing was put into effect by the county of Finnmark in 1960 it stipulated that the community nurses working in the medical districts of Kautokeino and Karasjok must know the Sami language.[35] Despite these initiatives, when the Finnmark Sami Council moved in 1963 that Sami youth should receive special economic support for education, the motion was rejected by the Ministry of Church and Education, which renewed its commitment to the social democratic ideal of equality and insisted that all Norwegian youth should be similarly treated with respect to educational grants.[36] In 1967, however, the Conservative-Liberal coalition that had followed the Labour Party government two years earlier established special educational grants for Sami youth.[37]

For the time being this was the end of reforms that targeted the particular problems of providing health care to the Sami population. Although certainly modest in scope and often targets of contestation, these reforms also symbolized a willingness to accept linguistic problems as 'real' problems in encounters between health professionals and Sami patients. To enhance cultural understanding within the health professions was, however, an aim that seemed too slippery to promote action. Under successive Labour governments, the Ministry of Health and Social Affairs was primarily concerned with establishing a viable health infrastructure throughout the country and the associated problems of attracting physicians to remote and rural areas and keeping them there. Specific Sami issues did not necessarily fit well into these larger concerns. Besides, factions among the Sami themselves protested vigorously against specific 'Sami measures' or 'Sami policies'. From the local government in Karasjok came the watchword that the Sami were Norwegians like anyone else in Norway. That these protests seem to have been organized by local members of the Labour Party implies that the party's stance on Sami issues was guided not only by an abstract ideology of equality but also by the opinions of party members in the north.[38]

Sami interests did, however, benefit from Labour's ambitious goal of equal health services for all, and we will now take a closer look at the equalizing process, which did not develop smoothly. In the post-war era, when the ambitions of health-care equality between regions were expanded from a basic system of medical officers to comprising the provision of general hospitals and specialist services, it became difficult to fill medical positions in rural and remote areas, as the historian Aina Schiøtz has discussed.[39] In addition, existing medical districts were often very large and communications were often poor. When in 1960 it was decided that each municipality should constitute its own medical district and that districts should be able to hire more than one medical officer, there were considerable increases in allotted health-care positions in Finnmark: twenty in 1959–60, twenty-nine in 1974–5. The difference between various regions was huge all the same: around 1964, there were fifteen physicians for every 10,000 inhabitants in the counties around Oslo, while in Finnmark, the ratio was 5.6:10,000.[40]

County officials repeatedly complained that many of the physicians who accepted appointments as district medical officers stayed for a very short time. For example, in 1959–60 all twenty medical officerships in the county were filled, but just two years later five of these were vacant.[41] To counteract these developments the government introduced a package of benefits in 1963 that included two weeks' additional vacation, economic support for heating, four months' paid leave every third year and a free air flight each year to Oslo (southern Norway).[42] In Finnmark, the immediate staffing crisis was alleviated, and for some years the situation was reported to be relatively good. The system, however, remained very fragile both in Finnmark and in other more remote parts of Norway. There were few applicants for empty positions, and many medical officers even questioned the use of paid leaves and holidays since it was impossible to get substitutes.[43] Thus, more reliable, long-term solutions for the staffing of the primary health-care system were demanded. They were sought in higher education.

The 1970s: Regionalization of Higher Education

As early as 1962, the Ministry for Church and Higher Education had floated the idea that a fourth university might be established in northern Norway. A committee was put to work to consider the question and it turned out in favour of the idea.[44] However, as the historian Narve Fulsås has demonstrated, rather than using the common 'national interest' as justification for the expansion, the committee argued for a fourth university on regional grounds: northern Norway needed a university to strengthen the educational level among the region's young people and to produce a well-qualified and professional workforce to work in the region.[45] The committee's reasoning was grounded in a specific understanding of the relationship between place of birth, place of education and place of work. Professor Torstein Bertelsen, a committee member whom we have seen playing a decisive role in introducing a Sami quota at the medical faculty in Bergen, had opined that the main reason why it was difficult to recruit qualified medical personnel to northern Norway was that very few youths from the region had ever been educated as physicians. He believed that the problem would disappear with a regionalized educational policy and underpinned his opinion with a survey of all physicians in Norway educated between 1937 and 1951. He found two decisive determinants for the location of physicians: where they were born and where they were educated. Bertelsen's evidence suggested the solution to a stable medical profession in northern Norway would be a medical school in the region.[46] In addition, he argued that even if a fourth university did not at all increase the number of physicians, much would be gained simply by educating physicians born in the north; to a much larger degree than others they would be willing to work in the region – and stay sufficiently long to get to know their patients and thus, provide them with better health services.[47] As Bertelsen argued, 'The medical community in a region must be based upon native physicians, and not least so in regions that offer work- and climatic conditions different from the rest of the country'.[48] The committee members followed Bertelsen's findings and even generalized them, asserting that similar factors were at play within all fields of higher education. They concluded that a new university with a medical faculty should be built in Tromsø.

A broad political opposition against a university in Tromsø manifested itself. The opposition was supported by yet another committee (*Brodal-utvalget*) that consisted of medical professionals, and not least by Karl Evang's Health Directorate and the medical faculty at the University of Oslo.[49] Evang believed that the population in northern Norway was too small to make up sufficient 'raw material' for medical education: 'the selection of diseases is simply too small'.[50] Furthermore, in Evang's opinion it would be impossible to fill the positions with well-qualified personnel, and he was unconvinced of the asserted close relationship between place of birth, place of education and place of work.[51] Even so, the committee's plan for a university in Tromsø was submitted to Parliament by the Conservative-Liberal government and legislated in 1968. The new university, its supporters argued, would function to equalize higher education in the country and to secure recruits for the medical profession in northern Norway and elsewhere. In 1973 the University of Tromsø opened its doors to the first cohort of medical students. A quota for youth born in the region was introduced to medical studies; in 1979 it was as high as 50 per cent.[52] In addition, there was a specific Sami quota that varied according to the total number of medical students admitted every year. In the mid-1990s the yearly intake was sixty students, at least two of whom had to be Sami-speaking Sami.[53] (Today, non-Sami students who speak Sami are given extra points in the admissions competition.)

In spite of these provisions, the establishment of medical education at the new University of Tromsø was not an implementation of the earlier effort to train Sami-speaking physicians; the recruitment of physicians to serve the Sami-speaking population was a side effect of the regionalization of higher education. But, moreover, the guiding philosophy of the University of Tromsø was to be 'regionally relevant', an aim which extended beyond formal instruction to the view that the university should take the pulse of local societies, solve local problems and promote wider awareness of local cultures.[54] Such aims naturally influenced the relationship between health care and minority cultures in the region. Generally they encouraged the development of an approach to medicine that incorporated cultural values; specifically they anchored the position of Sami issues. Sami language was to have an academic stronghold at the University of Tromsø, and Sami perspectives were as a rule integrated into social anthropology, sociology and history, as well as into medicine – and the field of medical research takes us back to issues concerning why Sami-ness mattered.

The first large-scale and regionally relevant investigation undertaken by the faculty of medicine in Tromsø was a study of coronary heart disease (CHD) in 1974. The investigating physicians reactivated the older term 'Lapp' – which by now was about to be considered politically incorrect. The study, which encompassed all men in the age group twenty to forty-nine years old in the county of Troms, revealed that it was difficult to limit the variable to 'culture' – the term 'origin' continued to pop up:

> Men reporting Finnish or Lappish origin had higher mean serum cholesterol values than the subjects of Norse origin ... Men of 'uncertain' ethnic origin occupied an

intermediate position. Men of Lappish origin had a significantly lower diastolic BP ... and a lower body height than those of Norse origin.[55]

The study found that 'the Lapps' had a much lower risk of coronary heart disease than the rest of the population in the county of Troms. Two explanations were suggested: first, that 'the Lappish social and cultural organization' protected against the 'deleterious effect of environmental factors operating in modern society'; second, that genetic differences 'known to exist between the groups' were largely responsible for the variation.[56] Significantly, genetic difference was presented as a proven fact, though references for this fact were not provided. Later CHD-studies always had 'Sami-ness' as one variable, even if the precise question might be formulated somewhat differently. In the CHD-study in Finnmark in 1987–8, for example, the question was put like this: 'Are two or more of your grandparents of Sami descent (ætt)?'[57] The concept of descent indicates a continued interest in biological inheritance – without any firm conclusions of its medical meaning.

But what about the anticipated 'Bertelsen effect' on the provision of medical professionals for the north – did it pass the test of time? In the late 1970s the prognosis did not look good; a new crisis in staffing health services in rural and remote areas was approaching.[58] A survey among physicians (*legestillingsundersøkelsen*) in 1990, however, showed that general practitioners in rural and remote districts most frequently came from the selfsame districts.[59] Being educated in Tromsø was almost as good as being born in northern Norway: students from other parts of the country who had been educated in Tromsø were likely to stay in the region after they had finished their education. It seemed as if at least one key to recruiting professionals to rural and remote areas had indeed been found.[60]

The quota programmes did produce Sami physicians who came to practise as medical officers and specialists, although the total number remained small. How many Sami physicians graduated from Bergen's medical faculty is uncertain: one source indicates that there were thirteen by the end of 1994; another says forty.[61] The number of Tromsø graduates is not available, but it is reasonable to believe it must be higher than in Bergen. Moreover, Sami have been admitted to medical schools elsewhere, and, indeed, the county of Finnmark has experienced an enormous increase in the percentage of its youth enrolled in higher studies. By the mid-1980s, Sami health professionals were sufficiently many to form their own organizations. In 1987 the Sami Medical Association counted around twenty members.[62] The Association turned out to be politically very influential.

The 1980s and 1990s: A Question of Rights

Around 1980 Sami organizations urged the Norwegian government to recognize their status as one of the world's indigenous peoples like, for example,
the Aboriginal peoples of Canada, and, eventually, to ratify ILO Convention
169 Concerning Indigenous and Tribal Peoples in Independent Countries.[63]
Issues concerning health were by no means the main issues, but Article 25 of
the Convention concerns health and social services.[64] It can be summarized in
three points: first, governments are responsible for providing health services of
'the highest attainable standard' in physical and mental health; secondly, these
services shall be developed in co-operation with the peoples concerned and 'take
into account their economic, geographic, social and cultural conditions' as well
as traditional preventive and healing practices; thirdly, the health care system
shall give preference to the training and employment of 'local community health
workers' and focus on primary health care.

When Norway ratified the Convention in 1990, a number of legal acts concerning Sami status had already passed Parliament. Of particular relevance to
health and health services are the Sami Act (1987) which entitled the population to communicate in Sami with government officials including those
belonging to the health and social sector; the Norwegian constitution (1988),
which inscribed the protection of the Sami as a people; and the elective Sami
Parliament established in 1989. Parliament gave the Sami 'one voice' towards
the authorities, and it recognized that health policies and health care practices
affecting the Sami should be developed in collaboration between Norwegian
authorities and the Sami Parliament.[65] These developments brought new arguments into the debate over health and health services, and served to put pressure
on the government to engage more actively: a linguistic and culturally adapted
health service to the Sami was no longer only an issue of how best to promote
health; it became a question of how to secure rights according to internal law
and international agreements.

The process to develop health and social services that were embedded in the
linguistic and cultural needs of the Sami population had started already in the
mid-1980s, instigated by Sami organizations and the Norwegian Sami Council
(Norsk Sameråd) that brought the initiative to the attention of the Ministry of
Health and Social Affairs.[66] The result was a process at the national as well as
the county level to determine the special needs of the Sami in regard to these
services, to organize such services and to fund them. A commission was set down
in 1991, which presented its report, entitled 'Plan for Health and Social Services
to the Sami Population in Norway', in 1995.

The 'Plan' was a voluminous document, counting 502 pages, and, obviously,
it did not simply repeat the same old claims from the 1950s and 1960s; there

were substantially new dimensions. From an *ethnic perspective*, the new feature was that it no longer sufficed to talk about health services to the municipalities in inner Finnmark: when the Sami Parliament entered the public debate over health care, it asserted that Sami all over the country had a right to be met as Sami and that a national plan for health services had to be developed. Seen from a *health care perspective*, the earlier concentration on primary health care was supplemented by a focus on specialist care, in tune with the overall developments within health care in Norway. In 1984 a state-run psychiatric policlinic for children and youth was opened in Karasjok in Finnmark, and other institutions had been given responsibilities in adult psychiatric care. A private specialist centre in somatic medicine, also located in Karasjok and initiated by Sami physicians, opened in 1987. The aim of both harkened back to the years around 1950 which was to provide the Sami-speaking public with services in their mother tongue. In the late 1980s and 1990s, public support for these centres, as well an expansion of specialist services, were on the agenda of the Sami medical profession.[67]

The new key phrase was *equality in access and results*, which was something quite different from the equal rights perspective of the 1950s.[68] The 'Plan' specified that health and social services must be equally accessible to the Sami and the Norwegian population; they should comprise primary health care as well as specialist treatment; they should reach the Sami population in the country as a whole; and they should not focus solely upon the Sami-speaking part of the Sami population but also deal with those Sami who had given up the Sami language in favour of Norwegian. This position pointed to an increasing emphasis on the interrelatedness of ethnic identity and health.

Alongside emerging new issues were long-standing ones. In order to provide the Sami population with equal services, Sami-speaking health personnel was a prerequisite. Thus, the 1995 'Plan' devoted much space to the recruitment of Sami and Sami-speaking persons to the various health professions.[69] An indication of how far perspectives had changed since this issue was raised by the Sami Committee is found in the way recruitment was connected not only to providing the Sami population with Sami-speaking health personnel, but to the Sami professional's future as Sami: 'A concentration upon local recruitment is in line with the wish of most Sami youths to live as Sami also after having finished their education. That means they want to live in Sami districts and use their education there'.[70] Thus, Sami-ness was linked to geography and a particular culture, while postings in rural Sami districts were conceived as a way to preserve Sami-ness for professionally educated persons.

However, for the foreseeable future it was not feasible that all physicians and other health personnel in contact with Sami patients would actually have mastered the Sami language; thus, a translation service specializing in medical language would have to be developed. The quality of services offered to the Sami population would have to be improved, and one of the major components of such improvement was to strengthen the health personnel's knowledge of Sami and transcultural issues. Finally, the crucial importance of providing health information in the Sami language was reaffirmed.

This adjustment of health and social services to Sami interests, however, did not mean that the Norwegian central authorities ceded political and administrative control. In this area the contrast between Norway and, for example, Canada has so far been strong. In Canada, the Aboriginal peoples have acquired considerable self-determination and established semi-independent health and social services.[71] In Norway, even if claims for an independent Sami health enterprise have recently been heard,[72] by common agreement between the Norwegian authorities, the Sami Parliament and the Sami Medical Association, health and social services have so far been developed within the framework of the country's general health and social policies: integrated and coordinated, but with consideration given to special Sami needs.[73] The different strategies adopted by indigenous minorities in Norway and Canada may be a function of the sizes of the populations involved. It is estimated that today's Sami population barely exceeds 40,000 (under 1 per cent of the country's population), whereas in 2001 there were over 1.3 million people in Canada (over 4 per cent of the country's population) who considered themselves to have Aboriginal ancestry.[74] But numbers do not explain everything; there are also political and cultural/religious reasons. On the political side, the equalizing efforts of Norwegian health and welfare policy have had broad support also from the Sami community. On the cultural/religious side, the spiritual health and traditional healing practices that seem to be so prominent among the First Nations and Aboriginal peoples in Canada have until recently played a peripheral role in public debates over health issues.[75] The main Sami claim was related to equal access to their country's health services, while traditional Sami medicine led an unofficial life alongside official health care. I will suggest that the increasing size and influence of the Sami medical profession since the mid-1980s has been crucial for this approach: Sami physicians have indeed been interested in developing a culturally competent and sensitive health service, but one firmly planted within academic medicine.

Sami traditional medicine became, however, more visible in the 1990s at the same time as healing and alternative medicine gained a stronger position in society at large. The 1995 'Plan' did, for example, contain an appendix concerned with Sami folk medicine, and offered the conclusion that 'renewed knowledge about the empirical use of folk medicine should be a part of a Sami cultural mobilization', proposing a broad research programme to be initiated concerning Sami custom and traditional knowledge.[76] This was launched primarily as a programme to strengthen Sami identity and pride, however, not to investigate traditional medicine's potential usefulness; nonetheless, it was conceded that knowledge of traditional medicine might be useful in health promotion. At that time alternative treatment had long since found its way into hospitals: in 2001 every fourth hospital in Norway offered some kind of alternative treatment. In 2000 a centre for alternative medicine (Nasjonalt forskningssenter innen komplementær og alternativ medisin) was established. Like the Centre for Sami health research, this centre is also based at the University of Tromsø.[77]

The 1995 'Plan' proposed that ethnic medicine be included in educational programmes for the health professions, in particular those offered in northern Norway. One might have thought folk medicine was included in the concept; however, that was not necessarily the case according to the Committee's definition:

> By ethnic medicine is meant cultural understanding, knowledge about multicultural societies, bilingualism, understanding of acculturation processes and the construction and managing of ethnic minority identity. Understanding ethnic medicine should enable health- and social professionals to see the development of sickness and the existence of social problems in relation to cultural and ethnic aspects. Such an understanding should inform the development of theories and research methods among ethnic minorities.[78]

The definition kept the focus on school medicine and treated ethnicity as a cultural variable; so defined, ethnic medicine stood firmly in the tradition of county medical officer Øyvind Jonassen in the 1950s (see Teemu Ryymin's essay in this collection).

The 1995 'Plan' did not result in any immediate large-scale initiatives, and in 1998 the Sami Medical Association applied for funding from the Ministry of Health and Social Affairs to pursue the leads laid out in the report. In particular, the Association emphasized the need to establish a centre of Sami medical competence to co-ordinate research and education within ethnic medicine, and it pointed out that such a centre could be conveniently located at the University of Tromsø. The proposal was acclaimed by both the Ministry and the University, and the University's Centre for Sami Research was commissioned to report on possible frameworks for research and education in ethnic medicine in Norway – with a focus on the Sami perspective.[79] The ready request for a report on ethnic medicine, not simply Sami medicine, indicated the growing awareness among Norwegian health authorities that the Sami-speaking population was not the only group who needed a culturally adapted health service. Another minority population in northern Norway, the Kvens (Finnish-speaking immigrants arriving in the nineteenth century and their descendants), had, for example, claimed similar rights to those the Sami had received concerning language. Authorities and health professionals had also begun to realize that the country's new immigrants had specific health problems as well as special needs.

Once again a committee, this time with heavy representation from the Sami Medical Association, was appointed to study the issue. Its conclusions were rapidly formulated and published in 1999. These included the redefinition of ethnic medicine to mean 'Sami medicine', a change the report justified by noting that 'ethnic' was too broad a concept to be useful, that it was often bandied about uncritically and that it had negative connotations.[80] Furthermore, the term 'ethnic medicine' did not signal strongly enough an emphasis on the Sami population. Consequently, the report argued against establishing a designated centre for ethnic medicine in Tromsø.[81] One of the members of the committee later explained this stance by saying that 'we did not want to let the focus on the Sami get lost in immigrant-issues'.[82]

Thus, the concept of ethnic medicine disappeared as far as the University of Tromsø was concerned.[83] Instead the Tromsø Committee recommended that the Ministry of Health and Social Affairs establish a centre devoted to research into differences between the Sami and the Norwegian population in health, sickness and treatment. The recommendation intoned the by now well-known litany: the need to recruit Sami-speaking health personnel and to increase the understanding of Sami culture among the health professions. But furthermore, the Committee held that equally important to the population who identified themselves as Sami were those 'with Sami background who had changed identity. This change might be accompanied by sufferings that make us realize how oppression from the majority may have caused certain patterns regarding health'. Thus, the 'Norwegianized' population was made a particular object for medical interest.[84] This marked a clear departure from the kind of culture-health concerns of the physicians of the 1950s or of the CHD researchers in the mid-1970s and early 1980s, but also pointed forward to an increased emphasis on identity and health.

Should interest in the 'Norwegianized' population be seen as evidence that the Tromsø Committee focused on genealogy *per se*? It was the cultural process of assimilation that was defined as possibly harmful to health, but in relating its discussion about ethnic medicine, the Committee conceded that its definition of the meaning of ethnicity was far from conclusive: 'Ethnic identity is ... concerned with signs related to different traditions, but it might also be related to kinship and genes'. It argued that ethnic differences might be studied as 'original and permanent differences or characteristics' or as 'relational or inter-subjective properties'.[85] Thus, the Committee appears to have sought to unite essentialist and constructivist definitions of ethnicity. Perhaps this was a compromise attempting to bridge unyielding differences of opinion, but the most likely interpretation is that it was influenced by genetics and related genes to ethnicity. In favour of this interpretation is that the Committee, for example, did refer to a study of genetic variations in chronic diseases between 'the three ethnic groups at the North calotte' and to a project on ethnic metabolic differences as relevant to Sami health research.[86] More importantly, as the report on ethnic medicine – or rather, Sami health – was being written, broadly based genetic research findings were published that showed the Sami to be a genetically distinct group who occupied a 'unique position ... in the genetic landscape of Europe'.[87] It might be suggested that the Tromsø Committee invoked genetic findings to mean that Sami-ness was also biology, not 'only' culture. Such a viewpoint could draw not only upon a particular interpretation of scientific research, but upon a long historical tradition that had been disrupted after 1945, but had spokespeople within the Sami community itself.[88] Even so, it was the linguistic and cultural situation, not genetic differences, that justified a centre for Sami health research, as it justified particular services to the Sami.

Conclusion: Why Sami-ness Mattered

Why should Sami-ness be relevant in designing health services? Since around 1990 the simple answer has been that Sami-ness matters because the Sami have a right to health services that are designed to meet their linguistic and cultural needs. Thus, at the heart of these rights are issues that have run through the postwar period; first of all, that Sami-ness matters as language and, second, that it matters as culture.

The Sami-speaking community in Norway is not large, and bilingualism is the rule. After the Second World War many believed, despite the turn in minority policies, that the Sami language was on its way to oblivion. Combined with the common trajectory of medical officers of occupying transient positions in Finnmark on their way to better opportunities in more central regions, and the strong belief in the power of expertise to transcend cultural issues, the efforts in particular to educate Sami health personnel were at first rather a small-scale venture: in the 1960s they were limited to some restricted quota-systems and special grants.

Since the 1980s, however, the measures have been expanded to encompass initiatives to broaden the knowledge of Sami culture among Norwegian health personnel. It was members of the medical profession in Finnmark who first argued that cultural knowledge was important in understanding the Sami patient and that Sami culture encompassed traditions that might be invoked by medical officers to improve Sami health. However, these contentions, first launched in the 1950s, were not generally accepted for some time. After a short 'pro-Sami period' there was a strong conviction that a Sami was a 'Sami-speaking Norwegian' with the same rights and duties as other citizens; the language barrier was considered a minor hindrance. To attain a more complete and lasting change regarding language and culture required a revision of official minority policy in the country, and it was only after the Sami medical profession had entered the scene that culture became a clear focus of interest in Norwegian public health work. At the same time policies emphasizing the equal rights of all citizens remained essential to establishing a health-care system that provided rural and remote regions with services of the same quality as those in more central parts of the country, and regionalization of higher education was a decisive step in creating the staff for these services. Moreover, this regionalization furthered the education of Sami youth into, among other areas, the health professions.

In the 1990s, attention to language was not only about present-day communication but also about understanding the impact of the assimilation policy in earlier times. Language shifts were regarded as important turning points for individuals and groups; they were seen to signal shifts in identity which in turn were conceived as experiences that might have impinged upon health conditions. Thus, health personnel were not only asked to be aware of Sami-ness, but indeed, of *past* Sami-ness. Thus, history, and in particular the assimilation of the Sami, was evoked as a socio-cultural factor pertinent to people's health. Not least, the linguistic competence of health personnel has become a yardstick of the state's acceptance of Sami citizens.

Before the Second World War, the Sami were believed to be racially different from other peoples in the north. In the 1950s, representatives of Norway's medical profession continued to hold that the Sami made up a distinctive race, but in their opinion racial issues were of no importance to the pressing health issues in post-war society. In more recent discussions of sickness and health-promoting factors, biological Sami-ness has resurfaced not as race, but as genes that might matter, even if one does not know how or what the practical implications are. In the late 1990s the Tromsø Committee, with representatives also from the Sami medical profession in Norway, in its theoretical posturing preferred to keep the door open for linking ethnicity to genes. Such open-mindedness is surely the result of (relatively) recent genetic research and indicates an inclination to let biology speak for itself. However, it should be remembered that genetics were not given a prominent place in the contemporary arguments for Sami health research. A major difference from the 1950s, though, is that at the threshold of the twenty-first century the Sami themselves were better positioned to define what should and should not count in defining Sami-ness and the provision of health services to them.

4 FORESHADOWING THE FUTURE: HEALTH SERVICES IN REMOTE AREAS, THE NATIONAL HEALTH SERVICE AND THE HIGHLANDS AND ISLANDS OF SCOTLAND, 1948–74

Marguerite Dupree

In the first three quarters of the twentieth century, contemporaries and historians have viewed the Highlands and Islands of Scotland as remote, whether measured by distance or accessibility.[1] Yet, the provision of medical services in this region was important to central authorities. In 1913 legislation established a unique Highlands and Islands Medical Service (HIMS) to meet the problems of access to medical services in the islands and northern half of Scotland. Both contemporary politicians and, more recently, historians have argued that the HIMS was a model that helped pave the way for the new National Health Service (NHS) introduced throughout Britain in 1948.[2] But, despite the role of the region in the establishment of the NHS, I will argue that discontent with the operation of the NHS in the area also later pointed the way to the first major reorganization of the NHS in 1974. The report of the Birsay Committee, a government committee investigating the medical services in the Highlands and Islands in the mid-1960s, highlights contemporary perceptions of the problems faced in providing medical services in remote areas of Scotland and responses to them. Notably, it was especially critical of the changes brought to the administration of medical services by the ending of the HIMS and advent of the NHS in 1948.[3] Once again the experience of this remote area foreshadowed wider change.

The Area

The Highlands and Islands area of Scotland is usually taken to mean the seven 'crofting' counties (Shetland, Orkney, Caithness, Sutherland, Ross and Cromarty, Inverness and Argyll), although a few other areas at the margins are sometimes included (Figure 4.1). It amounts to a little short of half of the area of Scotland (14,000 out of 30,000 square miles), including 118 islands with small populations. In 1961 it had fewer than 278,000 people, or about one twentieth of the Scottish population. As a result, this half of Scotland was nearly empty. The Registrar General's tables of population density show 0.0 persons per acre in these counties, compared with more than 1.8 million people (one third of the Scottish population) who lived within a radius of 15 miles from the centre of Glasgow.[4]

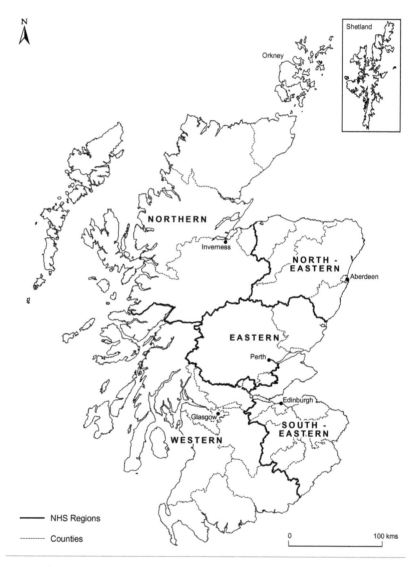

Figure 4.1: The National Health Service in Scotland, 1948–71. Source: Cartography by Mike Shand, based on J. S. Ross, *The National Health Service in Great Britain: an historical and descriptive study* (Oxford: Oxford University Press, 1952).

Several other features of the demography, geography and economy of the Highlands and Islands should be noted. First, there was a long-term absolute and relative decline in the population. Between 1851 and 1961 the total population dropped by about one third and its proportion dropped in relation to the rest of Scotland. In contrast to the settler areas described in other chapters in this volume, this was an area of emigration.[5] Also, within the seven counties there was considerable rural depopulation, with the proportion of the population of each county living in burghs increasing between 1931 and 1961. Second, by the 1960s the automobile had revolutionized travel in the Highlands (in 1961 there was one car for every six persons, compared with an average of one for every eight in Scotland as a whole), but many roads remained narrow and winding and, apart from the one main north–south road, the main roads followed the glens from east to west. State-supported ferry services were of major importance in western areas and Orkney and Shetland. There were also some regular airline services to the islands by the 1950s. Finally, the scattered population was poor. It was made up mainly of 'crofters', i.e., small farmers paying rent for their holdings, and some others who earned a living from fishing or from employment on estates.[6]

The Highlands and Islands Medical Service

In 1913 the government established the HIMS to meet the problems of the provision of medical services in the islands and remote northern half of Scotland. The HIMS was an expedient devised in the wake of national legislation in 1911 that introduced a compulsory insurance for the first time. The primary aim of the 1911 national insurance legislation was to protect groups of workers, particularly the industrial workforce, from the loss of income during periods of cyclical unemployment and sickness. Men and women aged between sixteen and seventy years old, employed under a contract of service whose annual income did not exceed £160 per annum, had to contribute four pence per week to an insurance pool, along with their employers (three pence) and the state (two pence). The scheme provided cash benefits for contributors during periods of unemployment and sickness, and it provided medical benefits for contributors, which took the form of medical attendance, treatment and medicines from a general practitioner, as well as a fixed sum of money paid out as a maternity benefit and a right to treatment for tuberculosis. Benefits did not include medical attendance for the contributors' family members, nor hospital treatment. The payments were paid out by 'approved societies' (friendly societies, trade unions, industrial insurance companies or the post office) on receipt of a sickness certificate from the general practitioner who treated the claimant. Doctors participated in the system as part of a 'panel' under contract to the approved societies and were paid by a capitation fee; they remained 'independent contractors' rather than salaried officials.

The government, when drawing up the legislation, realized the scheme would not be feasible in the Highlands and Islands because it was impossible for most of the population to pay weekly contributions. Most of the population was excluded from the scheme entirely, as crofters were self-employed and rarely had formal contracts for any employment; if they made voluntary payments their contribution would have had to include the employer's contribution as well: at seven pence per week such contributions would be impossible for most people. Even if the residents could pay, few would receive any medical benefit, because the necessary local general practitioner services did not exist in the area.

In 1912, after the passage of the legislation and before its implementation, the government set up a committee, chaired by Sir John Dewar (Figure 4.2), the Member of Parliament for Inverness, philanthropist and whisky manufacturer, to consider the provision of medical attention in the Highlands and Islands and to advise on the best method of securing a satisfactory medical service.[7] The Dewar Committee toured the area, took evidence from over 250 witnesses, and quickly produced a report that has become a classic of social investigation.[8]

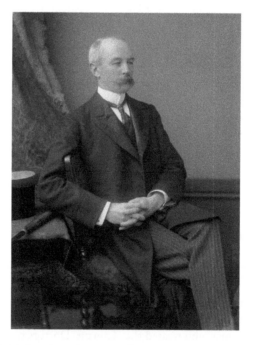

Figure 4.2: John Alexander Dewar, first Baron Forteviot (1856–1929); reproduced by permission of the National Portrait Gallery, London.

The Dewar Committee's report gave a gloomy picture of the health of the area, as judged by infant mortality rates and tuberculosis. It found the housing and nutrition of people were poor and noted reliance on patent medicines and the survival of witchcraft.[9] Moreover, it found the existing medical services very near to collapse and unable to support the National Health Insurance Scheme. In particular, the committee pointed to the large number of uncertified deaths, because a doctor did not attend the last illness: in many parishes the proportion was over 40 per cent and in one remote parish it reached 80 per cent.[10]

The report pointed out that the inadequacy of medical provision was not due to an absolute shortage in the total number of general practitioners, but to the geography of the region that made it impossible for this number of doctors to have effective access to such a scattered population. In addition, the report criticized the quality of the doctors' care, pointing out the rapid turnover in the more remote parishes and noting that those who remained had problems of some sort. Also, no doctor could easily afford to buy a car or a motor boat, although in many cases he needed both; there was no reliable telephone service; doctors' houses were unsatisfactory; doctors had no security of tenure; and incomes were so low that the average doctor could not take a holiday or take advantage of postgraduate courses because the cost of a locum was beyond his means. Furthermore, the report found the supply of trained nurses, provided through voluntary nursing associations, wholly inadequate and unorganized. Finally, the existing hospital services in Inverness, Kirkwall, Oban and Lerwick were inadequate. Travel to hospitals was difficult; patients were reluctant to leave home for treatment of uncertain benefit in an alien environment. If they did seek the most modern treatment, they faced long journeys to the Greenock or Glasgow Royal Infirmaries or to Aberdeen or Edinburgh. The committee concluded that the situation required further government intervention.[11]

Within eight months of the publication of the committee's report, Parliament passed legislation in 1913 implementing nearly all of the committee's proposals. It established the Highlands and Islands Medical Service Fund which provided grants to: 1) doctors; 2) nursing services; 3) specialist hospital and ambulance services; 4) telegraph and telephone services. The aim was to make it economically possible for everyone in the area to secure the services of a doctor and for the doctor in turn to render the services.[12]

The service was quickly implemented after the First World War, and attracted well-trained doctors and nurses returning from war service. Under the scheme the doctors were contracted to attend defined groups of patients and their families regardless of the distance of the patient from the doctor's place of residence.[13]

In return, the doctor could charge a limited fee if the patient could pay, but also received an annual grant from the HIMS Fund that provided an annual income that took account of the expense of travelling to attend patients, house rent and the cost of drugs provided.[14] In addition, the conditions of service of practitioners in the HIMS included a commitment to undertake the duties that the public health authorities of the district required, and they were expected to attend regularly at schools to treat diseases and defects disclosed by medical inspection.

Crucially, given the concerns of British general practitioners, these arrangements did not make the doctor a salaried servant of the state. In the exercise of professional duties he or she was as independent as general practitioners elsewhere. The contribution of the state was seen as relieving doctors of undue economic burdens, both by payments related to their professional commitments and by making financial resources available to provide suitable houses for renting, arrangements for holiday leave and for postgraduate courses at medical schools, and special assistance in the event of serious illness or other emergency. By the later 1920s the state and the doctors also participated in a superannuation scheme. In all these matters the practitioners dealt directly with a medical officer at the Scottish Board of Health in the central government at Edinburgh. About 150 doctors in the area were in contract under the scheme.[15]

Nursing services also expanded rapidly. After the legislation, county and district nursing associations were organized to provide locally residing district nurses, who in most cases combined home nursing duties with the functions of midwife, health visitor, school nurse and social worker. The local nursing association appointed the nurses and they were inspected by a national organization, the Queen's Nursing Institute of Scotland, but in these remote areas, working closely with the local medical practitioners, they had considerable autonomy. In many communities patients consulted the nurse first; if necessary, she referred the patient on to the doctor and she carried out any subsequent treatment under his or her instructions. The nursing associations were financed by local subscriptions, together with grants from the local health authorities, supplemented to a considerable and crucial extent by the HIMS Fund.[16]

Regarding hospital services, the HIMS Fund supplemented local efforts and made it possible to appoint full-time consultant surgeons to key hospitals on the Islands, beginning with Stornoway in 1924 and on the mainland; the Fund also supported substantial modernization of equipment and a considerable increase in nursing staff. Grants were made towards the salaries of surgeons and hospital personnel, and towards capital and maintenance expenditure for buildings and equipment. Other specialist services also developed. An ENT specialist was appointed in 1929 and grants from the Fund also made possible the development of diagnostic radiology and laboratory services at Inverness, as well as a postal service providing diagnostic facilities for the Northern mainland counties and Orkney and Shetland based on the laboratories at the Inverness and Aberdeen hospitals. The provision of the air ambulance service to the Western Isles started in 1936, linking them with Glasgow hospitals, and lifeboat journeys for medical emergencies to remote places were also paid for.[17]

An important review of the health services in Scotland was carried out in the mid-1930s and reported in 1936 (the Cathcart Report) that the provision of medical care had been revolutionized in the Highlands and Islands since the Dewar Committee's report.[18] From the patients' point of view better-trained doctors were more accessible and used. The proportion of uncertified deaths declined by 6 per cent during the first ten years of the new service, compared with 1 per cent in the rest of Scotland. In addition, patients' access to specialist diagnostic services and treatment increased. The increase in the number of trained nurses to over 200 and provision of local accommodation also meant that fewer illnesses went untreated and nearly all births were attended by a trained midwife or a 'double duty nurse', i.e., a nurse with midwifery training. By 1939 infant mortality in the Highlands and Islands had fallen below the rest of Scotland, though maternal mortality remained slightly higher.[19] It was the only area of the country in which the health services aimed to be administered as a whole, in which general practitioners, consultants, hospitals and nurses were seen as part of a comprehensive service, and where money was available for houses, telephones and transport. The central administration was admired for its simplicity and directness and the central staff of civil servants were familiar with the area served. The doctors were happy to deal directly with Edinburgh rather than being under the local political control they feared. Even the British Medical Association approved of the arrangements.[20] Furthermore, the HIMS had become 'a source of inspiration to other countries faced with similar difficulties'.[21]

The Coming of the National Health Service in 1948

In 1946, when introducing the National Health Service (Scotland) Bill to the House of Commons, the Secretary of State for Scotland singled out the HIMS for providing 'the necessary pointers towards ... a full and comprehensive service in Scotland'.[22] Yet, the coming of the NHS in 1948 removed one of the key features of the HIMS: its unified administration, directly by the Scottish Health Department of the central government in Edinburgh, funded by the single HIMS Fund. Looking back from the 1960s, this feature in particular was commended:

> [C]ontinuous personal professional contact was maintained between the central Department and the medical personnel in the field through one of the Department's headquarters medical staff experienced in problems of rural practice. Systematic visits to practices throughout the area were welcomed by the doctors, and the administrative handling of the scheme drew from the British Medical Association a special plea

to the Secretary of State that under the forthcoming National Health Service they should continue to serve under the aegis of the Department of Health for Scotland. They based their request on the fact that their relationship with the central Department over the previous thirty years had been one of complete confidence. In 1947 the Chief Medical Officer of the Department of Health for Scotland was able to say: 'we have no difficulty in obtaining doctors, specialists or nurses for any area within the scheme; indeed the numbers and calibre of applicants for vacancies are frequently embarrassing.'[23]

When the British NHS emerged on the Appointed Day, 5 July 1948, medical services throughout the UK became universal (i.e., available to all), comprehensive (i.e., all services both preventive and curative), and free at the point of delivery (i.e., financed primarily directly from the national exchequer with a small proportion from national insurance contributions). [24] However, unification of all health services under a single system of administration was regarded as impractical for political reasons; instead, the new service had a tripartite administrative structure. There were different forms of administration for hospitals, public health and independent contractor services for the NHS in England and Wales, and Scotland.

The dominant feature of the scheme lay in the nationalization and regionalization of the hospitals. It made possible the integration of all types of hospital under regional hospital boards appointed by the minister and responsible for the application of government policy, overall strategic planning, budgetary control and some specific duties such as the development of specialities and appointment of hospital consultant doctors. The municipal hospitals were taken away from the local authorities, but through their medical officer of health the local authorities remained in charge of functions such as maternity and child welfare, domiciliary midwifery, health visiting, home nursing, home helps, vaccination and immunization and other activities connected with public health and health education. Finally, the scheme also allowed for the separate administration of services provided by independent contractors, i.e., general medical practitioners, general dental practitioners, opticians and pharmacists. At the local level, committees, called executive councils, administered their services; they were essentially renamed committees inherited from the previous panel system under the 1911 National Insurance system. The executive councils in the main followed the geographic pattern of the local health authorities, but there were longstanding tensions between the two as the general practitioners adamantly resisted any suggestion that they become salaried employees of the local authorities.

Not only did the NHS have a tripartite structure, but the NHS in Scotland was introduced on the Appointed Day under separate legislation and although the administrative structure in Scotland was basically the same, there were some differences. In particular, the minister and department responsible for the service were the Secretary of State for Scotland and the relevant department in the Scottish Office, rather than the Minister of Health and his department.[25]

For patients in the rest of Scotland, England and Wales, the NHS brought free access to a doctor, nurse, hospital, dentist, other medical treatments and no charge initially for prescriptions, so patients no longer put off seeking treatment, and medical services were in great demand from the outset. Yet, for patients in the Highlands and Islands the advent of the NHS in 1948 meant little change in access to medical and other health services. The HIMS ended, and now those who had used medical services financed by the HIMS, like the rest of the country, had to register with a general practitioner. They did so rapidly. In Shetland, for example,

> after only one week under the new scheme, the news is that 11,000 people have sent cards in to the doctors of their choice; add to this the 7,000 already on the 'panel' and the total is 18,000: the Department's estimate of the population is 19,200, so that percentage is very high when compared with other areas ... It is early yet to say what the ultimate effect of the scheme will be, but everywhere in Shetland there seems to be the desire to make it work smoothly for the benefit of the people – which is as it should be.[26]

Among other changes under the NHS, nurses in the community were administered and paid by local authorities rather than local voluntary committees (funded by a combination of local charitable contributions and central HIMS funds), which improved their salaries and accommodation, provided a superannuation scheme, and led to those who qualified taking on the 'triple duties' of health visitor as well as district nurse and midwife. For patients, the latter meant continuity of care; for nurses it led to job satisfaction, as one nurse in the Outer Hebrides reflected on her work in the 1950 and 1960s:

> Being in the triple role was ideal. You knew the mother. You were usually the first to know if there was a baby coming and then you knew that baby, followed it up to 5 years and then at school. I had many years of the triple role and the continuity was marvellous. It was very rewarding and you felt you were part of the household. I lived in the nurse's house and drove the nurse's car. In the outer Hebrides it was an A30, then a Ford and finally a little blue Mini – new![27]

Although the change to local authority control reinforced the administrative distinction between the local district nurse and doctor, it did not seem to disrupt their existing collaboration and working relationships in most areas of the Highlands and Islands, foreshadowing the 'primary care team' and 'attachment' of district nurses, midwives and health visitors to GP practices encouraged widely in urban areas in the 1950s and 1960s. Also, in contrast to the HIMS, local authority medical officers undertook school medical inspections rather than subcontracting these to local general practitioners, thus disrupting the continuity of care for the patient and local general practitioner. Yet, infant and maternal mortality continued to fall in the Highlands and Islands in line with the rest of the country: in 1965 the number of births had increased by 15 per cent above the number in 1939, while infant deaths fell to half and maternal deaths to one sixth the number in 1939. By 1965 the issue for contemporaries was no longer how to catch up with the quality and access to medical services in the rest of the country, but how to maintain and improve quality and access to medical services within the tripartite framework of the NHS given the region's still exceptional difficulties of distance and isolation.[28]

The Birsay Committee

In 1964 the Secretary of State for Scotland appointed a committee 'to consider the arrangements for the provision of general medical services in the Highlands and Islands within the framework of the health services generally; and to make recommendations'.[29] Pressure for the appointment of the committee came from the Scottish branch of the British Medical Association in response to dissatisfaction among doctors in the Highlands and Islands resulting from the introduction of the NHS in 1948. The doctors' concerns focused on difficulties over remuneration and conditions which, although always present, became more acute around 1960 when proposals for improvements in the remuneration for all family doctors arose. The proposals applied to doctors in the Highlands and Islands on the same basis as those for the rest of the country, but doctors in the Highlands and Islands believed the changes put them at a serious disadvantage because the arrangements failed to take account of the geographic and other features peculiar to the Highlands and Islands. A memorandum to the BMA from a doctor in Orkney in September 1961 vividly set out the problems causing concern and prompted further investigation assisted by the Scottish Home and Health Department and eventually the appointment of the Committee on General Medical Services in the Highlands and Islands.[30]

Sir Harald Leslie (Figure 4.3), a notable Scottish lawyer, who became Lord Birsay in 1965 when appointed chairman of the Scottish Land Court, was an appropriate choice to chair the committee. A native of Orkney, he took his title, Birsay, from a village in Orkney. He stood unsuccessfully as the Labour candidate for Parliament for Orkney and Shetland in 1950. In 1961 he was appointed Sheriff of Caithness, Sutherland, Orkney and Zetland. Thus he was familiar with the region, particularly Orkney where complaints surfaced. Also, his wife, a native of Orkney, was a family doctor in the northern islands before their marriage in 1945.[31]

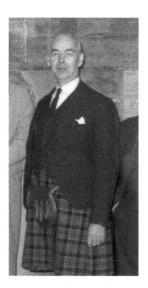

Figure 4.3: Harald John Leslie, Lord Birsay (1905–82); held within the W. H. Hourston collection, Orkney Library & Archive and reproduced by permission of Orkney Library & Archive.

There were eight members of the Birsay Committee apart from the chair. Three had wide experience of health service administration, including one woman who served on boards in all three parts of the administration – executive council, regional hospital board and local authority. Four members came from parts of the medical profession, including: one consultant physician from Raigmore Hospital, Inverness; two family doctors, one who had practised in two areas of the Highlands and whose father had been a family doctor in the Highlands, and the other who was active in the BMA; and one doctor who had just retired as Scottish Secretary of the BMA. The eighth member, the Professor of Modern History at Glasgow University, seems a curious addition, though he brought a broader perspective, having been a member of the UK National Commission for UNESCO and having extensive academic experience in the US.[32]

Beginning in November 1964 the Birsay Committee, like the Dewar Committee forty years earlier, held meetings throughout the Highlands and Islands and took written and oral evidence from over 150 representatives of relevant organizations, medical practitioners and individuals. A subcommittee also visited Norway for a week in September 1965 under the auspices of the Norwegian government to examine the provision of health services in rural areas and visit practices with problems similar to those in parts of north and west Scotland. Although aware of the dangers of attempting to apply the experience of one country to another, the committee found Norwegian administrative practices useful as models and attempted to incorporate some of their virtues into its major recommendations.[33]

The committee completed its report in March 1967 and it was published in June. The committee was quick to point out that although it followed in the footsteps of the Dewar Committee, its aims were more humble. The service in the Highlands and Islands was broadly satisfactory, so there was less scope 'for proposals having the scale and sweep of the Dewar recommendations'. The committee's aim was for conditions to be created 'in which decisions for the Highlands and Islands are taken in the Highlands and Islands'.[34]

The committee was particularly concerned with the increasing rural depopulation of the area and the high proportion of elderly among the remaining inhabitants. It found four themes emerging from its evidence: transport and communications; conditions of service; remuneration; and integration of services. The committee organized its report around chapters on transport and communications, the roles and deployment of general practitioners and locums, hospital and specialist services, local authority services, care of the elderly, methods of remuneration and administration.

The committee presented sixty-one conclusions and recommendations. Many of these were expected or relatively minor, but they highlight contemporary concerns and responses and are worth summarizing briefly. For example, the problem of communications was stressed by all witnesses, lay and professional. Long distances or sea passages raised barriers of time, money and feasibility and allied depopulation made domiciliary services expensive and sometimes impossible. Roads were still difficult.[35] The increase in car ownership since the war meant that rural bus services were not profitable and were shrinking. More patients were visiting their doctor's surgery, yet, 'many Highland doctors still expressed a preference for the old pattern of practice of the region, when the majority of patients were seen in their homes'.[36] The committee felt the trend would be toward patients attending well-equipped, purpose-built surgeries. The committee members were enthusiastic about the drive on/drive off ferries they saw in Norway, and welcomed their introduction in the Highlands, as they would make possible the redeployment of some general practitioners with small island practices among the seven practices with less than 200 patients and twenty-one with less than 500. Yet, it recognized that 'in the public mind the quality of the medical service tends to be equated with the proximity of a doctor ... so any attempt to reduce the number of small practices will be unpopular'.[37]

The committee concluded that the medical manpower devoted to the population of the Highlands and Islands was not disproportionately high and did not advocate any reduction in number, though the justification of small remote practices should be under continual scrutiny. It stressed the importance of refresher training for doctors working in isolation and pointed out the lack of close links between general practice and the universities in the same way as the hospital service. It also recommended the recognition of the special position of the rural doctor's wife in the form of payment for carrying out ancillary duties. It recommended that the powers to provide residential accommodation should be widened to permit the provision of separate main or branch surgeries. The committee pointed out the difficulties faced by doctors in the more remote parts of the Highlands and Islands in securing locums for holidays, illness or professional courses, and recommended the health service take responsibility for providing them 'without disturbing the "independent contractor" status of general practitioners', and particularly advocated extending the present provisions for providing locums from hospital staff.[38]

Regarding district nurses and patient referral, while the ultimate responsibility for deciding whether or not to visit a patient remained with the general practitioner, the committee concluded that the tradition in isolated areas of the patient first consulting the district nurse when in doubt about the need to call the doctor was reasonable.

The committee also recommended that the provision of a domestic help service should be converted from a permissive power into a statutory duty. There was room for improvement in the effectiveness of the measures taken to identify women willing to work as home helps and to ensure that all concerned knew where applications for help should be made. The employment of a relative as a home help should be specifically permitted in appropriate cases. Also, it pointed out that the shortage of hospital accommodation for old people was substantial on even the ordinary bed-ratio calculations and these underestimated the needs of the region.

Furthermore, the committee considered the remuneration of general practitioners in the Highlands and Islands and suggested that inducement payments to provide general practitioners in sparsely populated areas with a predetermined income no longer provided an adequate basis for remuneration. It recommended a new method.

One major theme, however, that emerged from the committee's evidence and its report was the difficulty of coordinating the health services across the boundaries of the tripartite administrative structure introduced in 1948.

The administrative structure for the Highlands and Islands after 1948 was essentially the same tripartite structure as in operation elsewhere in Britain, in contrast to the previous position under the HIMS with its centralized administration and financing, which was quite distinct from anything found elsewhere in the country. The HIMS Fund was concerned not only with payments and other grants to doctors, but also with the nursing service, hospital and ambulance services, the provision and improvement of doctors' and nurses' houses, specialist services, the extension of telegraphs and telephones and various other matters such as the special tuberculosis scheme. Very often the grants made in one field were conditional upon certain measures of coordination with others. There was therefore a substantially unified service, except for the services provided by local health authorities.[39]

The tripartite structure of the NHS was very much an innovation in the area and was not welcomed by the general practitioners, who made it clear that they would have preferred continued direct administration from the central department. The committee pointed out that in the Highlands and Islands, probably to a greater extent than anywhere else in the country, there was considerable overlapping in the membership of the various health service administrative agencies. Thus, insofar as shared membership of the administrative units could facilitate close co-operation, this advantage was available to the Highlands and Islands. Yet, no witness who came before the committee could reasonably be described as an enthusiastic defender of the present administrative structure, while many were extremely critical of it.[40]

The committee observed that from the time that the three separate branches of the NHS were established in 1948, it was recognized that ways of ensuring cooperation and coordination were necessary and that machinery should be evolved to provide for quick and effective discussion of common problems and agreement on solutions to them. The legislation made specific provisions for this, but by 1967 when the committee reported, none had proved lasting.[41]

The committee suggested that this disappointing state of affairs might have something to do with the marked differences which existed between executive councils, local health authorities and regional hospital boards in their organization and relationship with the service they provided: there were no 'opposite numbers' between the authorities' officials or professional personnel; the authorities were different in status; and they approached their work and problems from different, financial and statutory, angles.[42]

Many of the committee's other conclusions and recommendations reflected these administrative barriers. For example, the committee stressed that the general practitioner should have responsibility for a substantial element of public health work and school medical examinations, something which ceased with the end of the HIMS in 1948. It reported the frustration general practitioners and executive councils felt when hospital boards developed plans without consultation.[43] The ambulance service was strongly criticized for single manning and sometimes dirty vehicles, a situation attributed to the lack of clarity in the service's place in the administrative structure. Moreover, the committee was keen for doctors and district nurses to utilize the same premises, and it recommended that executive councils and local health authorities should consult each other before surgeries or other premises were built in order to ensure that multiple use of facilities was fully considered.

The evidence led the committee 'inescapably to the conclusion that a new way of administering the health service is urgently needed'.[44] It argued that 'the functional division of the service into separate sectors dealing with hospitals, general practitioner services and local authority services ... has at least in the Highlands and Islands outlived its usefulness'.[45]

The committee's final recommendation was the only one it made 'strongly'.[46] It recommended that general control of all health functions be concentrated in the hands of a single body covering the whole of the area (a Highlands and Islands Health Board to cover the existing crofting counties, together with Nairn), with day-to-day management being conducted by similar all-purpose area health boards, responsible for reasonably compact smaller areas. It stressed that this was not the same as the concept of area health boards favoured by the Porritt Committee appointed by the medical profession which reported in 1962 and advocated area health boards operating mainly through committees with functions closely related to each of the three main divisions of the existing services. Instead, it argued that a high level board with general powers of overseeing the area would not be helpful if at all lower levels matters proceeded as before. It argued for a unified administration in the local area with responsibility for resources relating to both hospital and general practitioner services, as well as certain local authority services, in order to give scope for local assessment of priorities.[47]

The committee pointed out that the idea of a unified service was by no means new, as it would have been at least as natural a development in the Highlands and Islands in 1948 as the tripartite structure that was created. And, the committee members believed it would be widely acceptable among those concerned with general practitioner and hospital services, though they recognized that there might be some reluctance on the part of local health authorities to relinquish their powers in health matters.[48]

The committee also recognized differences between the situation in Scotland and that in Norway, but drew for support of its proposals on the unified structure of the Norwegian system at the local level, and especially the Norwegian view of local knowledge as a reliable basis for decision-making and encouragement for local initiative and responsibility.[49]

Finally, the committee suggested that the Highlands and Islands region offered a place in which to experiment with a new structure or unified administration.[50]

Conclusion

In 1974 the first major reorganization of the NHS in Britain took place. A central feature was the replacement of the tripartite administrative structure with levels of organization by area.[51] Thus, the Birsay report's major recommendation in 1967 foreshadowed the future, and gave the most remote area of the United Kingdom – the Highlands and Islands of Scotland – a significant role in the movement that led to the first major reorganization of the NHS.

There is a certain irony in this since its predecessor, the Highlands and Islands Medical Service, in 1948 had been seen by contemporaries and more recently by historians as a precursor of the NHS that was originally introduced.

For patients the introduction of the HIMS after the First World War improved the quality of and access to medical services. By 1939 measures such as the proportion of uncertified deaths, and infant and maternal mortality rates approached those of the rest of the country. Given the existing access to medical services, the replacement of the HIMS by the NHS in 1948 did not lead to the surge in demand for services experienced in other parts of the country. The demise of the central administration of the HIMS and advent of the tripartite administrative structure of the NHS made continuity of care more difficult for local general practitioners, but increased the scope for nurses carrying out 'triple duties'. Infant and maternal mortality continued to fall in the Highlands and Islands in line with the rest of Scotland. The challenge for contemporaries in the mid-1960s was to maintain and improve quality and access to medical services, despite the continuing challenges of geography, demography and isolation characteristic of the region.

Also, remote areas provide examples of different forms of organization of the provision of medical services. The Birsay Committee in 1967 recommended that the Highlands and Islands be used to experiment with different types of reorganization on a regional basis. However, in this case, the remote area was not used to experiment, and historians have argued that if there had been such an experiment, it might have avoided some of the failings of the reorganization that took place in 1974.[52]

PART II: DOCTORS AND DOCTORING IN REMOTE AREAS

Introduction

This section examines physicians' efforts to practise medicine in widely diverse societies and the duties they envisioned for themselves. In the first case, Sören Edvinsson clearly shows that Dr Ellmin did not see himself as solely a purveyor of modern medicine to a remote area of nineteenth-century Sweden. There is no doubt that Ellmin also believed he was engaged in an adventure that he felt compelled to document. His mission was not only a 'civilizing' one; he also wanted his superiors in Stockholm and the Swedish public to learn about the hardships these residents of the north endured. Ellmin was a doctor, an adventurer and, to some degree, an advocate for the Sami people. As such he found himself in the liminal position between state employee with an obligation to introduce academic medicine as defined by his superiors in Stockholm, and social critic who believed that the government had an obligation to improve the physical and economic conditions in which the people lived. Øivind Larsen's contribution focuses more attention on the degree to which doctors were able to direct medical legislation particularly during periods of abnormal morbidity or mortality. He concludes that such legislation was often based upon perceptions held by distant physicians rather than cold scientific or statistical data. We find doctors asking whether certain patterns were unusual and, if so, were they markedly different than what had come before? Were the people themselves responsible for their ill-health or was their condition evidence of government neglect? Answers to these questions became part of the reports physicians submitted to state officials. In this way their perceptions and interpretations were instrumental to providing the type of medical care that people needed and the state sought to provide. If one is inclined to believe that there was something particularly European about the inability or unwillingness of local physicians to impose their will on distant populations, or that this was a characteristic of medical practice that has long since passed, the contributions to this volume by J. T. H. Connor and

Sasha Mullally will put any such thoughts to rest. Connor's study of the rural practice of Dr Ecke in northern Newfoundland proves that this physician also found himself negotiating between the type of medicine he had been trained to provide while at one of the most renowned medical schools in the United States of America, and the medical care his patients were prepared to accept. His practice in Twillingate was as peripheral to the medical world of twentieth-century North America as Ellmin's had been to that of Stockholm, and the practices of Norwegian doctors had been to the innovations found in Oslo. Similarly, Mullally illuminates the level of resistance directed against authorities in the Canadian province of New Brunswick who tried to dictate who could or could not provide medical care during the 1920s and 1930s. Popular demands for treatment from unlicensed practitioners, and in the case of Dr Leger even a licensed one, often trumped the best efforts of the province's College of Physicians and Surgeons to control access to the medical profession. Instead of meekly accepting the judgements of this medical body, the sick continued to seek out whoever they felt offered the best chance of relief regardless of whether that person had official approval or not.

5 A COUNTRY DOCTOR: HEALTH CARE IN A MID-NINETEENTH-CENTURY SWEDISH REMOTE AREA

Sören Edvinsson

The winter of 1851 was not a good time for the new doctor in Vemdalen, Johan Ellmin. He did not only have to adjust to life in a new environment, he also found his sleep disturbed. One night during Easter, he heard noise from the yard at the farm where he rented a room. A group of youngsters were trying to convince the young farm maid to leave the farm and come with them, and Ellmin soon found himself in a dispute with the intruders. This was neither the first nor the last time this happened, nor was it the only problem the doctor had to face. Placed in an unfamiliar and unfriendly environment, far away from family, friends and colleagues, it was perhaps not surprising that he was often ill at ease.

This article uses the experiences of Dr Johan Ellmin in the district of Härjedalen, Sweden, to shed light on some major themes of nineteenth-century medicine. By discussing how the health-care system was spread throughout Sweden, as well as outlining the obligations of *provinsialläkare* (district medical officers),[1] this text relates the activities of one doctor serving in a remote area to the development of medicine and medical organization in a significant historical period. The main sources used here are the reports that Ellmin sent to the *Sundhetskollegium* (National Board of Health) from 1851 to 1859.[2] These reports were very extensive and frequently exceeded what was expected, and for this reason they offer many interesting and exciting insights into the lives and minds of physicians in remote areas of Sweden in this period. They also reveal the local conditions in which Ellmin worked as well as his perception that the people in this 'foreign' territory needed civilizing.

Medicine in the Nineteenth Century

First, we need to describe the context within which district medical officers such as Ellmin acted. Much ambiguity about the causes of death and disease and about the role of medicine in society characterized nineteenth-century medical thought. The ancient humoralist traditions of Hippocrates and Galen still influenced medical thought. A central Hippocratic text during the eighteenth and nineteenth centuries was *On Airs, Waters and Places*, which emphasized the relationship between local environments and disease. It was also a time of confusion regarding medical theory and the most efficacious steps to be employed to combat disease. Contagionists claimed that personal contacts were the principal causes for the spread of diseases such as plague, cholera and yellow fever, thus favouring quarantine as a method to prevent disease, while the anti-contagionists looked at local conditions, usually through a miasma developed in filth, to explain the arrival of disease.[3]

There was a strong focus on geographical space in eighteenth- and nineteenth-century medicine. The Hippocratic tradition emphasized the impact of environment and both contagionism and miasma theories implied the importance of it. Medical topographies and reports played important roles in this medical context. National authorities as well as private persons took the initiative to collect statistics and different kinds of descriptions and the field of medical geography started to develop.[4] It was a time that witnessed the expansion of the medical realm.

The Linnaean tradition of categorizing and exploring the world was very influential in Sweden. One expression of this was the creation of national statistics through the so-called *Tabellverket* beginning in the mid-eighteenth century.[5] Another product was the medical topographies that the *Collegium Medicum* demanded of district medical officers during the latter half of the same century.[6] The statistics were, however, primarily descriptive and seldom used for analysis, and the medical topographies were only sporadically delivered. As such, neither resource did much to alter health politics or the provision of medicine.

More valuable health surveys were produced from the middle of the nineteenth century. Improvements in both statistics and the medical topographies resulted from the initiative of paediatrician Fredrik Th. Berg, who was a central figure in Swedish health politics for several decades. As Berg reflected, 'Ever since my first term of service as a doctor, the statistical method, or the collection and grouping of observations, in order, by a total survey thereof, to be led on the way of truth, had indeed been my hobby'.[7] In 1859, he became the first director of the newly created *Statistiska Centralbyrån* (Statistics Sweden) where he improved both the collection and the use of data. In contrast to the earlier, mainly descriptive, use of statistics, Berg and his colleagues used the collected data for analysis, often from a spatial perspective. One important finding was that mortality was much higher in urban environments than in the countryside. Statistical analysis also proved that there were large regional differences – for example, in infant mortality – that urged for an explanation.[8]

Medical topographies supplied additional information to state officials but it was not until 1851 when Berg took the initiative to request these reports that the district medical officers from all districts started to produce continuous reports, spurred on by officials at the *Sundhetskollegium* who now conducted yearly follow-ups to ensure that the doctors complied.[9] Berg described the purpose of the medical topographies in his first national report. To present a national description of the health of the population, Berg called for more knowledge about diseases prevalent in different parts of the country as well as on the influence of local conditions on health. To achieve this goal, he asserted that the national medical board should continue to collect the information for an extended period of time and for all parts of Sweden. Only comparisons made it possible to understand the importance of local characteristics. Through the reports from the district medical officers the National Board of Health would gain a 'complete material about the medical topography in the country'. More extensive reports were to be repeated every tenth year and included commentaries on a large variety of 'local conditions' that the medical authorities considered relevant for understanding disease, making them descriptions of very varied character. 'Local conditions' included two major types of explanations – one that focused on geographic or climatic conditions, and another that emphasized ways of living, local traditions and behaviours.[10]

The first paragraph of a typical annual report that adhered to Berg's instructions contained information about weather conditions and harvest results. This was followed by a description of the endemic, epidemic, sporadic, venereal and mental diseases that had appeared in the district. The following paragraph described the local health-care system, which included sections about local health-care organization (*sundhetspolis*), poor relief and prisons, charitable institutions, schools, spas, vaccination, pharmacies, midwifery and, finally, military conscription. The district medical officer also included information about his official duties, such as inspection visits, travels during outbreaks of epidemic diseases and medico-legal examinations. This was followed by information on the various groups practising medicine in the district, such as physicians, balneologists and dentists, veterinarians, pharmacists, midwives, vaccinators and quacks (unauthorized practitioners). In the last paragraph, the reporting physician had the opportunity to describe conditions and other observations he considered relevant to report.[11]

Physicians and their Role

During the eighteenth century, there was a great concern about population issues in Sweden. From a mercantilist perspective, a large and healthy population was important, and state-employed district medical officers were hired to help improve the health of Swedes. The royal decree from 1822 still regulated the obligations of the district medical officers at the middle of the nineteenth century.[12] They were responsible both for the general health of the population and for providing private health care in their districts regardless of the status or wealth of the patient. At the local level, the responsibility for health care was in the hands of the local church board.[13] The district medical officers were responsible for observing everything detrimental to health. In cases of epidemics, their duties were to visit the diseased and to prescribe pharmaceuticals. They also reported any cases of venereal diseases.

The responsibility for vaccination was often handed over to bell ringers and midwives.[14] Sweden was comparatively well equipped with authorized midwives who had more far-reaching responsibilities than their counterparts did in many other countries.[15] Swedish physicians accepted, sometimes reluctantly, that others might be required to perform some medical tasks. They could consider this as a practical arrangement due to the lack of physicians, especially in the sparsely populated parts of the country. However, the district medical officers controlled vaccination and the activities of midwives and pharmacists and, therefore, were primarily responsible for providing health care in their districts.

Thus, the district medical officers were publicly financed civil servants who oversaw health care and encouraged the introduction of measures that would prevent diseases from appearing. They were, however, also expected to provide treatment to the inhabitants of their districts. Many of them complained that this usually meant providing services to the most impoverished groups when a profitable practice relied on access to the upper classes, the presence of which varied substantially between different parts of the country.

Nineteenth-century physicians tried to find their role in society. Many felt disillusioned about their therapeutic capability. Officials at the *Sundhetskollegium* began discussing an alternative role for the health-care system. Some suggested that district medical officers should focus on public health and spend less time treating patients. To accomplish this change it would be necessary to substantially increase salaries,[16] a move not embraced by the estate parliament: 'This seems to me as an unnecessary luxury' as one parliamentarian put it.[17] Local parliamentarians expressed more interest in increasing the number of practising physicians than in appointing public health officials.

Access to Physicians in Sweden

Sweden is a large country with an area of approximately 450,000 km². Towns before the end of the nineteenth century were very small and most had populations of less than 2,000 inhabitants. Stockholm, with a population of 75,000 in 1850, was the only city of any size. The northern parts of the country were very sparsely populated and this low population density and the small size of urban environments presented important obstacles for the creation of a health-care system.

The history of official Swedish health care shows that it was of minor significance for most Swedes for a long time. There were only few physicians during the sixteenth and seventeenth centuries, and most of these were in the larger cities and at universities. The number of physicians increased during the 1800s but generally did not keep pace with population growth. It was not until the last decades of the century that access to physicians improved substantially, but they were still few in comparison with many other countries (see Table 5.1).

Table 5.1: Swedish physicians during the nineteenth century.[18]

Year	Physicians	Inhabitants per physician
1805	281	8,690
1850	463	7,522
1860	472	8,177
1870	599	6,959
1880	663	6,886
1890	884	5,413
1900	1,336	3,845

The first physicians using the title of *provinsialläkare* appeared in the late seventeenth century. While they were not state employed, their title gave them the right to receive compensation from the state for services they performed.[19] During the eighteenth century, scientists, higher state officials and politicians took up questions about the possibility of providing doctors in all Swedish provinces, something that eventually led to the first instructions for district medical officers in 1744. At that time, there were only nine district medical officers for all of Sweden. The government took the next step in 1772 when it made a financial commitment to providing at least one district medical officer in every province. This led to the appointment of a total of thirty-two district medical officers. However, even these measures did not help the population in the northern parts of Sweden, who continued to have very limited access to physicians. In Norrland, the part of Sweden composed of what are now the five northernmost provinces covering an area of 262,000 km² (more than one half of Sweden's total area), there were only four *provinsialläkare*. These were situated in Gävle, Söderhamn, Sundsvall and Umeå, so there was no district medical officer stationed north of

Umeå or in the interior of Norrland, which left almost half of Sweden without any professional medical care (see Table 5.2).

Table 5.2: Some categories of employed physicians in Sweden, 1744–1885.[20]

Year	District medical officers (*provinsialläkare*)	Extra district medical officers (*extra provinsialläkare*)	District physicians (*distriktsläkare*)
1744	9	0	0
1772	32	0	0
1816	40	0	0
1830	47	8	0
1835	47	15	0
1845	65	16	31
1852	66	17	30
1859	71	26	22
1885	137	0	56

The following decades saw no large improvements in the access to district medical officers. By 1816, there were only forty of them. In 1811, the interior of northern Sweden received its first district medical officer when the national health board appointed Pehr Rissler in the district of Jämtland (constituted by the two *landskap* Jämtland and Härjedalen). He had his practice in Östersund, which was the only town in the province and had a population of 221 in 1810 and 817 in 1850. Härjedalen was separated from the district in 1823 and received a district medical officer of its own who was initially stationed in the village of Sveg.

The two new categories of *extra provinsialläkare* and *distriktsläkare* appeared during the nineteenth century. In districts considered too large for a single physician to cover efficiently, the government provided a smaller salary to help support an *extra provinsialläkare*. Local initiatives at, for example, iron foundries and other industrial establishments resulted in the employment of *distriktsläkare*. These three categories of physicians were to follow the instructions for district medical officers.

District medical officers had a long history as part of the medical profession in Sweden. In towns and cities, *stadsläkare* (town physicians) fulfilled similar duties but were paid by local authorities. The majority of physicians were thus employed within the public sector. There were very few private practitioners and they had their practice mainly in the larger centres. Nonetheless, the majority of the different types of physicians earned a substantial part of their income by providing health care against a fixed fee or by agreement with individual patients. In that way, their daily work resembled that of the private practitioner.

The District of Härjedalen

The *provinsialläkaredistrikt* of Härjedalen was established by royal decree on 17 September 1823. The authorities decided to locate the medical station in the village of Sveg in the southern part of the district, where it remained until 1847 when it was moved to Vemdalen, a village situated more in the middle of the district but which had fewer inhabitants than Sveg. The district consisted of the *landskap* Härjedalen and the two southernmost parishes of Klövsjö and Rätan in Jämtland. These two parishes were later transferred from the district. The geographical area of the district was a little more than 13,000 km² and in 1823 the population reached approximately 5,000 inhabitants – all widely scattered, as there were no large villages in the district. The largest parish was Sveg with 1,298 inhabitants in 1850, while Vemdalen had only 723. The district is mountainous so there was very little grain production, and the population made its livelihood from animal husbandry. A Sami population lived in the mountains. An iron foundry, situated in Ljusnedal in western Härjedalen, was the only industrial establishment.

Despite the late appearance of physicians, Härjedalen offered a relatively healthy environment compared to other districts, according to available statistics. It had low mortality, with infant mortality levels between 50 and 130 per 1,000 live births from 1860–82, and the high life expectancy was similar to that found in the healthy neighbouring regions across the border in Norway. The exception to this picture of overall health was among the Sami, whose infant mortality rates were quite high.[21]

The frequent arrival and departure of physicians makes it difficult to reconstruct entirely the succession of physicians in the district.[22] The first medical officer, C. Krapp, arrived in 1824. He remained in Sveg until his death in December 1837. The next physician seems to have been in the district only a few months. His successor, S. E. Hallongren, stayed until he died in July 1846. For a couple of years there was a rapid turnover: Med. Dr J. A. Hedenström held the position from July 1846 to early June 1847, and Med. Dr O. F. Hallin came on 14 August 1847 and stayed through the autumn. In December that year Med. Dr C. O. Marin arrived but he too left within a year. The next district medical officer, Med. Dr P. O. Sjöstrand, arrived in mid-May 1849 but left in November. He was followed by Med. Lic. F. A. Lundberg, who requested to be dismissed from the position in September 1850.[23]

We can thus establish that medical authorities encountered severe difficulties finding a qualified physician to stay in the district. The only two (Krapp and Hallongren) who stayed for a long time before 1850 appear not to have been fully qualified. There was no medical exam mentioned in Krapp's biography (he was called student in medicine and surgery), and Hallongren was a candidate in surgery.[24] The others were mainly young physicians who soon left for better positions. There are several explanations for this rapid turnover and perhaps most important was the obvious difficulty in earning a living as a doctor in this area. When the *Sundhetskollegium* created the district in 1823, it argued that the salary offered to the district medical officers should be comparable to that provided to others in the country, especially as other incomes in the district could not be expected.[25] The problem of finding applicants for the position forced the *Sundhetskollegium* to propose increasing the salary to 666 Riksdaler and 32 Skilling Banco, i.e., a sum about 50 per cent higher than in other districts.[26] Physicians in seven districts, all of which were in northern Sweden or in the sparsely populated parts in the interior of mid-Sweden received salaries of 500 Riksdaler. All the others earned approximately 430 Riksdaler. The offer of higher salaries, however, did not improve the situation. With the exception of Ellmin, the rotation of physicians continued in the district for a long time, as seen in the fact that between 1859 and 1869 there were seven different district medical officers in Vemdalen.

In 1850, Härjedalen was without a physician. The position was announced several times during the first half of the year but did not attract any suitable applicants. One doctor indicated his interest after the application deadline, and even though the *Sundhetskollegium* was willing to accept it, the candidate withdrew his application shortly thereafter.[27] The board decided to try once again, and it is at this time that Dr Johan Ellmin entered the scene.

Johan Ellmin – A Physician in his Time

On the one hand, Ellmin has no large place in Swedish history or in the history of medicine. On the other, he is not completely anonymous. His life and career, especially throughout the 1840s, offer many insights into different aspects of nineteenth-century Sweden.

Ellmin was born in the parish of Varv in Skaraborg province in 1797.[28] His father was a soldier which might explain why he began his schooling relatively late. It was not until he was fourteen years of age that he first attended *trivialskolan* (a preparatory school) in Skara, and he was twenty when he started at *gymnasium*. In 1823, he arrived in Uppsala where he began by studying at the faculty of philosophy but soon changed his studies and went into medicine. He became a doctor of medicine in 1835 but, according to him, his economic problems made it impossible for him to continue in the scientific field. He worked as a physician for the poor in Stockholm from 1834 to 1844 but this did nothing to improve his finances.[29] He held various positions: he was one of the physicians in Stockholm during the first cholera epidemic in Sweden in 1834, a doctor at *Sjömanshuset* (sailors' office) from 1838 to 1850, and a doctor for the guild of tailors to name a few examples. He was in close contact with artisans and had good knowledge about the social circumstances confronting Stockholm's poor. In 1837, he married Johanna Christina Raumolin with whom he had three children.

His writings reveal a strong interest in ancient history and culture. In 1821, he published *Concert*, a book of poetry consisting of nine poems in which every poem represented an instrument. His second book came in 1834. He also had a keen interest in science and believed that it would help improve society.

We do not know whether it was his experiences as a doctor for the poor, his own simple background, or maybe his contacts with radical groups that made Ellmin become active as a reformer in the 1840s. For some years he was at the centre of events in Stockholm and was influenced by the radicalism of the time. He worked against considerable opposition to establish a local board devoted to eliminating poverty in Stockholm and supported the construction of a 'workhouse' for the poor.

At this time, the medical profession sought to make new findings known and to discuss scientific matters on both the national and international arenas. The third meeting of *Skandinaviska Naturforskarmötet* took place in Stockholm in 1842 with medical science as one of the main topics of discussion. Ellmin submitted a report in which he suggested that the three Nordic countries should collect information that would enable them to determine whether poverty was the cause of disease or if it was the other way around. Ellmin's proposal reflected contemporary interests in collecting more information that would help identify the causes of health problems. It was obvious that Ellmin was primarily interested in the social rather than the geographical explanations for disease and so his suggestion was very much a topic in the middle of medical debates.[30] It was also a question with strong political implications for the organization of society, the hot topic of poor relief and the desirable extent of state involvement in these issues. Within the sanitary movement, the reformers often emphasized that the local causes of disease must be addressed as this in turn would improve the economy and morality of society. We do not know Ellmin's point of view in this matter because the report was not published. The committee acknowledged the importance of his suggestion but thought that it would be too difficult to collect such data.[31]

In 1845, he took an initiative that had some impact on Swedish history but also resulted in some personal problems for him. He and two radical artisans created the *Bildningscirkeln* (Circle of education) and in this way, Ellmin became a pioneer for Swedish popular education.[32] The Circle invited every decent man to listen to lectures given by enlightened citizens sympathetic to the mission of the Circle. The statutes of the Circle furthermore established that the organization should stand on religious ground and that political polemics should be avoided. Though open to all citizens including labourers, the Circle primarily targeted artisans, who along with journeymen faced many problems owing to socio-economic changes at this time. The tradition of living with the master artisan had disappeared, and many journeymen were now frequenting bars and taverns while living in precarious circumstances. The solution favoured by the Circle was to strengthen the old patriarchal household in which the head of household took care of and educated those living under his roof.[33] The upper classes thus had a responsibility to educate the lower classes – they were to be lifted towards higher civilization through exposure to classical education and knowledge of new scientific findings.[34] Ellmin, who was known as *vattendoktorn*, the water doctor, was also opposed to the drinking of alcohol. After a year, however, Ellmin became out-manoeuvred as chairman of the Circle and it appears that he stopped attending meetings. Some members believed that the lower classes had too much say in the organization and it is likely that others were disappointed with his leadership.[35]

The Circle continued its activities but with more restrictions. Some of the initial founders formed a new group, *Skandinaviska sällskapet* (Scandinavian Society), which got its name and roots from Scandinavian societies found in places such as Paris, Berlin and London that attracted travelling journeymen from Scandinavia. Artisans and interested intellectuals or professionals such as Ellmin, in whose home many of the meetings took place, dominated the society. The more prominent role of artisans reflected a more radical tendency within *Skandinaviska sällskapet* compared to the *Bildningscirkeln*. Many of the journeymen had been in contact with radical movements in Europe and several members called themselves communists, though it is unclear whether Ellmin considered himself to be one. The first translation in any language of the Communist Manifesto was in fact produced within this network. However, the Christian foundations of the group are clearly visible in the subheading of this work, which the translator changed from 'Proletarians of the world unite' to '*Folkets röst är Guds röst*' (The voice of the people is the voice of God).[36]

Despite the idealistic and Christian beliefs of many of the founders, authorities watched the group's activities with suspicion.[37] In an effort to uncover a suspected communist cell within the society, the government sent spies to the meetings. Anxiety grew as a consequence of the numerous revolutionary outbreaks throughout much of Europe in 1848. Even Stockholm experienced some disturbances when riots occurred in March of that year. Troops were called in, eighteen people were killed, and many of the rioters were arrested. These events turned the attention of the police immediately towards the Scandinavian Society. Its leaders, Ellmin among them, were taken in for interrogation. Nothing substantial came of these interrogations, except that Ellmin and his friends became aware that they were under observation. From this time onwards, the radical groups met strong opposition. In the following years, many of the leading radicals left Stockholm; Pehr Götrek, for example, moved to Karlskrona.

Doctor Ellmin was also among those who left Stockholm. While it is possible that the troubles with the authorities had some impact on his decision, he would later state that his economic situation forced him to search for a more financially secure position, which would allow him to retire with a pension.[38] He was sent to southern Sweden as a cholera doctor during autumn of 1850 and next applied for a position in Eksjö but withdrew his application a couple of days before he applied for the position in Härjedalen. However, he must have been quite indecisive because he also withdrew this application a couple of weeks later. However, he changed his mind once again and finally got the position after the board commented on the difficulty there had been in finding someone interested in it.[39]

Ellmin in Vemdalen

Ellmin's reports stand out from all the preserved reports of other district medical officers because of their length and detailed descriptions of his surroundings. He wrote a rich report – one which exceeded all of Berg's requirements – for his first year in Vemdalen in 1851.[40] Much of his report was also printed in the first report from the *Sundhetskollegium*. Characterized by the flowery style of his language, many of Ellmin's reports were filled with references to antique history, religious texts and important political events. His description of how unashamed the people in Härjedalen were serves as one example of his style: 'In regard to the ways the inhabitants of Herjeådalen made their discrete businesses they are as unhampered as the mountaineers that Xenophon with his 10,000 met in the Caucasus on the way back to Greece'.[41] During his early years in the district, he was also eager to provide detailed descriptions of the local community. In this Ellmin referred to the instructions dating from 1822, which stated that the physicians should observe and report everything that might have an effect on health. He obviously took his obligations very seriously.

Through the 1850s, Ellmin submitted many different supplements to his annual reports. In 1851 he attached '*Utkast till Framställning af Herjeådalens ProvincialLäkare District, i anseende till Naturförhållanden, Sundhet och de olika, derinom boende, Folkstammarnes Bildning*' (Outline for a description of Härjedalen's physician's district, regarding the characteristics of the nature, health and the educational and mental levels of the different races living therein). In this work, he described a wide variety of local conditions including geography, economy, local traditions, population, health, and so on. In the following year, he continued the work with a description of one of the villages in the district. When Ellmin continued the outline again in 1854, it focused on the Sami population. The Sami were also the focus of a document from 1855 called '*Renländerne*' (Reindeer country). A second report entitled '*Herjeruna*' described different aspects of life in Härjedalen including poems, songs, games, and so on.

A third report entitled '*Mikael och Herje*' was a sort of historical description of the district. Attached in the 1856 report was a text titled '*Thule med Afseende på Ofred*' (Thule in regard of war). This, however, was the culmination of his extensive reporting, and from that time his reports became more modest in size.

Health in Härjedalen

We know from other sources that mortality was comparatively low in Härjedalen and was probably among the lowest in Sweden at this time.[42] Obviously, the health conditions, although relatively good for the time, were not ideal, especially if compared to the standards of today. Disease and premature death were quite common and this ambiguous image of general health conditions in Härjedalen is apparent in Ellmin's reports.

Ellmin concluded that health was comparatively good in his district and he attributed this partially to the fact that the people did not have time to be ill during the summers when they were herding their cattle in the *sätrar* (saeters) in the mountains. He also maintained that nowhere else in Sweden did people live so long as they did in Härjedalen. The combination of their good health and high life expectancy enabled the population to increase rapidly. Ellmin argued that the mountain air was very healthy (and certainly much better than around the Mediterranean), and identified two additional reasons for the population's good overall health: the people lived simple lives without excesses, and finally, but not least 'the *festina lente*, that is the main characteristic of the people of Herjeådalen, and where he as a consequence is extremely good at sparing his physical strengths during work. When in other places, one person does a work, here always two are needed'. In short, eating and resting took up the most of their days.[43]

Epidemics occurred from time to time but the population seems to have avoided the most devastating consequences of them. The most common diseases among the Swedish population were what the locals called *magschvi*, a gastro-intestinal disease the cause of which Ellmin considered to be dietary, and *krimen*, a respiratory disease.

Topography – The Geographical Dimension

Ellmin's explanations for the high life expectancy in Härjedalen suggest some characteristics that were considered healthy at the time. Much of these revolved around the importance of climate. Every annual report included a discussion of weather conditions during the year. Fresh and open air was essential, while foul and stagnant air was dangerous.[44] Medical expertise believed that wind and ventilation were essential for avoiding disease. Good weather conditions were also important for ensuring a good harvest and allowing people to leave their crowded and unventilated houses. Therefore, inclement weather could easily be linked to the presence of certain diseases.

In his first medical topography, Ellmin provided an extensive description of Härjedalen. It contained purely geographical information such as the size of the district, altitude levels, and the names of the main villages and hamlets. He also provided a description of the local economy. Despite offering these detailed descriptions, Ellmin did not always suggest how the conditions affected the population's health. Instead, they appear rather as general background descriptions of the geography in which he included everything that might possibly have some impact on health. Indeed, he may have viewed them as valuable in their own right because they were continuing the Linnaean tradition of collecting data. They also were not out of keeping with the interests that contemporary Europeans had for foreign countries and peoples during this era of imperialism.

Topography – The People, their Economic Condition, Moral Standards and Way of Life

Ellmin's reports suggest that he at least partially attributed the relative good health of the local inhabitants to their laziness. This is not particularly surprising because in his earlier writings and his activities in the *Bildningscirkeln* he emphasized the socio-economic and behavioural causes of disease more so than the geographical. This corresponded to a general shift in the medical topographies that no longer focused on airs, waters and places but rather began to include a variety of factors that were considered relevant to health. As C. Hannaway writes, 'social and hygienic aspects of the environment had now come into play'.[45] How does this relate to Ellmin's understanding of disease and what were his conclusions when it came to remedies?

One aspect of the lives of people that was directly related to disease and bad health was food preparation and diet. The common food in Härjedalen consisted largely of sour milk, rotten and inadequately salted fish, and tainted meat. According to Ellmin, a stranger not accustomed to local food would think that it tasted awful and was inedible. As if this was not enough, local inhabitants drank large amounts of bad aquavit and coffee. All this resulted in numerous gastro-intestinal diseases.[46]

One recurrent complaint in Ellmin's reports was the abuse of alcohol, which was not surprising considering his negative attitude towards drinking and was something he was not alone to observe. The prominent Swedish physician, Magnus Huss, described alcoholism as a common disease and many doctors considered the abuse of alcohol to be one of the most devastating causes of diseases in Sweden.[47] Alcohol consumption was considered very high in Sweden and some researchers have suggested this as an important explanation for the high male mortality during this period.[48] According to Ellmin, in Härjedalen this problem took the form of drinking large amounts of 'Hoffman's *droppar*', which was a medicine containing alcohol.

Although Ellmin filled his reports with numerous comments regarding the different habits of people in his district, he presented only a few other examples of how the population's way of life and social conditions affected health. He stated that there certainly were famines but that the people managed quite well. They had great skill at preparing their meals from almost nothing and could from time to time make something tasty from it. In this way, Ellmin contradicted his otherwise negative opinion of the local food. Parents told their children to eat less bread and more *sofvelrätten* (meat and fish), something that Ellmin himself had difficulty affording.

Ellmin occasionally offered a positive image of the local people. He wrote that they helped each other in times of crisis and on other occasions. They were hospitable when meeting strangers and could leave their things outside and keep their doors unlocked without fearing that thieves would steal their valuables. Their physical appearances were often quite pleasant. However, these statements were not representative of his overall perceptions. He filled his reports with negative descriptions of the people of Härjedalen, and of Vemdalen in particular. Even when he recognized the people's beauty, he quickly went on to describe how they dressed in a way that destroyed their looks. Women put cloths around their heads, which they tied on the forehead. Ellmin remarked that the knot left two wings resembling the wings of a bat that changed the most beautiful face into one of fury. Moreover, hospitality aside, the local people had no problems with cheating a stranger.[49]

Ellmin was even more critical of the care of the poor who were passed around from farm to farm. Often they had to live with the cattle in order to stay warm, and he had several complaints about the lack of hygiene caused by living so close to the animals. The practice of leaving carcasses of horses lying outside to rot in the sun also greatly disturbed him. This suggests that although medical theories were beginning to focus attention on the individual, the belief in the detrimental effects of bad air and odours remained.

Ellmin directed his harshest criticisms towards the behaviour and attitudes of the people. He was particularly annoyed with their laziness and lack of ambition, their total lack of respect for authority, and finally their preferences for hedonism and simple pleasures. Their laziness and lack of ambition was apparent in many ways. They ate their meals leisurely in a quiet and restful atmosphere. Their relaxed attitude made Ellmin doubt the possibility of there ever being any industrial development of importance. Furthermore, he was annoyed that many people seemed to have difficulties understanding the simplest thing. When explanations were offered, the common reply was a stupid 'Häää?', something

Ellmin suspected was used when they did not want to understand. He described their lack of ambition in a rather peculiar way:

> When people from other places in northern Sweden confidently walk with swift steps as the Castilian on the roads with their gun and their mare ... the man from Herjeådalen strides along with bended knees, bowed head and clumsy hands ... [50]

The laziness and backwardness of the people became apparent in how they treated and used their horses. Covered in dirt, the horses were frequently used together with oxen to pull farm equipment, which made the pace of the horse resemble that of the oxen.

Ellmin was furthermore annoyed at the people's disrespect for those in authority. They did not have any sense for social hierarchies and called everyone the personal '*du*' instead of the more respectful (in the opinion of urban and higher class Sweden) '*ni*'. Even the children were accustomed to saying '*du*' to their teachers. Parents told their children that if the teacher were too hard on them, they simply could leave for the day and go home. Such attitudes followed people through their adolescence to adult age. It was very difficult for household heads to discipline their servants who often took days off whenever they felt like it. If a young maid was serving on a weekend evening, her friends could intrude to convince or force her to join them because they felt that she did not have to stay there and work. The local people directed their lack of respect towards government officials or other members of the higher classes in particular. People did not respect the law and instead abided by their own old traditions. Although such behaviour was endemic throughout the district, Ellmin did notice some local differences. He claimed that while the character of the people was rough and proud but gentle in most places, the people in Vemdalen presented all the worst characteristics. Hoards of drunken, violent youth terrorized respectable people and particularly state representatives and other officials. Even those responsible for enforcing the law were afraid of them.[51]

Ellmin also complained about the hedonism and simple pleasures that the people of Härjedalen pursued. They were never in a hurry and this meant that they took long breaks from work for more pleasurable activities:

> People of both sexes go to rest under the skin rug without any other effort in the morning than with the breakfast porridge. With extreme pleasure they also fulfil their marital duties, and it is a fact from the days of the bondage of the Hebrews under the Pharaohs, that people struggling with misfortunes and distress are more fertile than more favoured nations.[52]

Ellmin suggested that the hard climate and unfertile soil made the people in Härjedalen seek these pleasures. He strongly disapproved of the local tradition of night courting and suspected that it was not the decent and innocent practice he had been led to believe. Young loving couples used the barns as meeting places. The long summers when people stayed in the *saeters* were another opportunity for immoral behaviour. They lived far away from any control from the authorities, and the youngsters spent their time playing, singing and dancing.

Ellmin obviously showed great interest in the behaviour of the population and generally described it in a very negative way. Seldom relating his comments directly to health, he was more concerned about the general morality of the, for him, foreign people. Ellmin described them as unknowing and primitive savages that the authorities had a particular responsibility to educate and civilize. While he foresaw the potential for conflict, he suggested a way to deal with the local population:

> If the Härjedaling lets his despotic attitude some time confront the law, but on these occasions is met with a severe reprimand, he will turn manageable, even pleading and completely sincere when asked for a confession. For this three things are demanded: strength, fairness and benevolence.[53]

The Sami Population

If Ellmin described the people he most frequently met in Härjedalen as a foreign and sometimes exotic group, he perceived the Sami as even more exotic. There were approximately 800 of them living in the western mountainous parts of the district, relying mainly on reindeer herding for survival. Ellmin showed considerable interest in them during his time in Härjedalen and wrote extensively about them.

Although Ellmin was aware of several health problems among the Sami, he emphasized eye diseases as something characteristic of them. Other observers had also reported the same type of diseases in the northern interior of Sweden. Ellmin attributed these problems to the smoky interiors of their primitive dwellings, the so-called *kåta* (lapp cot). Another explanation was related to their outdoor life in the bright snow-covered mountains.

A large problem that Ellmin identified was the lack of health care provided to the Sami. He wrote that he had proposed to visit the Sami population in order to reinforce the importance of vaccination. However, he was unsure whether the authorities were obliged to compensate him for the costs of providing free health care to poor Samis or for his travel if he decided to undertake such a trip. He waited for an answer but the conditions under which health care could be offered to the Sami population remained unclear. In his report of 1851, he stated that no parish had organized for the health care of the impoverished Sami.[54]

The problem with vaccination seems to have prevailed for several years but changed at the end of the decade. When Ellmin left his position in 1859, he considered it his main achievement that the rights of Sami to vaccination and health care had been established.[55] Although the Sami certainly had reasons to complain about the poor level of health care they had received, Ellmin gave examples of their positive attitudes towards professional medicine. In one of his later reports, for example, Ellmin attached a signed statement from a Sami expressing his gratitude for Ellmin's treatment and help when his family was sick.[56]

Ellmin repeated a perception of contemporary and later observers that the Sami tended to drink too much alcohol. Ellmin referred to one informant who said that the Sami could easily spend 400–500 Riksdaler a year on aquavit and '[t]hen tell us that they are poor!' The way Ellmin and his informant described the Sami had many similarities with colonialists' descriptions of their encounters with native people in other parts of the world: 'The Laps', he pronounced, 'are the Hottentots of the North, and resemble them completely in their relation to alcohol'.[57]

The doctor's 'colonial gaze' is also obvious from other statements in his reports, in which he frequently described the Sami as savages. There was a great deal of hostility between the Sami and the rest of the population of Härjedalen, and conflicts sometimes arose. Ellmin thought it to be a sad observation that these uncivilized peoples 'seemingly remnants of vanishing tribes, can't get on and live together with the more developed people coming from the mountains of Asia, where we consider ourselves to have our origin'. Ellmin, however, did not solely blame the Sami. He pointed out that Swedes and the Swedish authorities often ill-treated them and that the clergy and government officials had not always provided adequate protection for them.[58]

Disagreements between the Sami and the rest of the population were often rooted in conflicting interests brought about by their different economies. According to one informant whose opinion Ellmin apparently accepted without any hesitation, the Sami had no respect for individual rights of ownership: 'The Laps often drive their reindeer to regions, where they obviously have no right to let them graze'.[59]

For Ellmin, the Sami economy belonged to the past – or at least ought to belong to the past. In his opinion, these people were at a very low level of civilization due to their lack of care, education and religion. Missionaries were sent to China, but the Samis were largely left to fend for themselves. Ellmin felt that he had the answer that would bring civilization to them: 'Give them Christianity, righteous laws and definite borders, wherein they safely could let their herds graze, and they would repay the Swedish society by becoming decent and law observing citizens, that both had the will and the ability to pay taxes to the government'.[60] He also felt that the Sami economy must be changed and that the Sami must be made to conform to Swedish society. They could even make good contributions to Sweden as their great ability to survive in harsh conditions could be of value to the Swedish army in times of war.[61]

Practical Problems and the Role of Professional Medicine

Ellmin reported several obstacles that he faced as he performed his duties as district medical officer in Vemdalen and many of these were of a practical nature. The few roads were in bad shape. The long distances and the remote character of the district also hampered the postal services. Deliveries were made once a week and outgoing post was picked up at the same time, which meant that Ellmin's replies to incoming letters had to wait a week. These delays were critical for the sick who were waiting for medicine.

A larger problem, according to Ellmin, was that his station was in the wrong place. Vemdalen was certainly more in the middle of the district than was Sveg, but it was an inconvenient place in many ways. It was a small village and not on the normal travel routes of the people of Härjedalen. The former station in Sveg had been a much better choice because the population was larger and it was a more natural centre of the district. In addition to this, Ellmin had a negative opinion of the people in Vemdalen, while he felt that the people in Sveg were much more civilized. When the station was moved to Vemdalen, people in eastern Härjedalen often preferred to visit the physician in Järvsö in the neighbouring province, and people in western Härjedalen often went across the border to Röros in Norway.[62]

A combination of these problems made it almost impossible for a doctor in the district to earn a living. Salaries that district medical officers received were intended only to cover the costs of their official duties and it was expected that income from their own practices would be sufficient for them to make a decent living. However, there simply were not enough patients for the doctor in Vemdalen. Unlike in towns and cities where people commonly asked for assistance from doctors, in large districts people often refrained from making the long journey to the doctor in cases of illness. This was a frequent complaint by Ellmin. Another problem, and one which he reported during his first year in Härjedalen, was that many diseases did not come to his knowledge because he had to rely on the people of Vemdalen to tell him about them but they rarely used his services. Instead, he was financially dependent as a doctor on the few officials and civil servants residing in Vemdalen. For long periods, he had no patients to care for at all because the people relied more on the mercy of God and continued to follow the practices of their ancestors.[63] In 1856, he complained that the population in Vemdalen still had no interest in using his services and he remained primarily a physician for the poor. Among them, he encountered their low level of civilization and education, which made it difficult to perform his duties. A practical example of this was that his patients did not understand prescriptions that involved taking a half glass or a spoonful of medicine. If, however, the prescription was changed so that the patients were told to take a 'brännvinstumlare' (glass for aquavit) or a coffee cup of medicine they understood immediately.[64]

Many people continued to use the services of quacks, and Ellmin seemed resigned to this practice. He claimed that there was a quack in almost every single village and hamlet. It was easy for them to continue their activities because the doctor and legal officials were located in the relatively isolated village of Vemdalen.[65] It seems that only one person created problems severe enough to annoy Ellmin: a quack who used the noble name Tigerhjelm and declared that he had completed a medical exam. Ellmin finally confronted Tigerhjelm and asked about his background and studies. According to Ellmin, the quack responded with obvious lies about both his name and education and even presented a fake diploma. There was even physical violence between the men on a later occasion.[66]

Many parishes had no authorized midwife because they were unable or unwilling to assume the cost of hiring one. Ellmin described a peculiar practice that he claimed an unauthorized midwife used to perform when it was necessary to turn the foetus. A couple of strong men were called to assist the delivering mother out of bed and onto her feet after which time she was turned upside down. The men repeated this several times and 'in this manner the childbearing woman is turned like a grindstone or as the wings of a windmill caught in a storm'.[67]

From Ellmin's descriptions, he was quite unsuccessful in establishing a market as a physician in his district. Except from the purely practical problems related to the location of the station and other complexities, some other circumstances may have caused his self-reported failure. Professional medicine was something new and unknown in Härjedalen, with the exception of the work of some midwives and a pharmacist. In such an environment without previous experiences of professional medicine, the local population was suspicious about what the appointed doctor could offer and the physicians had to prove their competence. Unfortunately, for many or most diseases, the nineteenth-century physician did not have much to offer. Furthermore, Ellmin was a stranger and represented an official sphere that was very distant for people in Härjedalen, which was a rural, quite egalitarian society with freeholding peasants and no upper class except for the clergy, a foundry owner and a few state officials. That the problems became larger because of the physician's own attitude and possible difficulties in integrating himself into the local community is also quite possible.

From Ellmin's reports, it is obvious that people largely still relied on folk medicine and that there were apparently quite a few individuals practising it. These folk healers had several advantages: they were well known to the people among whom they lived, they did not represent any outside authority and they probably shared many of the same ideas as the patients. We do not, however, have to make too large a distinction between folk medicine and professional medicine. People used what was most readily available, whether the official district medical officer, the local folk healer or a visiting quack who presented himself as an educated physician. Some of these folk healers picked up their knowledge from medical books – and some from physicians themselves. The most famous folk healer in Härjedalen towards the end of the century, Anders Wallström, or Soln-Anders as he became known, used to drive with Ellmin during sick visits when he was a young boy, something that inspired him to learn more about medicine.[68]

Epilogue on Ellmin and his Later Life

In this article, we have paid little attention to several features of Ellmin's time in Vemdalen. He apparently had many personal problems during these years, including loneliness (he lived far away from his family) and ill-health. A sometimes difficult man, he had many conflicts with the local population. There were also signs of mental problems. Ellmin wrote that he found his greatest joy when he was writing his reports. Unfortunately, these descriptions became increasingly strange. In 1856, a colleague at *Sundhetskollegium* made a note on his annual report that expressed concern about the confused character of Ellmin's report as well as several of his previous documents. The board decided that someone should contact Ellmin and ask him if it would be possible to write more sensibly: '*om möjl. Skrifva klokare*'.[69] Following this rebuke, Ellmin's writing was more restrained.

Ellmin finally left Vemdalen in 1859 due to health problems and stayed for a while in a small village in the neighbouring province of Hälsingland. He does not seem to have rejoined his wife in Stockholm until the early 1860s, not long before she died in 1862. In 1863, the medical board granted him full pension, allowing him to resign from his position as district medical officer in Vemdalen. He moved together with a young woman who was about to divorce and they married in 1864. Unfortunately, they did not have a long time together as Ellmin died the following year due to what was described as an accidental overdose of opium.

Conclusion

In the early nineteenth century, large parts of Sweden had insufficient health care. This was especially the case in northern Sweden. The present article describes how health care was extended to some remote parts of the nation, the ambitions of the medical authorities and some of the problems that physicians met with in districts where there was minimal tradition of and knowledge about professional health care. The fate of the district medical officer of Vemdalen, Johan Ellmin, who certainly was a colourful person, partly illustrates many of these issues. His life and work illuminate many of the conditions of contemporary physicians. Even if in many ways he was an exception, his interest in reforms, his civilizing ambition and his eagerness to investigate all parts of the lives of the people in his district situate him in the ideological currents of his time, notably the increasing interest in how social conditions determine health. The extension of health care to all parts of Sweden was a part of the nation-building process. Health politics that followed in the mercantilist tradition had already begun in the eighteenth century and demonstrated the state's interest in improving the population's health and combating premature death and disease. In an attempt to provide health care for all Swedish citizens, parliamentarians wanted to provide salaried physicians in the districts they were representing. The central medical authorities also had other priorities. The appointed district medical officers were to observe everything that might have had an impact on health, to take initiatives that would eradicate unhealthy conditions and to collect information about such conditions to increase knowledge about health and disease.

One important characteristic of medicine at this time was its focus on the geographical dimension of disease. Medical geography developed in different countries sometimes in connection to imperial politics. The interest in geographic space could take the form of gathering statistics, but it also involved studying local conditions and the impact of 'airs, waters and places' in the tradition of Hippocratic medicine. The nineteenth century also witnessed the gradual medicalization of society as physicians began paying more attention to social conditions and common practice and traditions as causes of disease. Physicians became the eyes of the central authorities and they fulfilled their responsibilities in the medical topographies they wrote.

Ellmin took his obligations of writing medical topographies about his district seriously. He presented a detailed topography during his first year in Vemdalen. He expressed some peculiar thoughts, but generally his reports fulfilled the requirements demanded by the *Sundhetskollegium*. Moreover, other contemporary medical topographies reveal that his views were not markedly different from those expressed by other physicians. He continued to write his detailed and increasingly voluminous descriptions of the area in the following years. Although his reports continued to include the mandatory information, his emphasis was on the society and behavioural characteristics of the people he encountered. It is likely that this owes much to the ideas he had developed during his early radical years in Stockholm when his mission was to improve living conditions for all citizens. He was particularly interested in the question of whether poverty caused disease or if the reverse was true, something that implicitly or explicitly was an important part of the mid-nineteenth-century medical discourse.

In one way, Ellmin's views of the lower classes could be considered compassionate and positive. He believed that their lives could be improved and sincerely wanted to bring this about. He did not stop at simply addressing matters related to health but aimed at changing all aspects of their lives as part of his 'civilizing mission'. Ellmin's medical topographies clearly reveal his 'colonial gaze'. The collection of these topographies was a way to explore unknown parts of Sweden in the same way that colonialists and missionaries explore foreign continents. Ellmin's goal was to compile a complete description of his district, which he believed was largely unknown. His description of the people of Härjedalen, and particularly the Sami, as savages lacking education and civilization resembles popular attitudes of foreign people. To him it was the responsibility of upper-class Swedish society to educate and civilize the Sami because their way of life was doomed to disappear.

6 MEDICAL REPORTS FROM THE 1800s AND WHAT THEY TELL ABOUT HEALTH CONDITIONS, POPULATION AND THE WORK OF DOCTORS IN PERIPHERAL NORWAY

Øivind Larsen

Summary

Reports of Norwegian medical officers from the nineteenth and twentieth centuries provide detailed information for the entire country down to the level of individual health districts. The nineteenth-century reports are of special medical historical interest. The design of the reports makes it possible to compare the real health situation to the perception of it held by health personnel. Data on epidemic diseases from the period 1868–1900 have been excerpted and compared to the written descriptions in the reports and interpreted in relation to the overarching medical and social contexts. This analysis illustrates the importance of health perception as an independent historical agent.

Diseases, Perceptions and Health Services

The main argument here is that a relationship exists between the health conditions in a population, how this health situation is perceived and the function of the health services. This relationship is more the result of shifting perceptions than the actual health of the population and the conditions in which the people live.

These perceptions are held by people at different levels in the medical hierarchy from the lay patients, through various categories of health personnel, up to the central national authorities.[1] These ideas and beliefs make up the basis for attitudes in health matters which exert influence when setting priorities.[2] Therefore perceptions and attitudes are key to the understanding of developments in medicine, health and health services.

The Norwegian medical reports from the public health officers provide information on both the epidemiological situation and the perceptions of it held by the district physicians. As such they can be used to illustrate how actual circumstances and perceptions work together to influence the type of medical care provided.

The Medical Reports

On 20 December 1803 the Medical College (Collegium Medicum), a body responsible for health matters, issued a circular which gave practising doctors in the dual kingdom of Denmark and Norway the new responsibility of submitting annual reports.[3] According to the instructions, doctors should provide information about topics provided on a specified list. The reports were to be sent without delay to the Medical College, which would convey the contents to the King through the Danish Chancellery.

The state of war at the beginning of the nineteenth century severely hampered the administration of the twin kingdom. Hostile Swedish and English naval vessels blocked the seas between Denmark and Norway, and in 1809 a separate Norwegian Medical College had to be established. Local Norwegian authorities assumed responsibility for its function in 1815. Various ministries were responsible for this institution thereafter until 1891 when a national board of health assumed this role. The general idea behind the reporting system was to gather information for practical use in health planning, preventive medicine and health care.

In principle, annual reports from every district, which by and large corresponded to the municipalities, exist in the Norwegian National Archive for every year although there are some holes, such as for the periods 1805–13 and 1831–4. The reports that have been retained represent an enormous amount of material about local conditions in Norway in the nineteenth century. The doctors were asked not only to provide information regarding diseases and health services, but also to write more generally about their impressions of local life. Despite variations in the quality of the material over the years, these sources are a goldmine for local historians.

Authorities from the medical administration edited the individual reports and from 1853 onwards they were printed as part of the Norwegian official statistics. These official documents provided both a survey over the whole country and individual reports at the county level. Excerpts from especially interesting individual district-level reports were often published as appendices. Written descriptions of the health situation, health care and living conditions were accompanied by a set of tables containing quantitative information. The editorial process and organizational principles remained more or less the same for long periods, and this makes longitudinal studies possible. However, the edited and printed reports only very occasionally included longitudinal data, and even if it was present it only covered a few years.

Wilderness, Nation-Building and Health
– Norway on the Outskirts of Europe

Situated at the top of the European continent and covering the western part of the Scandinavian peninsula, mainland Norway, whose borders were established in 1814, is the sixth largest country in Europe.[4] It is a very long country stretching from a latitude of approximately 58 degrees north at Lindesnes in the southernmost county of Vest-Agder to a little more than 71 degrees north at Kinnarodden in the far northern county of Finnmark. However, despite its northern latitude the climate and living conditions are largely quite favourable in most of the country. This is due to a combination of warm ocean currents along the long coast and prevailing wind systems. Heavy and frequent rainfalls occur in the coastal districts west of the mountains, while the rolling hill landscapes in eastern Norway are drier.

Modern Norway achieved relative political independence in 1814 when the union with Denmark was replaced by a rather loose union with Sweden that lasted until 1905. The country is subdivided into numerous counties to aid administration. There was a maximum of twenty counties between 1866 and 1972 and nineteen counties from 1972 onwards.

However, in 1837 the more important subdivision of the 'kommune' was introduced. These were municipalities with wide self-governing authority. By 1838 there were 392 such municipalities and this number increased to a maximum of 747 in 1930 before declining to 430 in 2008. This administrative structure is important for the provision of primary health care because such care has for a long time been the responsibility of the municipality. Most of the second-line hospital services were administered by the counties until the state assumed responsibility for them in 2002.

The municipalities varied widely in the number of inhabitants found within them. The population of Norway was 883,487 in 1801, 2,814,194 in 1930 and 4,606,363 in 2005. In 1837 this meant that the average number of inhabitants in a municipality was around 3,000. This rose in 1930 to 3,767 and to 10,614 in 2005. Admittedly, even today there are large variations in municipality size from around 200 individuals in Utsira to more than half a million in Oslo.

Even if considerable urbanization has occurred, the Norwegian population is still widely scattered around the whole country. In 1801, 44.7 per cent were living in the central counties around the capital in the south-east. This percentage increased only slightly to 48.2 in 1930 and to 49.6 in 2005. At the beginning of the nineteenth century, 9 per cent of the population lived in the three northern-most counties that cover approximately half the length of Norway. These same counties accounted for 12 per cent of the population in 1930. This percentage remained relatively constant until 1970 when it was 11.7 per cent before falling to 10.0 per cent in 2005.

The rough terrain makes it difficult to earn a living. Only 3 per cent of the land area can be used for agriculture while 18 per cent is fit for forestry. For this reason traditional Norwegian farming, the dominant way of living prior to the late nineteenth century, still mostly occurs on independent, separate, self-contained farms. Large estates were, and still are, very few. The continental village system was never established in Norway in areas other than where geography, for example at closed ends of fjords or along shore plains, made it logical for farms to be located close to each other. Several towns developed along the coast as a result of the important fisheries. These small settlements fulfilled a wide range of social and administrative functions disproportionate to their size. Industrialization took place rather late in Norway as it was largely restricted to the last third of the nineteenth century. The fact remains that large parts of the country consisted of mountains and wilderness which, among other things, made communication throughout the country difficult.

A demographic transition occurred in nineteenth-century Norway. The population surplus that appeared after 1815 when mortality began to decline caused internal migration, especially to the regions in the south-east and, after the 1860s, a substantial emigration mainly to the US.

The nineteenth century also marked the main period of nation-building in Norway. A modern state emerged after its early dependence on Denmark at the beginning of the 1800s. Part of this nation-building involved the creation of a modern medical and national health services. Until 1811, Norway had no university and thus no medical school to train doctors, and there was almost no functioning health-care system. Both were in place a century later having been developed in a period when diseases such as cholera and tuberculosis had shocked society.

Norway Portrayed with Medical Eyes

The medical reports reflect the situation as seen through the eyes of the district physicians. The Sanitation Act of 1860, passed mainly as a consequence of the cholera epidemics which had ravaged the country from 1832 to 1833 and again in 1853, strengthened the provision of public health activities and gave district physicians extensive authority especially in cases of epidemic diseases. The district physician chaired the so-called Sanitation Commission or Board of Health in the municipality[5] and could, for example, implement rather harsh measures if deemed medically appropriate.[6] As Norway had few large cities until the end of the nineteenth century, most of these physicians worked in municipalities with only a few inhabitants but which covered large areas. The nineteenth-century district physician normally represented an extension of the central administration in the municipalities together with the vicar and the *lensmann*, who was the local representative of the police authority.

The medical reports dating from 1860 onwards became more informative than their predecessors, and this is particularly true after 1868 when they were full of details and well structured. At this time the texts that accompanied figures and tables were rather more objective and scientific than they had been. However, these were the words of the elite. The practical implication of this was that the judgments that district physicians made regarding what was bad or good, acceptable or unacceptable, had direct bearings for the medical care of the local population. That is to say, the activities of the Sanitation Commission were largely dependent upon the initiatives and opinions that the district physician expressed.

The medical reports contain extensive information about hospitals, cottage hospitals and other medical institutions. However, these sources also show that the hallmark of Norwegian medicine in the nineteenth century was that of primary care and particularly the home visit. Even surgical operations were performed in the patients' homes.

The problem of communicable diseases dominated the minds of nineteenth-century medical officials. After all, the Sanitation Commissions had been established against a backdrop of rising mortality from infectious diseases. It is no surprise that discussions of this group of diseases occupy considerable space in the medical reports and represent a valuable source for researchers.[7]

Aggregate county level data found in the medical reports provides information about incidence (yearly occurrence in the population), mortality (yearly deaths in the population), and lethality (deaths among the affected in the particular year) and these were used to calculate long-term trends (see Figure 6.1).

From 1868 to 1900 the country experienced considerable demographic upheaval as a result of substantial population growth, urbanization and emigration.

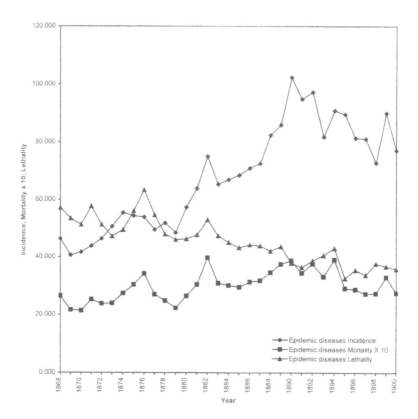

**Figure 6.1: Epidemic diseases: incidence, mortality and lethality:
Norway 1868–1900.**

Figure 6.1 clearly shows that the incidence of epidemic diseases increased remarkably until the 1890s when it first began to slow and then fall slightly. The collective group 'Epidemic diseases' in the terminology of Statistics Norway for this period included: typhus, typhoid, simple fever, meningitis, puerperal fever, smallpox, chickenpox, scarlet fever, rubella, measles, erysipelas, pyemia and septicaemia, whooping cough, diphtheria, croup, mumps, acute catarrhs in the respiratory tract, catharral and follicular angina of the throat, influenza, pneumonia, pleuritis, rheumatic fever, coldfever (ague = malaria), acute diarrhoea, bloody diarrhoea and scurvy. The same list was used, with only minor and insignificant revisions, throughout the time period covered here.

Mortality followed a similar pattern, while lethality fell throughout the entire period. The reports also reveal geographical differences as shown in Figure 6.2. For example, one can see the 'urban penalty' phenomenon in the contrasting incidence of epidemic diseases between the rapidly growing capital of Christiania and the two rural counties of nearby Smaalenene and the more remote Finnmark.

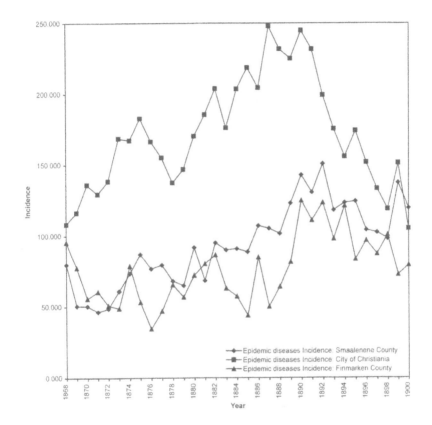

Figure 6.2: Epidemic diseases: incidence for Smaalenene County, the city of Christiania and Finnmark County, 1868–1900.

Figure 6.3, a map showing the incidence of epidemic diseases for 1886 confirms this pattern but also points to the even larger gradients seen between other counties and the urbanized areas of the south-east and around Bergen in western Norway. These places were important transit harbours for the west-bound emigration, which was especially high during the later 1800s.

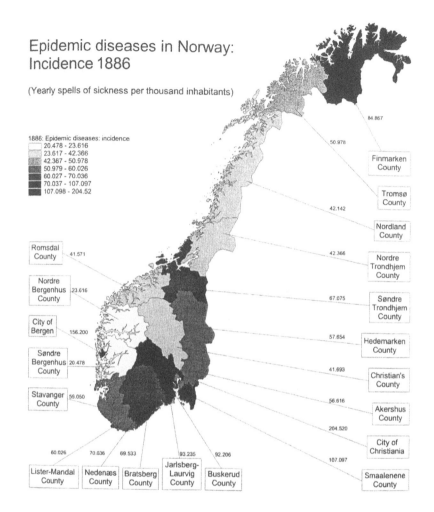

Figure 6.3: Epidemic diseases in Norway: incidence 1886.

Figures in the medical reports also allow for comparison of different diagnoses. Diphtheria ravaged Norway in the last half of the nineteenth century and typhoid fever was also present throughout the period (see Figure 6.4). More interesting are the cases of acute diarrhoeas (often named 'cholera nostras' in the reports) which followed patterns of social upheaval and probably simply reflected the prevailing standards of hygiene.[8]

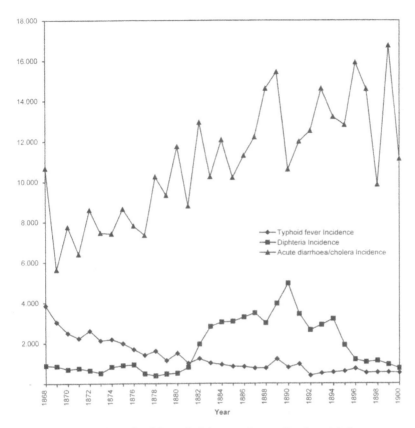

**Figure 6.4: Typhoid fever, diphtheria and acute diarrhoea/cholera:
incidence, Norway, 1868–1900.**

Medicine and Physicians in the Nineteenth Century

It has been claimed that public health services in Norway started in 1603 when
a physician in Bergen, Dr Villads Nielsen (*c.* 1564–1616), was publicly commissioned with a royal salary.[9] However, real public health work, understood as the
public concern for the health of the population, is an offspring of the nineteenth
century. It is marked by the creation and expansion of a system of district physicians and the introduction of the Sanitation Act of 1860 as its core components.

In 1814 there were only approximately 100 doctors in Norway, but this figure increased to 1,000 by the end of the century. The population only doubled
over the same period so the increase in coverage by medical professionals was
remarkable. Doctors of the early nineteenth century had mostly received their
training in Copenhagen. At the end of the century, all Norwegian doctors had

been educated at the New Norwegian University (Det kongelige Frederiks Universitet) in the capital of Christiania. This institution had been founded in 1811 as part of Norway's attempt to gain independence. The medical faculty commenced its teaching in 1814 and the first medical candidates passed their final examinations in 1817.[10]

Medical teaching in Norway was started against all practical odds as a political issue. The tasks of the new national university were to educate national elites so that the official posts in the municipalities could be filled with Norwegians rather than Danes as had been the case. Therefore, the doctors of the nineteenth century were conscious of their role as nation-builders and this was implicit in their training and service.

The new university was mostly a teaching institution until the 1870s after which time research activities increased. This is shown by the low number of doctoral degrees in the first decades of its operation. However, the very first academic thesis in Norway was defended in 1817 by Frederik Holst (1791–1871) who was to become a professor in hygiene. It examined the public health issue of 'radesyge', a disease of still unclear nature which was then a big problem in Norway.[11]

The growth of a professional community of doctors with responsibility for the maintenance of knowledge and skills also took place outside the academic circles. Already in 1826 the medical journal *Eyr* was founded,[12] a medical society saw daylight,[13] and many doctors embarked on study tours, with or without public grants, to foreign hospitals and universities to improve their knowledge.[14]

There were only a few small hospitals outside the capital which meant that practising physicians often had long and strenuous days with dangerous travels on land and sea. The risk of getting infected from their patients added to the difficulties. The occupational hazards of the medical profession were well recognized. The editor of the two first editions of the encyclopaedia *Norges Læger*, Dr Frantz Caspar Kiær (1835–93), collected questionnaires from Norwegian doctors on this topic in 1886. Although his death prevented him from completing his analysis of the results, this work was later completed by another individual who was able to demonstrate the presence of extreme working conditions.[15]

However unhealthy the situation in the rural districts, the more extreme medical conditions took place in the cities in the years of massive urbanization. Access to proper medical services was often unsatisfactory and to be cared for at home if a person was sick was often impossible in the crowded cities. An emergency medical station to which anyone could call in case of accident or disease was first established in the large city of Kristiania (as Christiania became officially known in 1877) in 1900.[16]

Norwegian medicine had attained European standards by the end of the nineteenth century. The capital had a large municipal hospital, Ullevål sykehus,[17] which had gradually expanded into a general hospital from its construction in

1887 as an institution for the treatment of epidemic diseases. Other cities soon followed suit.

The period covered by the district physicians' medical reports referred to here, is a time when population, disease pattern, medical knowledge, health service and national infrastructure changed simultaneously.

A Key to Understanding Physicians' Perceptions

In their medical reports the physicians expressed opinions about the prevailing health situation and discussed whether it was good, bad, or better or worse than in the previous year. However, more concrete data can be taken out of the tables in the same reports.

Codifying written expressions and relating them to the quantitative data provided in the reports makes it possible to calculate a 'concern index' that illuminates a doctor's perception of the seriousness of local health conditions.[18] On the one hand, if the physicians deemed the situation as being good when many outbreaks of sickness occurred, the index value is low. On the other hand, if there were many outbreaks and the wording expressed concern, the index will be high. Figure 6.5 reveals long-term trends in the degree to which some physicians envisioned the health situation to be serious.

Although the latter half of the nineteenth century saw rather profound changes in Norwegian society, there is no reason to believe that the diagnostics performed by the doctors should be influenced by the socio-economic status or gender of the patient.

The race issue in Norway of the latter half of the nineteenth century almost only applies to the Sami population of the far north. This group is very interesting from a theoretical point of view, but the size of the group was small. As race is not recorded in the statistics, one has to estimate the proportion of Sami of the total number of inhabitants in the Sami districts, which typically are in the county of Finnmark. In 1891 the total number of inhabitants in this county was 29,341, a mere 1.47 per cent of Norway's population of 1,988,674. Obviously the Sami population was only a fraction of those living in Finnmark; the rest were mostly ethnic Norwegians or of some other (e.g., Finnish) descent. Therefore, for the topics addressed in this article, the influence of the Sami on of the statistics is miniscule at the national level and small on the county level, but of course is important at the level of municipalities where the Sami lived. However, even here only to a minor degree when it comes to the perceptions held by the doctor. Of course there are a lot of social factors affecting the perception of disease in general, but the perception of disease appearing as the *perception* held by the doctors, not by the patients or the population, should have been quite uniform. For the period covered here, all doctors had their training from the only

Norwegian university (in Christiania) and thus had the same professional background. In addition, in this period knowledge about the microbial causes behind most contagious diseases was well established among most medical personnel.

The concern expressed by the district physicians for Norway as a whole was quite high at the beginning of the period stretching from the 1860s to the 1890s. There then appears to have been a gradual adjustment to the generally increasing number of cases of epidemic disease (see Figure 6.5) before concern rose again towards the end of this period.

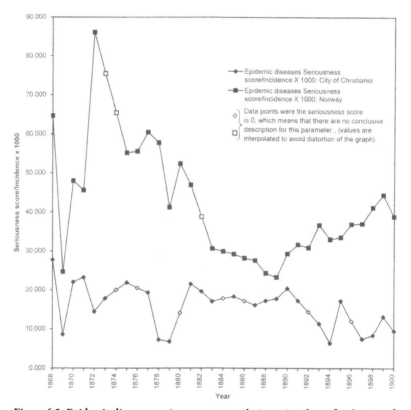

Figure 6.5: Epidemic diseases: seriousness score relative to incidence for the city of Christiana and Norway, 1868–1900.

Figure 6.5 also demonstrates another interesting pattern. The concern index is much lower for the capital of Christiania than for rural areas and this relative difference does not appear to vary over time. This may indicate that the 'urban penalty' was a more or less accepted situation already at the time when it occurred. However, the study indicates that changes in the statistical figures over time reveal that the incidence of epidemic diseases increased steadily until the 1890s, at which time the trend began to fall. This development was most pronounced for the densely populated capital of Kristiania. The pattern was the same but at a lower level in the countryside, regardless of where the region was in Norway. The level of 'concern', which expresses the separation between 'normal' and 'exceptional', was inverse: in general it rose at the same time as the incidence went down. It is most likely that the conditions in Kristiania were the most important in triggering medical initiatives and public health work.

Discussion: A Delicate Balance

Information provided in the Norwegian medical reports seem to support our hypothesis that it is important to recognize how perceptions of levels of disease and health influence state behaviour. The method used here demonstrates that we can infer that the perceptions held by local medical practitioners gradually changed and that this shift had implications for the provision of health care. For example, if a physician reported the situation as being quite good, his report did not require or initiate any immediate action upon submission. A balance between actual health conditions and perception may explain why medicine and health services functioned in a way which was regarded as more or less satisfactory, even though at a level which in later periods would be perceived as inadequate.[19] The opinions expressed through the textual comments in the medical reports reflect, on the one hand, the prevailing expectations and, on the other, the prevailing priorities and possibilities.

These medical reports deserve attention because they are official documents that were tailored to provide guidance to central authorities. The disease *perception* and the *attitude* towards health and disease held by district physicians were clearly key to the development of national medicine and to the health services. They are also vital to our understanding of the historical processes at play.

7 'MEDICINE IS HERE TO STAY': RURAL MEDICAL PRACTICE, THE NORTHERN FRONTIER AND MODERNIZATION IN 1930s' NEWFOUNDLAND

J. T. H. Connor

The 'country doctor' in the twentieth century has been analysed from numerous perspectives,[1] but it is only recently that historians and other scholars have begun to problematize the concept of 'rural medicine'. But what constitutes rural or remote medicine as a historical sub-specialty of the history of medicine and health? Even those who currently practice, promote and study health care in the hinterlands remain unclear about the definition of 'rural'; while proponents may disagree, however, there seems to be a consensus that simply being 'non-urban' or 'agricultural' is not a satisfactory definition. Sparse population density and isolation are clearly factors to be considered, but so too are social and community mores and conventions (perhaps 'the people' and the sense of 'place' would be a convenient shorthand for such factors) as well as climatic extremes.[2] The economy (or its collapse) in a region is another element that helps define rural – especially if it is/was derived primarily from the exploitation of natural resources rather than from an industrialized manufacturing base or mixed market economy.[3] Historians, therefore, should consider local culture, climate, geography and the economy in understanding rural medicine along with the usual staples of technology, changing techniques and practice patterns, institutions, and the treatment of disease and injuries. Through study of the isolated Newfoundland outport of Twillingate located in the eastern archipelago of Notre Dame Bay, this paper considers these social and physical factors by focusing on one practitioner and his personal and professional interactions with this community during the 1930s. Basing this study on the detailed and sensitive diary of a young American doctor, Robert S. Ecke, in addition to supplementary archival materials pertaining to the small rural hospital that he was based in, a narrative emerges that is much larger than its individual parts. Although this analysis can be categorized as a micro history and perhaps as biography, it also is useful for exploring the broader evolution of rural or 'frontier' medicine and its relations to 'modernization'.

The 'Northernism' of Newfoundland (and Labrador) is more pronounced than a glance at an atlas indicates. Heavy glaciation, which removed soil and exposed much rock, along with the effects of the cold northern Labrador Current have left tundra-like vegetation to survive in an almost subarctic climate. The eastern coastline is craggy while that of the west is spectacular with its fjords (in the early twentieth century, Newfoundland was promoted as the 'Norway of the New World'). Traditionally, the everyday life, strong culture and identity, and intermittent prosperity of Newfoundlanders were based primarily on exploiting the surrounding North Atlantic Ocean – in particular through the cod fishery, until its collapse in the early 1990s. Throughout most of the island's history, the primary urban area was the City of St John's located in the most southern peninsular region. Twillingate (the anglicization of the original seventeenth-century French name of Toulinguet), the location of the subject of this paper, was one of a handful of other established settlements of any size, which can best be described as a village in the European sense. The remainder of the island is a sparsely populated area with scattered pockets of people living in *outports* that quite literally often cling to the coastline. By any definition Newfoundland and Labrador must be described as rural, if not remote or even isolated. Even by the mid-twentieth century, the vast majority of the population was inaccessible by land transport; travel by coastal steamer and other smaller vessels remained the order of the day. Telecommunication and rural electrification systems became widespread and commonplace only well after Confederation with Canada in 1949.[4]

Muscular Medicine, Socialized Medicine, and the Notre Dame Bay Memorial Hospital

Medical services and health care, while problematic and spotty in their delivery, were surprisingly better developed and better organized than might be first assumed given the physical and economic challenges that had to be continually faced. Indeed, rural and remote medicine in Newfoundland and Labrador can be seen as an early colonial success story. Central to this historical claim was the man who cast a long shadow: (Sir) Dr Wilfred Grenfell (1865–1940). Sponsored by London's Royal National Mission to Deep Sea Fishermen as a missionary doctor, Grenfell took up his permanent charge in the early 1890s at the northernmost tip of the island in St Anthony and in adjoining Labrador. Within a decade, Grenfell's reputation for daring exploits, dedicated medical care, evangelism and charisma were becoming legendary. Later, as an active self-promoter through numerous international speaking engagements and articles and books,

Grenfell and his blend of 'muscular Christianity' and (muscular) medicine became a phenomenon. The founding of his own American-style charitable organization (the International Grenfell Association (IGA) created in 1914), his marriage to a wealthy American socialite and his admittance to affluent circles in New York and New England all but guaranteed him the financial stability to continue to deliver relatively high quality health care to remote settlements. His chain of small hospitals and nursing stations in northern Newfoundland and along the Labrador coast were staffed by engaged, energetic and well-trained British and American doctors and nurses establishing a tradition of migration and medical practice that outlived Grenfell. It is probably not an exaggeration to say that Sir Wilfred became the medical czar of the north as he had the freedom and resources to do what no government health agency ever could.[5]

When people in the east-coast settlement of Twillingate in Notre Dame Bay decided to build their own hospital, they naturally turned to Grenfell for organizational advice rather than to the government in St John's which was geographically closer. Planned as an enduring tribute to those local men who died during the First World War, the Notre Dame Bay Memorial Hospital (NDBMH) was funded in innovative and unique ways – a North American pioneering model of sorts that has gone unrecognized historically. As we shall see, it was also the reason why Robert Ecke and other young American men headed north. Although the NDBMH was never part of the IGA enterprise, it did initially fall within Grenfell's sphere of influence. Grenfell was the most prominent and only non-Twillingate member of the NDBMH Association founded in 1924 to oversee the governance of this institution.[6] Grenfell was also instrumental in securing tens of thousands of dollars from the US to augment local contributions to build and expand the hospital through the Commonwealth Fund (CF), a philanthropic foundation started in New York City by the Harkness family, which gained its staggering wealth from oil production. The retention of the one of the most prominent architectural firms in North America to design the new Twillingate hospital can also be traced to Grenfell. William Adams Delano, senior partner of Delano and Aldrich of New York City, had admired Grenfell since their first meeting in the early 1900s; he also visited Newfoundland in 1926 and travelled on the IGA hospital ship *Strathcona*. Not surprisingly, Delano was also appointed to the Board of Directors of the IGA.

Despite the critical technical and financial support obtained from the US, the actual building of the hospital was an intensely community-driven project. For three years, local tradesmen – often trained on the job site in the skills of masonry, concrete technology and plastering – created a monument to commemorate the past as well as an edifice that ushered in the future. The CF annual report for 1925 drew attention to the inordinate efforts of the people of Notre Dame Bay in this regard. The 'remote location' led to protracted problems, but the 'devotion of the people of Twillingate' and their 'generous giving of their time and labor in transporting freight, digging roads, installing the water system ... working nights throughout the summer ... [and] undergoing every discomfort' culminated in the opening of a fully functioning hospital in September 1924.

Five years later, an additional $50,000 was forthcoming from the New York philanthropists to add a new wing, including a children's ward. The CF executive 'took special satisfaction' in their support of the NDBMH owing to its impressive success and its mission. Not only was it the only hospital to serve the 50,000 fishermen and their families along 300 miles of seacoast, but area residents had repeatedly demonstrated their whole-hearted commitment to the institution through their free labour along with over $80,000 that they themselves had raised. One incident recounted that clearly underscored the spirit of community voluntarism, to say nothing of illustrating the remote and exotic nature of this northern colonial land, was a house launch. Although a fairly commonplace event in Newfoundland outports, the event was marvelled at in the 1929 CF annual report, which noted, almost incredulously, how 600 men dragged a frame house for two days over three miles of snow and ocean ice in order to provide a home for hospital nurses. The continuing philanthropic support enjoyed by the hospital is noteworthy in several ways. First, this expression of generosity by the CF had previously gone unnoticed by both American and Canadian historians. Secondly, it appears that supporting projects outside of the continental US was not typical for the CF, so this gesture is all the more significant. Finally, the initial financial contribution to the NDBMH took place several years before the CF formally decided to fund rural hospitals; the highly successful Newfoundland experience which was grounded in its demonstrable community support appears to have been used as a pilot project for the CF's Division of Rural Hospitals. This programme operated from 1926 to 1948 and saw funding for fifteen institutions located in the southern and north-eastern US.[7]

Wilfred Grenfell also orchestrated the appointment of Dr Charles Parsons as the hospital's founding Medical Director. Parsons, a 1919 graduate of Baltimore's Johns Hopkins University, the leading medical school in the US, had previously served the IGA in Labrador at its Battle Harbour Hospital. Beginning in 1924 he would steer the newly opened Twillingate hospital for the next ten years.[8] Succeeding him was John Olds, another Hopkins medical doctor who had graduated in 1931. Olds had spent the previous summer at NDBMH as a senior medical student when he took part in a Hopkins-Newfoundland training experience initiated by Parsons, but then returned in 1933 for a year to replace Parsons who took leave. In 1934, Parsons formally resigned his position ostensibly for health reasons. (Later Parsons travelled to China with Canadian Dr Norman Bethune, where they planned to aid the communist cause of Mao Tse-tung. Although Bethune would stay and eventually die while serving, Parsons was requested to leave China; Bethune described him in a private letter as a 'drunken bum'.[9])

The timing of Olds' appointment as the hospital's new Medical Director coincided with the onset of the Depression and that of the era of Commission Government when the colony of Newfoundland gave up democracy and responsible government in favour of an appointed governing board of commissioners – both events demanded continued funding for the support of rural medicine to be both immediate and innovative.[10] Olds had a reputation for being a mechanical tinkerer or inventor of sorts, but perhaps his single most significant invention was his introduction of a localized style of socialized medicine. Olds' scheme was, if not entirely to replace 'fee for service' with a new plan based on a blanket prepaid contract, at least to complement and supplement the standard mode of payment for medical and hospital care. The people of Twillingate and surrounding areas had a tradition of sharing and working communally, not only out of necessity along with their rural temperament to do so, but also out of political astuteness, for the Notre Dame Bay area of Newfoundland was also the birthplace in 1908 of the activist and highly successful Fisherman's Protective Union (FPU) along with its founder and long-time leader (Sir) William Coaker.[11] Thus, when Olds canvassed the many families and individuals around the numerous rural outports and isolated settlements that the hospital served, his plea was seriously listened to.

In a circular letter Olds explained how a subscriber under the 'Individual' contract system costing $10 would guarantee 'him [sic] and all members of his family Hospital care for one year at no further expenses than half price for an operation if needed'. (At this time in Newfoundland's history, a family typically would consist of both parents, perhaps as many as fifteen children, and probably grandparents too.) A second 'Community or Blanket' contract was as generous but more complex to reckon as it was based on population settlement patterns. Olds had divided Notre Dame Bay into thirty-nine districts, each of which would elect a hospital committee that would be responsible for raising funds equivalent to $44 per hundred people in any one district; thus, if a district had a population of 500, then a total of $220 per year would cover their hospital care, excepting the 'half price' operation rider. Under this version of the plan, a flat rate of forty-four cents for each person was calculated but need not be followed if extreme poverty existed. Similarly, if owing to unequal wealth distribution some people were better off than others, then they might wish to pay more than their fair share. 'In this way', Olds emphasized,

> everyone will be pooling a small amount to pay the Hospital bills of everyone in the community. It will be a tremendous saving to anyone requiring treatment and yet the Hospital will have enough money to meet its expenses. If you all stick together and do

your bit the cost will pinch no one. If you do not the sick will have to pay large bills ... The only answer is to this is that you cannot afford NOT TO.[12]

Hospital annual reports from the 1930s indicate that this plan was successful in generating revenue. Just under $10,000 was derived annually from direct patient receipts and contract payments, with the remaining $20,000 coming from regular and special government grants (for the care of the tuberculosis along with official medical officer of health duties). Based on figures available for the period it appears that there were perhaps about 8,400 subscribers annually. This socialized medical income model helped offset the running expenses, allowing the NDBMH to keep its doors open.[13]

When contextualized within the historiography of rural medicine in North America, the 'mixed economy' of the Twillingate payment plan can be seen as one of several pioneering socialized medicine efforts. Southern rural agricultural regions in the US benefited from medical and financial relief under the New Deal initiatives of the Roosevelt administration owing to the establishment of the Resettlement Administration (RA) and its successor, the Farm Security Administration (FSA). Similarly, the efforts of individual physicians who soldiered on during extremely tough times have been recognized for the doctors' sense of duty and caring service. Held up as a model in both contemporary and historical contexts was the Farmers' Union Hospital Association co-operative of Elk City, Oklahoma, formed at the beginning of the Depression years. With the support of the Oklahoma Farmers' Union, a local physician devised a coverage plan in which, for a one-time sign-up fee followed up by annual dues, farmers became shareholders and were entitled to medical and hospital care; by 1939 there were about 10,000 subscribers.[14]

Could Olds have been inspired to do for Newfoundland fishers what he knew had been done for Oklahoma farmers? Perhaps. But what might be more likely is a linkage to his *alma mater*, the Johns Hopkins University medical school. In 1932, Hopkins, the premier American medical school, appointed the physician-historian of medicine Henry Sigerist as director of its recently founded Institute of the History of Medicine. Through his own historical writing, teaching, editorial work, tireless public speaking schedule and organizational skills, Sigerist created the professional discipline of medical history in the US. For him, medical history was not the study of great doctors and the march of medical progress as it had been pursued in the US; rather it was the study of the social organization of medical knowledge and practice – for Sigerist, the study of the medical past was to help generate a better medical present and future. Thus Sigerist's second legacy was his fervent advocacy of socialized medicine (or as he referred to it, the sociology of medicine) across the US and Canada. Formal and informal networks of prominent like-minded physician-historians, medical practitioners, government administrators and other policy personnel soon formed, with Sigerist becoming their erudite and respected spokesperson. Within the medical school, Sigerist also spread the word to a younger generation, as his diary for April 1934 attests: 'I started a new seminar on the Social Aspects of Medicine. There seems to be much interest in it, the room was crowded with third and fourth year medical students ... I will repeat this course every year and develop it'.[15] A major plank in this platform of social medicine was the pursuit and practice of rural medicine.[16]

The dream of socialized medicine in the US would fade during the 1940s and after (but not in Canada). Meanwhile, there was Twillingate, Newfoundland – the colonial outpost in the Atlantic Ocean that no one really knew about it, but, ironically, could have become the 'poster child' for American-style social/rural medicine in the 1930s! We may surmise that John Olds learned of the American rural/social medicine agenda either by osmosis and/or from his many fresh associations with Hopkins as a graduate of the medical class of '31 and then 'translated' it for use in his own unique rural situation. But a more definite historical connection between Hopkins and Twillingate and rural medicine *qua* socialist-inspired activity can drawn for his slightly junior Hopkins colleague, Robert Skidmore Ecke, who attended medical school in Baltimore from 1931–5, then actively engaged in Hopkins medical life for some time after that when he was not practising at the NDBMH. In all likelihood Ecke was one of the third- and fourth-year medical students who had 'crowded' Sigerist's social medicine seminar to imbibe what the new European professor had to say.

Certainly, following one of his working trips to Twillingate, Ecke wanted to know more about socialized medicine. In spring of 1937 Ecke contacted William Lockwood, research director for the American Council Institute of Pacific Relations (ACIPR) in New York City, who advised him to get in touch with Frederick D. Mott who was assistant to the medical director of the US federal Resettlement Administration (forerunner of the FSA) based in Washington, DC. Lockwood told Ecke that Mott was an

> enterprising young fellow who is determined to pioneer in the development of socialized medicine. He has investigated the problem rather thoroughly throught [*sic*] the country, and probably knows as much as anyone about the opportunities in that field. His work at the R. A. concerns the development of medical services in the several Green-Belt projects of that organization.

Certainly, Lockwood sensed *simpatico* between these two young doctors and urged Ecke to look Mott up because he thought they 'ought to know each other'.[17] Mott was one of the leaders of American socialized medicine who, along with colleague Milton I. Roemer, would write the pioneering and definitive monograph *Rural Health and Medical Care* in 1948. Both were among Sigerist's 'social medicine enthusiasts' who later moved to Saskatchewan in the Canadian rural west to establish that province's pioneering socialized health-care plan.[18]

'Doc Hackie' of Notre Dame Bay

That Robert 'Bob' Ecke was left-leaning and supportive of socialized medicine as a young man (one of his Hopkins medical superiors once referred to him as Bolshevik) is ironic because later in his career he became a ranking US army officer, an employee of the Central Intelligence Agency (CIA), and a staunch, lifelong Republican Party supporter. Because of these facts, and also that the rest of this discussion is devoted to Ecke's experiences and perspective on rural medical practice, he demands more of a biographical introduction. Born in New York City in 1909, Ecke grew up under supportive parents of Dutch Lutheran background. His father fought in that 'splendid little' Spanish-American War (remaining an army reservist) and then became a lawyer; his mother maintained their genteel and cultured middle-class home. His brother (known as Albert Dekker – after his mother's family name) became a Hollywood movie actor of some note but died under suspicious circumstances (related to an auto-erotic suicide or murder); his sister had a successful career as a military officer. Ecke studied chemistry and German at prestigious Bowdoin College in Maine, where he was an excellent student; he also played college football and was much involved in amateur theatrics. He graduated *cum laude* in 1931, whereupon he entered Hopkins medical school, becoming a doctor four years later.[19]

Despite the demands of the Hopkins programme, Ecke managed to find time to maintain his acting and to lead a balanced social life through his association with the Pithotomy Club (a medical students' group established in 1897 that engaged in scurrilous and scatological humour and theatrics at the expense of their teachers and colleagues). Ecke's Hopkins training, including a term at Harvard Medical School in his final year, was well rounded; he was also among the first to be exposed to a new curriculum that tried to balance biomedical science subjects with a more humanistic/holistic approach to health and disease and which identified the need for physicians to co-operate with social and other allied workers and to recognize the merits of preventive medicine. Another facet of the new approach at Hopkins was training in Baltimore City Hospitals which Ecke undertook just after he graduated – this experience exposed him to a range of social conditions that poorer (predominantly black) patients faced. Ecke was also awarded a one-year research fellowship in 1936 which allowed him to work with the Hopkins poliomyelitis pioneer, Dr Howard A. Howe; this collaboration resulted in the first of many important publications.[20]

A stint as an ambulance doctor working in the tenements of New York City's Brooklyn district, as well as forty days (a much shorter period than originally planned) at the Manhattan General Hospital where Ecke became thoroughly disgusted with medical practice based on the American capitalist model of medical care, all added to his early experience. Throughout many summers of his college days and also for a short while after, Ecke was a councillor at the well-established Camp Winona in Maine. This activity not only stood him in good stead for the rugged outdoors life he would have to lead in Newfoundland, but, as Ecke later recalled, it brought him in contact with some up-and-coming Americans such as a young Bobbie Kennedy, whom he remembered reprimanding; John Olds had also previously been a councillor at this camp. Ecke volunteered for service in the US Army at the beginning of the Second World War; he was first posted to Canada's high north at Fort Chimo, Ungava Bay, then to North Africa and southern Europe where he was an important research member of the presidential-appointed United States Typhus Commission. Several more important publications also came from this work.[21] For the period from shortly after the war's end until the mid-1960s, Ecke served in the newly created CIA. Although he would not comment on his assignments, it appears that some of his duties focused on studying Soviet medicine. In the later 1960s, he returned to research and also undertook private medical practice; he retired in 1979. He never married, but had an almost fifty-year partnership with his companion, Robert Olson. Dr Bob Ecke died in Maine in 2001.

It is unlikely that the people of Notre Dame Bay ever fully knew the dimensions of the person or completely appreciated the man, they would call 'Doc Hackie' (the regional dialect adds an 'h' before a word beginning with a vowel, which also becomes pronounced in a way as was done several hundred years ago). In contrast with their local hero, John Olds (or rather '*H*olds'), who spent his entire professional life with them, Ecke made only five visits to Twillingate totalling a few years. During his days at the NDBMH, first as a visiting Hopkins medical student in the summer of 1934, then as junior hospital doctor intermittently for the period 1937–41, and finally as acting medical director from 1947–8 (to relieve Olds temporarily), however, he was an astute observer and recorder of people's medical troubles as well as their lives and times. His diary provides a wonderful written account of events, which includes much introspection about his own professional development as a rural doctor. This textual material is supplemented by other extensive archival materials, including extant colour movie footage (extremely rare for this time and place) as well as black-and-white still photographs now held at Memorial University.

Unlike many medical memoirists who write at the end of their careers when memories can fail, stories can become embellished or events become filtered through later life experiences, Ecke's documented the beginning of his career as physician and surgeon in a detailed and candid journal, in which he logged events and his opinions more or less as they occurred.[22] It remains a problematic historical source owing to its quotidian format, and that occasionally when he was too busy he would 'catch up' after a few days or a week, perhaps allowing inaccuracies to creep in. Owing to its chronological not thematic organization, with entries not arranged in any 'useful' analytical way, it was necessary first to prepare, in effect, a subject index of this material. In so doing, several patterns begin to appear from which we can draw some general conclusions.[23]

Most sweeping are the following results: That the rural medical practice that Ecke and his co-workers undertook was of immense breadth and depth, embracing almost every facet of interventionist and preventive medical care imaginable at the time. Ecke worked in the hospital operating room (theatre), the outpatient department and the wards, made house calls around the clock and spent weeks on end in the floating clinic that attended patients around 300 miles (500 km) of coastline and countless islands. He travelled by foot (with and without snowshoes), dog team, horseback, skis, dog and skis (*skijoring*), horse and sled, motorbike, motor boats, dories, and larger vessels, motorized snowmobile and the occasional automobile. He feared for his life many times as he got lost in blizzards, fell through semi-frozen ice, got tossed around in North Atlantic storms and crashed vehicles he was driving. When necessary he would sleep in the homes of patients on a spare bed, a chair or on the floor. Often on these occasions he shared their food, drink and hospitality; often he would bring food to them. Typically, any formality and protocol quickly gave way to common sense and/or survival. As such, Ecke can readily be described as a 'country doctor' or rural practitioner, but given the physical challenges he often had to overcome he may also be described as a practitioner of 'extreme medicine'.

More specifically, his journal illustrates the importance of varying clinical aspects of his practice as reflected in the relative frequency of their being mentioned. The overwhelming majority of Ecke's time was spent dealing with pregnancy and obstetric cases, including a number of caesarean sections – perhaps not surprising since Newfoundland had one of the highest birth rates across North America and northern Europe. A close second was surgical procedures, which included sophisticated abdominal operations, as well as more routine tonsillectomies (very common), dental extractions (extremely common), and a very high relative frequency of appendectomies. The treatment of infectious and communicable diseases (tuberculosis, typhoid and other fevers, poliomyelitis, meningitis, syphilis) as well as the promotion of public health measures and preventive medicine also figured prominently. Punctuating these general classes of cases was a host of others involving dermatological, neurological, cardiac, gynaecological, urological and mental illness conditions. Accident and occasional cancer cases rounded out this picture of an all-encompassing general rural medical practice. Very infrequently were patients referred to St John's or elsewhere for additional or more advanced treatment; more typical was the transfer of difficult cases from more northern settlements to Twillingate (and often these were lost causes involving extremely sick people who would die shortly after their arrival at the NDBMH). In addition to the duties attached to medical and surgical treatment were the concomitant tasks associated with their diagnosis. The hospital was adequately equipped to undertake bacteriological and radiological testing, basic blood work and, commencing in 1939, when it acquired an ECG machine, cardiac examinations.[24] The ECG in particular put the NDBMH at the forefront among sister institutions.[25]

Ecke's comments illustrate how in certain situations rural practice could differ from that in the city or other less remote locales. Owing to the isolation of people and difficulty of travel, surgery might be performed for preventative reasons. Clearly, one had to play the odds: Better to have your appendix removed if there was a chance of a problem, for if it flared up and ruptured when neither patient nor doctor could travel death was probably inevitable. 'Tonsils and things in the morning and I took out another appendix. Tonsils – tonsils – I wish I had never heard the word', declaimed Ecke in a fit of frustration on 11 November 1938. Two weeks later on 24 November, he was still reflecting on rural surgical practice, but was a little more philosophic:

> I was brought up in the school where the time to operate for appendicitis was when you made the diagnosis. I still cleave to that belief, but we had to make concessions at Twillingate. We became a little liberal on that score. Many of our patients lived in outlying islands and exposed parts of the rocky coast where in the winter or because of storm they would not be able to reach us for weeks at a time. If one such gave a story of an appendix-like attack during the winter before, even though there might be a minimum of trouble at the moment we were inclined to remove the appendix. As matter of fact, given no rupture, I figured out that one of the safest places you could be was on our operating table with a diagnosis of appendicitis.

Accounts of Ecke's numerous obstetric escapades, however, are the most illuminating with respect to the challenges occasionally facing both rural doctor and patient. As the following excerpts demonstrate, the clinical, social, ethical and economic issues faced by this young practitioner and the people he cared for were often difficult and extreme, but occasionally humorous and uplifting. In these latter respects they reflected the land and the people of the rural North. On 1 June 1938, after Ecke had performed a gastrointestinal operation on one woman he travelled to Manuel's Cove to see another, Mrs Gillard, who was in labour. 'The name didn't mean anything to me. I wandered down and it seems she has been pregnant for years', Ecke at first noted in a professional, but offhand way. But his demeanour soon changed on seeing the patient and her situation:

> She has been in a kind of mild labor for three days ... They must be the poorest people in Twillingate, but their house is the one where I would take a visitor to see a really

> lovely fisherman's home. Clean, neat, attractive garish wallpaper. Curtains of bleached flour bags with colorful bits of cloth appliquéd to make borders. The kitchen has lots of hooked rugs, a well-shined low stove, a few homemade chairs, and a good-looking sideboard, also homemade.

Further inquiry revealed that Mrs Gillard was missing a leg due to an amputation performed four years previously owing to tuberculosis of the knee. He continued to note that she was a hard-working, honest woman, but no merchant would advance the family food; there was not a crust of bread in the house. Ecke continued his physical examination, noting that the baby 'seemed to be huge'. He went on to comment:

> I felt we would never be able to do anything in the house. In fact, I was sure she would need a caesarean. I explained to her that she couldn't have a baby without an operation. There was none of the frequently encountered hysteria. She was silent for a moment while her eyes became moist. 'All right, doctor', she said quietly, 'do what you can to help me but remember, life is sweet'. I was deeply stirred by this woman's plain faith in the world – in the face of the little it had done for her. I got out of the house quickly, so her husband wouldn't wonder why my eyes were wet.

The result of the caesarean procedure was the birth of an extremely hydrocephalic baby that forced Ecke to wonder what would have been the outcome had he attempted a home birth as was usual. But the family situation pushed him to reflect further on the child's chances of subsequent survival. 'I told the nurses not to urge it to breathe but, of course, it came to life at once and thrives', he entered in his diary. Ecke further noted how a little later he 'leaned over it in the nursery several times and wondered if I should pop a morphine tablet into its mouth. But it is not nursing too well, so I don't believe it will really survive'. Ecke's contemplation of active euthanasia in this case may reasonably be viewed as an example of the paternalistic nature of medicine at this time, but by the same token his potential action was grounded in the ultimate well-being of a destitute fisher family. In some respects his intimate knowledge of economic and social matters due to his access to this tight rural community was a drawback as it ensnared him in this moral dilemma. Presumably, nature resolved this situation as there are no more entries about this case.

Rural social conditions and mores also played out unfavourably in, or complicated, other obstetric situations. As several oral history collections that relate to health customs and attitudes of older generations of Newfoundlanders note, talk of 'women's troubles' was taboo. Topics such as pregnancy were rarely mentioned in public. If it became known that a woman was pregnant she apparently was referred to as just being sick; similarly, when in labour she may be described as having been 'took sick'.[26] Ecke's experiences would support this observation. In one, noted in a 28 November 1938 entry, a hospital employee wished to suppress knowledge of her pregnancy as she was unmarried and 'her man' was working in the woods. Despite the fact that she had been in labour for some time, she resisted seeking medical attention – it was only as a result of relatives calling for Ecke that he arrived at the cold, decrepit, dark, dismal dwelling. The bed sagged to the floor with the two-week overdue patient 'way down in the gulch'. Because of these totally unsatisfactory conditions Ecke had the woman removed to the kitchen table in order that he might examine her and where she was chloroformed by a 'lusty neighbor'. Owing to her peculiar anatomy which obviated a full examination as well as the fact that several house cats had wandered over Ecke's once sterile obstetric kit, he realized that he could do nothing more in the house and thus persuaded the woman's mother to allow him to take her anesthetized daughter to hospital. The woman's stay in hospital lasted ten days, during which time she lay with 'her head turned towards the wall, not saying a word and frequently weeping'. There was also the case of a young girl brought into hospital accompanied by her father who complained that she was unable to dig the family potato patch because of a pain in her belly. Upon examination, the head of the baby she was carrying was on the perineum; she gave birth right away (19 June 1938). And Ecke could not help but comment when on 30 April 1941, Twillingate's 'spinster post mistress astounded the village last night' when she gave birth. Family shame and embarrassment may have been at the root of some of these reactions, but staying silent or being ignorant about pregnancy was not uncommon.

Ecke's journal accounts of his childbirth attendance also allow us another novel window on a prominent feature of rural healthcare in the North – the practice of lay midwives. The demise of lay midwifery in Newfoundland happened comparatively late in the twentieth century (not until well after Confederation with Canada), thus on numerous occasions Ecke and midwives collaborated during births. Midwives' professional relationships with medical men in Newfoundland always appear to have been harmonious; doctors and midwives would frequently consult each other, share duties at the bedside or give way to the other's experience and skill when necessary to the benefit of the pregnant woman and baby. Professional competition or petty jealousies seem not to have arisen. The majority of Newfoundland midwives learned their skills at the bedside from their mothers who, in turn, had also learned them from their mothers. Thus midwifery was very much a tradition embedded within island oral culture; other women might have engaged in formal training most often in hospitals in St John's. Another apparent quality uniting all these women was their phenomenal success as midwives. While evidence to support this assertion is admittedly often anecdotal and non-verifiable, midwives delivered (or 'borned') between several hundred to a thousand babies each during their careers – which adds up to tens of thousands of babies! Even more spectacular is the fact that a mother never seems to have been lost – hardly any babies too, even though they ranged from tiny, sickly premature ones (fed through eye droppers and sustained in boxes kept near the kitchen stove) to twenty-pound bruisers. Infant mortality during the first five years of life may have been high due to childhood killers such as diphtheria, typhoid and diarrhoea, but for their part in bringing in new lives Newfoundland midwives delivered.[27]

In most instances that Ecke cited his relationship with midwives was harmonious and the company convivial. A favourite of Ecke's was Mrs Oxford, who always referred to him as 'sweetheart'. On one occasion (4 November 1940) after an arduous, cold trip by motorcycle and motor boat to Herring Neck to attend a birth that was labelled by local men as a matter of 'life and death', Ecke arrived to find that the baby had been born with Mrs Oxford catching it. 'The mother was fine, without even a tear', Ecke recorded, 'but the baby was moaning and all agreed that babies always died when they moaned. It looked alright to me. I fixed the eyes, the cord, and the foreskin'. All being well, a

> jolly cup of tea was ready in the comfortable heavy gloom downstairs. The woman joked about why we had babies and is it the men's fault entirely or not. One of the men spoke of cutting wood by moonlight and a woman said if he didn't spend so long in bed with his wife he would have more time to do his work by daylight. The logic was obscure, the humor was clear and well received.

One final, long but excerpted journal entry for the twenty-four-hour period for 5/6 January 1939 captures vividly the unique social and demanding medical life of this locale. The full entry is written episodically illustrating the haphazard events and pace of this special day, but in it Ecke displays his vulnerabilities and is also highly reflective about his isolated, yet satisfying situation. 'The best time I ever had in the snow today', wrote Ecke.

> Hitched [dogs] Dudley up with Sport and it worked perfectly. All the dogs came along but the two in harness pulled like the devil up and down hill, over anything. I just followed them and we went way into the interior of the island. It was beautiful and lonely with all the hills looking alike as the sun went down.

Later, after a 'tub and tea', he went on a house call to Bluff Head Cove 'where the whale washed ashore yesterday with a harpoon in him. They have been cutting it up all day for the dogs'. Yet another obstetrical house call during the evening, which was also a natural delight as the 'moon was so bright you could tell bright colors by it'. Ecke further recounted that upon his arrival at this patient's house he found it in an uproar:

> 'Something is coming out!' shouted the midwife. I looked and sure enough, something was. I thought for a moment it was a prolapsed uterus, but after getting some pituitrin and ergotoxin ready, and putting on some gloves, I saw it was a fetus held in by the cord around its neck. I unwound it and drew the offender alive and quickly

after it the placenta. It was about six months. No bleeding but didn't think all the
membranes were out so I left a long course of ergot.

Although Ecke handled many maternity cases in hospital, he seems to have been
quite adept at home births. This situation appears to contrast somewhat to a
roughly contemporary medical colleague on the other side of Newfoundland.
During the mid-to-late 1940s at the Bonne Bay Cottage Hospital located on the
north-west coast of the island, Dr Noel Murphy did undertake confinements in
patients' homes, but it is clear that over time he encouraged pregnant women to
give birth in the cottage hospital (on average about 100 cases a year).[28]

If dog-sled teams, beached harpooned whales, and snowy terrain failed to
remind the American doctor that he was in a different place and different culture
from his native New York City, his return trip to his hospital-home ought to
have confirmed it. First, his travelling companion was a local man who had 'been
down on the arm mummering'. The seasonal tradition of mummering dating
to medieval England had villagers dress themselves in bizarre outfits to dis-
guise their identity, while they visited neighbours' homes to drink, dance, sing
and engage in all sorts of good-natured mischief and revelry; Newfoundland
remains, along with parts of Ireland and England, one of the last bastions of this
practice. Secondly, the evening of 5 January was then celebrated as Christmas
Eve (not 24 December) – another ancient tradition observed. Thus, that night
there was a 'good party' at which Ecke 'took Benzedrine and drank very little'.
He continued, 'My tuxedo looked swell. The girls were all dressed up. Marianne
was particularly beautiful in a new, black velvet, off-the-shoulder business. There
was a lot of lipstick spread around. I left early and couldn't sleep'. This description
has a surreal overtone to it: Men in tuxedos, women in black dresses dining in
the frozen and barren, northern hinterland. Ecke's lack of consumption of alcohol was unusual for him, but his pill-popping was not. Indeed, frequent drinking
and the liberal use of prescription drugs were common at the NDBMH as Ecke's
diary often makes alarmingly clear. (Later that day, Santa Claus, a medical colleague from Virginia, wandered the hospital wards 'pretty tight'. The hospital
eggnog was known for its potency.)

In addition to the seasonal dining activities described, others were pursued
throughout the rest of the year such as bridge, chess, reading, listening to classical
music and opera on the gramophone and American radio stations as well as the
empire service of the British Broadcasting Company (BBC), playing Beethoven
on the piano and intense conversation. All considered, a depiction of a bourgeois
existence within the enclave of the hospital and its micro-environment emerges.
Such an evaluation along with the fact that these men and women practised their
brand of 1930s socialized medicine suggests a sense of a community within a
community. As non-Newfoundlanders, American, educated, urbanites and doc-

tors, they were simultaneously a part of and yet apart from those they treated and truly cared for. Again, returning to Ecke's journal for 'Christmas Eve/Day' of 5 January 1939, it appears that he would share this interpretation; he was also aware of the tenuous nature of the situation: 'At this moment we are all good friends', he wrote.

> There is no feud or grudge afoot. Everyone is speaking to everyone but to this inquiring eye reservations are apparent ... Everyone of us here at various times has revealed rather ugly sentiments to any three of four others. Yet there is no doubt that it is necessary of course that we all be friends. Our group is small and we are in desperate need of one another yet it would be hard to detect any false note in the present relationships.

Recovering the Patient's Voice

Just as Newfoundland was a colonial outpost on the margins, so too can we portray Ecke and his colleagues as creating and inhabiting yet another 'sub-colonial' outpost. The extent of the general social and intellectual gulf between hospital life and that of patients in this northern, rural setting is evident from Ecke's writing, but he further distinguishes the gap by noting how people living on isolated islands were different yet again from those of Twillingate, who had 'been spoiled a little by the near civilization we have here' (23 February 1939). The writings of patients themselves, which have miraculously survived owing to Ecke's obsessive habit of sorting and storing his personal records, also cast light on rural doctor–patient relations at the margins. These documents by patients give historical voice to them as a group which is often silent or ignored; they also cast more light on health-care practice in the NDBMH/contract catchment area.[29] All of the twenty-five or so letters available are handwritten in script (none are printed), many in pencil by hands that suggest a basic but functional education; several are quite literate and well produced. (Literacy in this region of the island was probably higher than other parts as educational opportunities were more available owing to its predominantly Protestant – Church of England – orientation.) They are respectful and variously addressed to 'Dear Dr', 'Dear sir', 'Dear Doctor', 'Robert S. Ecke M.D'. 'Dr Hicky', 'Dr Heckey', 'Dr E' or occasionally to 'Dr Holds'. As they are signed and mostly dated, and identify their point of origin, these letters appear to be representative of the patients from the hospital's expansive service area.

These letters were written by men and women from outports across the Notre Dame Bay area such as Carmanville, Norris Arm, Change Islands and Victoria Cove. While there are differences in the literacy levels of their authors, common to all of them is the need of the writers or family members to be informed about health matters. They were often responses to letters sent by Ecke or perhaps his colleagues to patients, illustrating that diagnosis and/or treatment by mail was another facet of medicine in the North. While slow and maybe unreliable owing to the vagaries of the shipping schedules of the coastal steamers that transported the mail, this form of communication was often the only one available to most people owing to the absence of any radio/telephone/telegraph communications network. As the following excerpts also show, the letters were often written in local dialect. My *verbatim* transcription has been undertaken not to be judgmental or condescending, but to try to capture the 'oral culture' of this region with its orthographic markers and vocabulary – the people wrote in the style and register they spoke.

About a month ago I examine in the Hospatle and I have taken the medicane that the Doctor has given me Also find it a great help.

But I find my back quit a lot some time and now I am sending you my water for you to test again because some time the water seems to be all right But most all the time tick cloudy or of Dark coler and the Pain that I find in my Back his a quick pain and Doctor Sometime I am onely three weeks when my monthly operate come on if I goes on Long Walking or on Boat and it is Blowing its makes Diferns right away and I feel week on them time like I short Breathing hot flashes But I find the Mediciane great help and would like get more if Possall

[Mrs WH, 6 September 1939]

I have been troubled lately with a pain in my left side, about six inches below my armpit, and rather more in front than behind.

It hurts most when I breath, or as some one expressed it, I have a 'catch' in my breath. This may not be the medical term for it, but it seems to suit very well.

I am painting it with iodine, and am drinking cod-liver-oil what would you advise?

Please give this letter a little consideration and oblige.

[Mr WF, 20 January 1939]

Would you please come up as I want couple of teeth pulled and are unable to walk down to the boat. Please come sometime during the evening.

Contract payed. [SB]

I am sending Gertie along to the Hospital please try and do your best for her please advise me after Opration also drope me a word two weeks before coming home and maybe her father will come down to come home with her I am not giving her the mony just now but let me know when you want it and should there be any obstical in that way I would not have the mony at the time would a few days make any diffirince please let me know

[Mrs JL, 30 October 1938]

I am writing you to let you know I received your letter and parcel

So you think its neuritis I have in my face yes I think it is or some thing worse the pain of it is terrible. I am no better and not so well as I was last fall and no better appetite what I eats is only a force in.

I am not sending the money as I know I will get a good chance to send it or will be coming myself in some boat when the ice get away clearly
[Mrs GW, 22 March 1941]

I am sending over Hettie Belle She has been trouble this last two years with gass & her mounthly appearance stopped on her in June first She was always a hearthy girl & never complain to be sick I am sending a note because she may be backward in telling you She will be seventeen the fourteen of September we are on the Blanket[-contract?] forms
[Mr JL, 31 August 1941]

I am very sick my bowels is bad and my water is like blood i am wonderful sick cant get no rest night-time att all and my stomach is full of pluss will you come down and see me again
    I ham week right down Could you give me Something to Strant me or any thing to ase my pains I ham coculing all over my and stin[g]ing my [h]ands and fingers his cutting and Stingen wonderful Come has quick has you can
    And my feet his wonderful bad with puss in them
    [Mrs B]

I have been quite worried regarding lumps behind baby's ears. They are hard and seem to move. The one behind his left ear is on the bone, but behind his right ear its farther down behind the lobe. They do get any larger and have been there about a month. I do not think they give any pain as baby is not troublesome. What do you think is the cause of them?
    Baby is four months old and weighs 16lbs, Is bottle-fed and so far has only had the milk. Would it be advisable to give him cereal now. What time in the day & how much?
    Would be relieved to hear from you as soon as possible,
    [Mrs RC, 3 March 1939]

In general, the letters discuss symptoms, aches, pains and ailments in the hope this information might assist in diagnosis. Discussions of laboratory tests appear, perhaps accompanied by a 'water' (urine) sample from the patient. The use of the term *water* for urine and its production is noteworthy. Such descriptive observations by patients about their bodies while simplistic would nonetheless be useful diagnostic clues for Ecke. Also revealed in these documents are traditional ways of expressing the folk aetiology of ailments and their symptomology. Phrases such as '"catch" in my breath', 'my feet his wonderful bad with puss in them', and 'i am wonderful sick … my [h]ands and fingers his cutting and Stingen wonderful', very much point to the local dialect. In particular, the use of 'wonderful' in this context means *awful* and is Elizabethan in origin; it is not meant to connote something good or positive. The practice of self-help by topical applications and ingestion for example, is also evident through actions such as painting areas with iodine and the consumption of cod-liver oil. Requests for medicine, tonics and treatment are also commonplace. The candour about menstruation is surprising ('I am onely three weeks when my monthly operate come on', 'her mounthly appearance stopped on her in June') as such a matter was apparently little discussed in outport culture. Presumably any mention of it in these letters was deemed appropriate as in this context there was direct communication with a physician.[30]

Finally, even from this small sample of patients' letters, the concern over payment for medical services rendered is quite evident. In one instance, Mr J. L. informed Ecke that his family was covered under the 'blanket' contract thus no additional payment ought to be expected, while several other patients expressed hesitancy about paying. Although the two such examples quoted above suggest that medical bills would be paid, Ecke's memoirs relate the trouble he often had extracting payments from people, especially from those he believed were not facing financial hardship. Arrangements for house or shore calls and hospital stays are also discussed, especially the logistics of travel to and from isolated areas. The limiting effect of harsh climatic conditions on transportation and communications arrangements ('will be coming myself in some boat when the ice get away clearly') underscore the difficulties of rural medical practice.

Modernity, Newfoundland and the North as 'Frontier'

When Ecke finally published his Twillingate medical experiences six decades later at the turn of the twenty-first century, he referred to them as the 'memoirs of a frontier Newfoundland doctor'. The term *frontier* is evocative, but is generally not one applied to a British colonial context or for that matter to a Canadian one. It is very much an Americanism that conjures up thoughts of the opening of the West in the nineteenth century, or more recently of outer space – that final frontier. Historically, it originates with Fredrick Jackson Turner and his 'thesis' (or 'myth') of how America expanded as its civilization inexorably galloped westward.[31] But it is ironic that the term is not misapplied to the NDBMH for this institution, although located in a Newfoundland outport, was *de facto* an *American* outpost. As this paper has shown, funds from the US were essential to the building and subsequent expansion of the hospital, American architects designed it, an American doctor directed this institution at its inception, other American medical students and doctors were essential support staff until the era of Canadian Confederation and during the early decades of the hospital American trained nurses occupied key roles in its operation. Further as Ecke's journal repeatedly noted, observation of the Thanksgiving holiday in November (the quintessential American holiday celebration) was *de rigueur*, and as his colour home movies displayed vividly, flying on the hospital's flagpole below the British Union Jack (then Newfoundland's official flag) was the American Stars and Stripes!

Yet was this medical community in the wilderness? Did its creation impose order and bring 'civilization'? The answer to these questions is both yes and no. And the ambivalent nature of this answer makes the study of Twillingate instructive for our exploration of rural medicine in the North. Before the hospital was built, Twillingate was a well-functioning small settlement whose economy depended on the north-east and Labrador coastal schooner trade, the seal hunt and the cod fishery. The area was definitely rural, while some of those living in outports in the Notre Dame Bay archipelago would certainly be described as being remote, if not isolated. For the period under study, homes and businesses had no electrical power or running water and sanitation; luxury goods and comestibles were rare. Subsistence living was often the order of the day, especially in the days of the Depression. Thus life and living conditions could be likened to that of an American frontier Western town (but certainly without the wanton lawlessness). In many respects the founding and subsequent functioning of the NDBMH did not drastically alter this situation, but nevertheless the hospital *qua* institution, which not only symbolized the 'modern' through scientific medicine but also was a material culture monument to it, did exert a civilizing influence.

How? Hospitals, as those who write their history know and those who work in them appreciate, are not just purpose-built physical structures – merely bricks and mortar. No matter how impersonal they might appear, they are actually micro-communities with collective personalities that often impress themselves on their host environment. The NDBMH was the largest and only non-wooden structure in Twillingate; it had its own internal plumbing system, which was unusual for the region; electricity was supplied through a hydro-electric plant on hospital grounds, which was exceptional; it was centrally heated, again out of the ordinary; it housed exotic, complex and sophisticated scientific apparatus; and life-saving events happened inside its walls. In short it was a technological palace that announced that modernity had arrived. Similarly, those in white coats who ran the hospital symbolized the new and the progressive. These men and women were highly educated, hailed from bustling metropolitan centres, ate different foods, engaged in cultured activities, even dressed formally for dinner on occasions. In short, they were urban, urbane and civilized. It can be concluded then, that a civilizing or modernizing influence was brought to bear on the 'frontier'.

However, the brand of the 'modern' that was introduced to Notre Dame Bay through the medium of the hospital and its imported medical personnel was not condescending to the local rural community, nor did it exert a corrupting influence. It would have been easy to see this rural – frontier – community as 'backward', but Ecke and his colleagues who may have been considered by some as being socially 'superior' were not imbued with the missionary spirit to convert or uplift the native population (as were Grenfell and colleagues). They had a strong desire to build, to help and to improve, but such benevolent motives were infused with a socialistic ideology that made their American idealism palatable and workable in this outport community on the margins. The hospital at Twillingate and the extended health care it provided throughout the region, was in many respects 'high tech' for such a rural institution of the era – but its culture was grounded in that of the people it served. Curiously, it was the medical community of St John's (if not the rest of the island) that believed that their Twillingate colleagues were 'high hat', not the local residents.[32]

An undated section of Ecke's journal, perhaps written during the fall of 1940 (but before 1942), that is especially reflective in tone and intent, explores these issues of mixed social status and society, rural medical practice, personal motivation and the 'frontier-civilization' dichotomy.[33] These 'Ruminations' as Ecke called them, while they dealt with his attempt to make sense of his own life, were grounded in evaluations of the local context of Twillingate, the hospital and Newfoundland. Although he often begins with generalities, typically his thoughts end up focusing on rural and remote medical practice in the North. While musing over the 'fun' of eating in patients' homes no matter what was served (but Newfoundland hot, black tea along with clotted or Devonshire cream on local berries were among Ecke's favourites), he recorded his impressions of the position of the doctor, the practice of medicine and the hospital in the community: 'The people respond in the same way they would in any American rural area'. But, notwithstanding this observation, Ecke conceded, 'It does happen that our standard of living at the hospital is rather higher than that of our neighbors. We have running water and steam heat.' This privileged lifestyle, augmented by the fact of being the only hospital and doctors available for 'most of the bay people' meant that they were all but indispensable. The total effect was that it gave 'our ensemble a slight "manor" quality'. But keeping everyone grounded was the local system of social and community values which held that

> [u]nearned income or even large, earned income does not especially increase a man's stature ... The man who is respected is the man who works hard, who fishes well, who can build a house or a boat. The true aristocrat is the man who has skippered a ship well or is a good pilot.

Within this framework of social distinctions, how did the doctor and medicine fare? Here, too, the journal guides us, for Ecke discerned generational (and perceived gender) differences that reflected a larger shifting social landscape as 'civilization' slowly displaced the 'frontier'. 'Those older rugged characters tended rather to look on doctors and gentlemen of the cloth as people you had to call in once in a while, but on the whole were luxuries that the women folk seemed to demand', Ecke observed. He concluded:

> Their tolerant humor with regard to us was never irritating. I enjoyed their hospital joshing. If you traveled thirty or forty miles by dog team to visit their 'weak nerved' granddaughter or their son, 'spoiled too much by reading', they respected your having come much more than they did what you could do when you got there. Often enough, they themselves claimed our services in extremes.

Finally, a particularly prophetic statement: 'These older fellows who didn't take the doctor too seriously are heavily outnumbered by the younger folk who have come to realize that *medicine is here to stay* [emphasis added]'. Ecke's highlighting of this realization was only one of several manifestations that the modern age had arrived (albeit a bit behind schedule compared to other areas). The hospital was at the forefront of this movement – something that Ecke was ambivalent about, for his relationship with the North and its people was connected to their idyllic remoteness. He admitted to having a 'strange yearning for the remote and the wild and the lonely inaccessible' and took a 'perverse delight in circumstances that make travel impossible'. Moreover, while admitting to liking the comforts of a hot bath and a comfortable bed, Ecke lamented that the 'frontier keeps retreating though'. Thus he reflected that when he first came to Newfoundland in the summer of 1934, 'there wasn't an operating radio on this island [Twillingate]'. This, however, soon changed:

> Gradually refinement has crept up on us. We used to have poor lights in the hospital, the diesel had to be conserved and was always getting cut off in the middle of a poker game ... Now we have an efficient gasoline generator ready at all times. I feel threatened by 'efficient' machinery and somehow it makes me feel inferior. We used to have to settle down to very plain food in the winter. Now [the local merchant] ... imports fancy canned goods and takes the risk of bringing in fresh tomatoes in the middle of winter.

The collective effects of geographic locale and social situation led to a final rumination about 'frontier' medicine in the North. Doctors there were put 'in a spot'. A 'good deed' by a doctor like Ecke reflected well on all, conversely a 'bad act on our part means for them that doctors are bad'. Twillingate's experience with its rural doctors is instructive in this regard, for it highlights a darker facet of medical practice in the North. The founding medical director of the NDBMH, Dr Charles Parsons, eventually resigned for 'medical reasons' after a decade in Twillingate, and it is generally accepted that alcohol was at the root of this situation; Norman Bethune (himself no stranger to drinking) perhaps unkindly but accurately evaluated his character on the boat to China (recall Bethune's phrase 'drunken bum'). Similarly, his successor, Dr John Olds, a physician who is still revered in the region, also had to take time off to recuperate from his excessive alcohol consumption. And, Ecke, if he had totally committed himself for an extended stay in the North might easily have ended up in like manner; certainly, his regular consumption of liquor along with popping various 'uppers' and 'downers' suggests a possible path.

The abuse of addictive substances by doctors is not unique to the North. But what maybe sets such rural and remote regions apart from their urban counterparts is the people's ability to overlook (for some time) and/or forgive such transgressive behaviour – perhaps out of necessity, or from prevailing social mores. In Newfoundland, this attitude may be even more culturally programmed than elsewhere. On the one hand, the 'doctor' (by definition both rural and male) in Newfoundland culture enjoys a positive image owing to legend and fact. Observe, for example, the tradition of the mummers' play as performed by the folk which has as one of its stock characters a doctor who brings another character back to life – he is heroic. In this regard, Sir Wilfred Grenfell and his larger-than-life nature and record of good deeds personified this ideal. (Grenfell was also a ferocious advocate of abstinence from alcohol.) On the other hand, the 'local doc as drunk' is also recognizable as a regional stereotype in popular fiction and culture.[34] Medical life in Twillingate during Ecke's time seems to have captured both sides of this picture. By comparison, during the late 1940s Dr Noel Murphy of the Bonne Bay cottage hospital who, too, was often accorded a place of honour at wedding tables and other social events would usually diplo-matically excuse himself from such festivities before they got too boisterous. As the only doctor for hundreds miles he was conscious of maintaining his profes-sional demeanour and 'distance', thus he did not publicly imbibe alcohol or revel with his patients.[35]

In total, the NDBMH from its very inception through to the era of its lit-eral rebuilding and reinvention towards the close of the twentieth century had a galvanizing effect on the community that built it and which it served.[36] Ecke's journal along with other primary documents of the era has allowed a scholarly window on rural medical practice in the North and the concomitant process of 'modernization' in this rural and remote area. Medicine in this part of the North was here to stay.

8 POLICING PRACTITIONERS ON THE PERIPHERY: ELITE PHYSICIANS AND PROFESSION-BUILDING IN A BICULTURAL PROVINCE, 1920–39[1]

Sasha Mullally

Over the course of the interwar decades, the College of Physicians and Surgeons in the Canadian Province of New Brunswick began a programme of significant organizational reform. The Medical Council, a body that set and enforced licensing standards on behalf of the College, dramatically stepped up efforts to seek out unlicensed practitioners within their provincial borders and require them to supply proof of their credentials. This process turned out to be anything but straightforward. In the prosecution of its most intransigent cases, members of the Medical Council would find themselves drawn into a frustrating, drawn-out, merry-go-round of litigation. The medical registrar, J. M. Barry, complained in 1934 that when the Medical Council tried to enforce licensing legislation in the rural districts in the province, it found itself having to 'fight with every interest in the County' to do so.[2] The rural frontiers of medical practice did not succumb to central authority easily, or willingly.

A case in point is their difficulty in policing one illegal physician, Dr Alfred Leger.[3] Between 1927 and 1931, this American-trained doctor had moved around several northern towns and villages avoiding prosecution from the College. On two occasions, he had written to the Medical Council assuring them he had proper qualifications (although not presenting a diploma or other formal credentials). In these letters he had communicated both the desire and a commitment to practice in a rural area where the residents had little access to health care. A Francophone and native New Brunswicker, Dr Leger seemed to believe that his dedication to the underserved Acadian regions of the province would provide sufficient grounds to let him continue in the profession. On both occasions, however, the Medical Council denied his request for formal registration.[4] On October of 1931, Dr Leger took the unusual step of appearing before the Medical Council in person. The minutes of the Medical Council meeting record he made a very impassioned plea for formal licence. While the members entertained his presentation and questioned him at length, upon his departure, they resolved to stand by their original decision.[5] Appearing in person before the licensing body simply drew more attention to his illegal practice, and the Medical Council stepped up their surveillance of the physician's activities.

In 1932 the Medical Council received news that Leger had surfaced again and, in defiance of the law, had set up a practice in Northumberland County. Medical Council minutes record considerable discussion of his case. Council members noted, with some concern, how some new correspondence from the medical registrar for the state of Maine confirmed their suspicions that his medical education was actually incomplete. However, there was also evidence of local backing for Dr Leger. A letter sent in by a Northumberland County parish priest apparently supported his practice.[6] Nonetheless, the Medical Council decided to move forward and take legal action against Leger and struck a special prosecuting committee to gather evidence against him.[7] Eventually, they would be successful in ousting the doctor from the province, but only after years of effort, four of which would be taken up by a lengthy and costly legal conflict. We will return to the case of Dr Leger later in this paper. But in the pages to follow we will also see how the New Brunswick Medical Council's failure to stop the illegal practice of a single unlicensed rural physician, among many other illegal practitioners who persisted in rural regions of the province, is a largely untold side of the story of medical professionalization.

In his classic study of medical profession-building in the US, Paul Starr has characterized the interwar period as one where American physician organizations consolidated their medical power, building on the profession's previous successes with the creation and passage of medical licensing laws.[8] Canadian historiography has for the most part accepted and applied this interpretation and this timeline to the history of physician organization on this side of the border. The 1920s and 1930s have been called an 'age of equipoise' for rank-and-file physicians in Canada, decades where they enjoyed comfortable practices, protected by licensing legislation that granted them hegemony among other healers and practitioners and secured the centrality of scientific medicine within the medical marketplace.[9] This paper argues that it is time to reconsider the history of medical professionalization in Canada. A closer look at rural medicine, rural doctors and medical relations between 'the country and the city', for instance, complicates this picture of interwar medicine.

Based on an analysis of the corporate records of the Medical Council of the College of Physicians and Surgeons, this paper will reveal how elites on the Medical Council tried, with little success, to effectively police medical practices in rural regions of the province. At a time when professional medicine was meant to be in its ascendancy, irregular healers continued to operate, drawing from the support of some rural communities. The story of Alfred Leger and other practitioners who operated in the liminal, 'unpoliceable' rural frontiers of organized medicine throws light on the gap between professional, urban understandings of 'medical expertise' and 'adequate service' and understandings held by those in rural communities. By placing these practices within the particular political, social and professional context of New Brunswick, this paper will also draw attention to the importance of place as an influence on the organization of health services.

Elite Physicians and Medical Governance

During the first half of the twentieth century, provincial medical societies and Colleges of Physicians and Surgeons in Canada did build on the legislative efforts of previous medical generations and consolidated their role as gate-keepers of the practice of medicine. In the Province of Ontario, for instance, the 'regular' doctors incrementally took control of provincial licensing boards and gradually marginalized medical sectarians, such as homeopaths and eclectics, as the call to improve and standardize medical education and medical practice gained ground.[10]

This process took shape in myriad ways across the country because healthcare services in Canada are governed by provincial legislation. In recognition of this, the past decade has witnessed a resurgence in the use of region as a category of analysis in the history of medicine.[11] Megan Davies has shown how public health services and medical practices in nineteenth-century British Columbia were defined by the needs and customs of care already established at the community level.[12] In his study of laboratory workers in the Maritime Provinces, Peter Twohig has, likewise, argued that local variation in the terms and contours of both professional organization and service delivery was the rule, not the exception.[13] These studies point to a need for more work that takes into account the importance of place, using place to reveal the different ways that physician elites managed the professionalization process among provincial jurisdictions.[14]

In New Brunswick, the provincial College's ability to effectively prosecute unlicensed physicians was a relatively new power, one vested in the Medical Council by the Medical Act of 1920.[15] With this Act, the New Brunswick College's Council exerted, on paper at least, a great deal of control over the provincial medical marketplace. Unlike many other Canadian jurisdictions, the New Brunswick Medical Council had decided not to participate in international or interprovincial licensing reciprocity agreements. With no medical school within its provincial borders, New Brunswick relied on medical graduates trained in other jurisdictions to supply their communities, at least, those who could pass muster with the College of Physicians and Surgeons. It was up to the Medical Council of the College to review these credentials and to set terms for examination and licence. Council minutes reveal the inner workings of this body and allow for historical analysis of these policing activities. Because these interwar decades were the first occasion when the Council could wield the threat of substantial fines against those who flouted the law,[16] it focused its gaze on managing rural professional hinterland.

Professionalization could not be considered complete without control of the medical practices in rural areas. Peter Mitham has argued that medical professionalization in New Brunswick in the late nineteenth century was based on building and maintaining the kind of education and practice standards that would uphold 'the honour and dignity of the profession'.[17] Professionalization also promised practical benefits for 'regular' physicians, allowing them to manage standards of care and limit the activities of potential professional rivals. For rural physicians these rivals were sometimes midwives, sometimes lay practitioners and sometimes other physicians. Rural physicians sometimes felt as if they were on the 'front lines' of scientific medicine's expansion. In New Brunswick, there was an uneasy relationship between medical elites and medical rank-and-file, and between centre and periphery.[18]

'Rural' and 'Urban' in a Bicultural Province

Biculturalism is a key factor when considering health politics and health care in New Brunswick. A small province by Canadian geographic standards, New Brunswick comprises a territory slightly larger than that of Ireland and is situated on the Atlantic coast. It shares a land border with Quebec on its forested north-west boundary, and another with Nova Scotia across a marshy isthmus to the south-east. It shares a third borderland with the American state of Maine to the west and south-west. As one of the three Maritime Provinces,[19] New Brunswick also has two coastal areas – the Bay of Fundy to the south and the Gulf of St Lawrence to the east and north-east, which spills out into the Atlantic Ocean.

Although it is small, the province encompasses both English- and French-speaking communities. A geographic divide between the rural districts in the northern areas of the province and the more populous municipalities of the south also marks the linguistic and cultural boundary between French-speaking Acadian communities and Anglo-Celtic, English-speaking populations. Among Canadian provinces, New Brunswick is the only officially bilingual and bicultural jurisdiction.[20] Although dominated numerically, economically and socially by an Anglophone majority, rural Francophone communities across New Brunswick have endured with a distinct identity, especially those populations clustered to the north and north-east on the 'Acadian peninsula'.

Bilingualism and biculturalism in New Brunswick influenced the demographic distribution of physicians; for most of the twentieth century, Francophone communities have had access to fewer doctors. Problems recruiting physicians to this region seems to be the reason Dr Alfred Leger, among other alternative and 'lay' practitioners, continued to work as rural healers despite increased medical regulation from the central, city-based licensing authorities. While the presence of unlicensed practitioners was not limited to the Francophone regions of the province, the bicultural divide in New Brunswick seems to have made some rural communities in the province more 'remote' than others, at least in the eyes of the provincial Medical Council, an organization dominated by urban Anglophone physicians. This meant the politics of rural medicine in New Brunswick would be heavily informed by place and region, and these were at once spatially, politically and culturally determined.

Medicine along the French–English Divide

By the 1920s the Medical Council had established a formalized process whereby physicians could register to practice in New Brunswick. The process focused on the standards of medical education, and the Medical Council sought to enact measures that would, in the future, open the roster only for graduates of 'Class A' medical schools.[21] This was partly motivated in response to efforts of the Canadian Medical Association to raise and standardize licensing credentials among provinces and to encourage interprovincial licensing reciprocity. Licensing reciprocity was something the New Brunswick College of Physicians and Surgeons resisted. The Medical Council decided not to take part in any licensing reciprocity agreements with other provinces and even reserved the right to veto any applicant regardless of their training. They did, however, informally adopt the License of the Medical Council of Canada (LMCC) as the 'gold standard' of licensing qualifications.[22]

While recognizing the importance of keeping unlicensed healers out of the medical field, the actual policing role of the College of Physicians and Surgeons, at whose behest the Council Members acted, was in a state of flux throughout the interwar period. Local law enforcement and legal authorities, organized at the county or municipal level, were also sometimes slow to implement and utilize the new legislation, apparently because they found it too difficult to recruit and retain health-care professionals. If the licensing legislation was to be enforced, the Medical Council would in most cases have to launch the suit itself.

Interference in local medical affairs was politically risky for the central authority. The geographic divide between French-speaking and English-speaking parts of the province was mirrored in the geographic distribution of physicians. Apart from economic factors, it is unclear why northern Francophone districts had such difficulty recruiting and retaining doctors. But they did, and the disparity was stark. The northern New Brunswick counties of Madawaska and Restigouche, for example, had a physician per population ratio of 1:1,800 by the end of the Depression, and nearby Gloucester County on the Acadian peninsula had an even higher ratio of 1:3,000.[23] At this time, ratio for the entire province was approximately 1:1,500[24] and for Canada was approximately 1:1,000.[25] Northern rural communities were very concerned by this state of affairs. Throughout the interwar period, the Medical Council received and tabled the receipt of letters from northern small towns and rural regions of the province that sought to recruit doctors, but the Council, for its part, considered these problems to be local ones. Only occasionally would the registrar forward community concerns to medical school officials in nearby Nova Scotia and Quebec. Throughout the 1920s and 1930s, the Medical Council maintained, contentedly, that 'the number of practising physicians in this province is sufficient'.[26]

The health of rural residents could not have figured into their calculus. Infant mortality, long a key marker of population health, remained high in New Brunswick, especially in the northern counties. Between 1920 and 1924, the five-year mean infant mortality rate for the province hovered close to 112 deaths per 1,000 live births. Between 1920 and 1924, by contrast, the mean infant mortality rate for Madawaska County was 175.[27] The unfortunate residents of the north-western county reported infant mortality rates between 50 and 75 per cent higher than the province as a whole. In fact, counties with the four highest infant mortality rates in rural districts were located in the Francophone reaches of the province. In comparison, rural areas with largely Anglophone populations saw infant mortality rates below the average for all rural districts, and below rates for the province as a whole.[28]

Practitioners on the Periphery

With the dearth of doctors in the province approaching a famine in rural and remote regions, and a troublingly high infant mortality rate, rural communities were perhaps not in a position to worry about the formal credentials of their health-care providers. Numerous unregistered and alternative practitioners from a variety of traditions, disciplines and training backgrounds flourished in the resulting vacuum. The Medical Council records are very rich sources of information on such practitioners, whose itinerant, unlicensed and/or 'lay' status often renders them otherwise invisible in the historical record. The Council minutes tabled many complaints from physicians who competed with these practitioners, general practitioners who clearly expected the College to prosecute and protect their sphere of practice.

General practitioners usually had a sympathetic hearing from Council members, and the matter of 'prosecuting the irregulars' generally occupied a good deal of time from the Medical Council over these years. Reflecting on the medical marketplace in 1935, the Council was pleased to note that '[t]he naturopath and chiropractor are gradually dying a natural death'[29] – though osteopaths presented a more challenging problem. In the fall of 1931, for instance, a travelling osteopath and chiropractor named Talbot had made his way through rural districts of the province, 'curing all chronic diseases and complaints'. The Council had debated whether direct action against the 'charlatan' was well-advised. Dr Clowes Van Wart noted with approval that the College of Physicians and Surgeons in Ontario employed an investigator and prosecutor on a full-time basis to pursue these cases. Members present ultimately felt, however, that this kind of expense was 'beyond the means' of the New Brunswick Council and 'it was decided, as in the past, that no action be taken'.[30] During this decade and a half, the Council took action to limit the practice of only one osteopathic practitioner, and he was based in the capital city of Fredericton. In fact, during the years under investigation here, with this one exception, all practitioners pursued, warned or prosecuted by the Council for breaching scope of practice, illegal activity or 'infamous conduct' were located in rural and remote regions of the province.

The practitioners who caused the Medical Council most concern were midwives. These caregivers raised the ire of many rural physicians throughout the 1920s and 1930s.[31] Some of these individuals appeared to be traditional midwives engaged in a full-time childbirth practice, while others were trained nurses who provided occasional midwifery services. Physician complaints came in from all rural regions of the province, indicating a widespread patronage of midwives in many regions of New Brunswick.

Most complaints were merely noted by the Council, and the conflicts they represented seemed to be resolved without Council interference.[32] Some physicians, on the other hand, were determined to end the practice of 'lay obstetrics'. Dr B of the Kedgewick area wrote in regularly over the 1920s and 1930s to complain about 'certain midwives' practising in 'his district' of Restigouche County, part of a decade-long correspondence campaign to convince the medical registrar and Medical Council to take legal action to curtail their activities.[33] The Medical Council's responses to Dr B and other physicians who wrote on this matter varied. It seems that only in cases where the caregivers were well known to use anaesthesia or give other medication in labour that the Council would take any action, which usually took the form of a warning letter. These seem to have carried sufficient weight in most cases to curtail illegal scope of practice, or at least to satisfy the local physician who made the complaint. In 1936, for instance, the Council responded to reports that a Mrs S was allegedly practising medicine in Perth. The minutes suggest a medical rumour mill about midwives and other 'irregulars' was circulating incriminating information about this particular birth attendant. The 'information received' indicated that Mrs S not only delivered babies without a physician present, but that she 'gives ether and uses pituitrin' in her regular midwifery practice. The Council instructed the registrar to deal with the matter in the short term by writing a letter threatening prosecution.[34] The Council made no further reference to Mrs S of Perth again, and she seems to have ceased her activity, or at least became more discreet about using drugs in her practice.

Other midwives were more difficult to stop. The same year, the registrar tabled a letter from a midwife Miss C of Bath. Miss C had training as a registered nurse. She explained to the Council that she had practised for some time with her late father, who had been a local country doctor. She was writing to enquire whether there were any legal barriers to her carrying on the obstetric cases for which her father had been engaged before his death. It seems from this correspondence that Miss C felt responsible for her deceased father's patients and felt duty-bound to provide continuity of care and see their cases through to successful parturition. The wording of Miss C's letter, as related by the registrar, indicates that this woman felt quite confident in her ability to step in and fill in for her physician father. Her letter is wondering about legal qualification, not asking for advice on skill or capacity, and it provoked considerable discussion among members of the Medical Council. Although they could do little legally to stop her from freely offering her services, the registrar was instructed to write her and urge her to 'back out gracefully and allow the regular practitioners to earn their livelihood'.[35] How ever they felt about Miss C's capabilities, the Council had a duty to protect the interests of registered physicians.

The Council minutes often depict rural medicine as an intensely competitive environment, but one that also witnessed a good deal of co-operation and collaboration among practitioners. In late 1935, the Council received a complaint from Dr S of Carleton County, who complained of the activities of 'two midwives in his district' and asked for action from the College. Miss C practised out of Bath, so she might have been one of the midwives against whom Dr S spoke. But at the same meeting, a letter sent in from another physician in the area offered a different view. Dr L, also from Bath, explained to the Medical Council that the midwives in his area, and elsewhere in Carleton County, were filling a much-needed health-care need. This sympathetic physician alleged that Dr S 'was influenced exclusively for financial reasons' in opposing their good work. The Council members took no action against the women. But they did write back to the midwives' local supporter. In his letter, Dr L had extolled the skills of one midwife in particular, who could even 'safely use chloroform' in her work delivering babies. The physician, we learn, 'had supplied it to her' for this use. In their response, the Council members made it clear that his 'attitude' was problematic and 'not in the best interests of the Profession'.[36] It does not seem as though this practice stopped. A year later, they had to chastise him a second time for not providing stricter supervision of the midwives' activities and the physician 'was warned not to supply a midwife with chloroform again'.[37]

Elite physicians tried to impose limitations on these informal rural collaborators but, except in the case where physicians supplied midwives with drugs, they relied on local members of the profession to sort out their own affairs. The Council had little tolerance, however, for more independent midwives, especially if they were 'chronic offenders' who regularly stepped outside the legal boundaries of their medical work. In the autumn of 1930, the Medical Council records show that their solicitor, Mr Harrison, actively prosecuted a woman named Ms D, a midwife based in the Nash Creek area. Ms D was arrested, convicted and fined twenty dollars for practising medicine without a licence. Nonetheless, at the next Council meeting a physician from nearby Jacquet River reported to the Council that, once again, 'the lady is active'.[38] The Medical Council took no further action against her. Although elite physicians imposed limitations, their ultimate effectiveness was sometimes limited. Council discussion indicates it was difficult to prove these individuals accepted payment and were actually operating a regular 'practice' in the same way a physician would, such as with the case of Ms D.

Apart from showing patterns of prosecution, these Medical Council minutes suggest considerable service overlap between physician and midwifery care in rural areas of New Brunswick. While some rural physicians wanted to drive midwives out of practice, others helped midwives by supplying them with anaesthesia and other drugs only legally allowed by physician-*accoucheurs*. Recent work by Canadian historians, such as Wendy Mitchinson, has noted the persistence of women midwives in rural areas well into the twentieth century.[39] Miss C's correspondence with the Council reveals how midwifery caseloads could be shared, in this case between a father doctor and a nurse daughter. The New Brunswick Medical Council minutes not only support the revisionist view of recent scholarship on childbirth,[40] but illustrate the many forms this partnership might take, and the technologies that might be shared, in servicing rural communities. For midwives and nurse midwives of the interwar decades, association with and support from a physician colleague seems to have been a critical component of their ability to work at the bedside, however circumscribed. The discourse on 'lay obstetrics' in the Medical Council's minutes indicate very few physicians in the medical elite found lay midwifery an acceptable form of medical practice, but the varied responses of local doctors show individual physicians had many different ideas about what were acceptable forms of medical authority, even in the rural and remote peripheries of the province.

Who is the 'Laity' in Rural Medical Care?

Almost ten years after he tabled his first complaint, Dr B was still complaining about midwives in the Kedgewick area. One reason that might explain why the Council made no effort to control the spread of 'lay obstetrics' in Carleton County, is its regular correspondence with the area priest, who weighed in on the issue of health services in his district. Fr M gave his support to the two local women who were often Dr B's targets. One of the priest's letters included statements from the two midwives outlining their qualifications and training as registered nurses. Priests like Fr M often got involved in rural health matters. Their participation in these discussions illustrated variable definitions of 'good work' and 'good service' held by community members at this time.

When parish priests featured in the Medical Council minutes, they are generally writing in as community advocates and interlocutors. It was especially common for priests from the Acadian communities of the province, whose populations were overwhelmingly Catholic, to act as their representatives before the Council. Priests most often corresponded with the Council asking its assistance in securing a community physician. They would also, on some occasions, complain about individuals they considered to be poor practitioners, or those setting a bad moral example.

Some surveillance supported medical professionalization. Priests monitored the activities of travelling healers in the district, who might take advantage of parish residents. In 1931, for instance, the Council had received another complaint from Fr M, who wrote because he was concerned of 'the professional activities' of an 'Indian' healer. He enclosed a printed notice circulated by this practitioner advertising the services of a 'Dr. Michael'. The minutes do not specify the nature of this practice, but whatever it was, it was unacceptable to the Medical Council. The Council sent a letter warning the itinerant 'of the danger of his position'.[41] At the same time, the registrar requested Fr M keep an eye open for this travelling medicine man, and immediately 'report any further activity of this so-called physician'.[42]

Parish priests were useful in medical policing, providing the Medical Council with a local, community-based authority to regulate rural medical practice. However, there appeared to be limits to the influence and discretion of the Catholic clergy in the medical field. In 1929, it came to the attention of the Medical Council that two priests were practising medicine themselves as part of their pastoral work in the rural Acadian reaches of the province. A letter sent in by a physician reported that one Fr W, 'although a graduate in medicine from some medical school', was practising medicine, even though the priest was obviously 'not legally registered'.[43] The registrar also reported that a Fr R was also attempting to practice medicine in a nearby district in north-eastern New Brunswick, also without any medical qualifications to his name. It is worth noting here that Fr R and Fr W were providing medical services in regions that had the dubious distinction, outlined in previous pages, of the worst physician-population ratios in the province. Although these priests would not be working in direct competition with local medical doctors, since those were in very short supply, their work did not escape censure by the provincial College. These violations were not resolved in the courts, however, but solved by appealing to a parallel authority structure. The Council instructed the registrar to 'write to his Lordship the Bishop of Chatham and call to his attention the activities of these two clergymen'.[44] It is unclear whether this had the desired effect, but after this action was taken, the activities of Fr W and Fr R are not mentioned again in the Council Minutes.

Policing Rural and Remote Physicians

How does the regulation of physicians fit into the monitoring of midwives, itinerant healers and priest-medics? And how do repeated offenders, such as Leger, fit into these emerging practices of professional regulation by central physician elites? Leger's case was not closed where we left it in 1932, with the Medical Council deciding to build and pursue a legal action against him. To this date, he had been caught practising medicine without a licence in three different rural communities in north-eastern New Brunswick. In 1933, when the Council reviewed its progress in its suits against Leger, the results were decidedly mixed. Their solicitor was sorry to report that the case was brought to the Chatham Court in December of 1932, but summarily thrown out. The Council's solicitor recommended in the future 'it would be advisable to have a lawyer from the Chatham district take over the prosecution' and engaged the services of Mr W. H. Davidson to represent the Medical Council. Davidson quickly built a case and it went to trial in Chatham on 21 February. The registrar, Dr S. H. McDonald, took the time to travel to the northern capital of Northumberland County to testify against Leger. This time, the Council won a small victory. The magistrate found Leger guilty and fined him twenty dollars for practising medicine without a licence, as well as the cost of the court and mileage for the witnesses. In default of payment, Leger was sentenced to two months in jail.[45]

The Council's success was short-lived. The doctor's lawyer, Mr George McDade, gave immediate notice of appeal.[46] One year later, Judge J. L. Ryan of the Northumberland County Court set aside the conviction on a technicality (the court stenographer had not been sworn in).[47] Further, Leger's solicitor sent a long letter to the New Brunswick Medical Society, asking them to lobby the Council members to reconsider their position on Leger and make an exception for him in the enforcement of medical licensing. We do not know what rationale Leger 's lawyer put forward, but this correspondence to the Society included a letter from Judge Ryan which, judging from the minutes, praised Dr Leger's community work and supported his position.

The Judge's letter was 'the subject of much discussion' among the Medical Council members present at their spring meeting in 1934. Far from being moved, the members made it clear they found Leger's continued legal contest of their authority unacceptable, and this stiffened their resolve. They sent a complaint about the conduct of Judge Ryan to the federal Minister of Justice in Ottawa and instructed their solicitor to pursue building another case against Leger.[48] The next time a case against Leger was brought to trial, Judge Ryan found against the accused man. However, the Council recounted that 'the Judge reduced the [fine] by $17.15 and no reason was given for this'.[49] The Council was also surprised and chagrined to receive, as part of its expense account from the trial, a charge of $15.50 from the RCMP corporal who served the summons, incurred mileage, served subpoenas and was required to attend court.[50]

The Council would have to wait another year to achieve real success in their case against Alfred Leger, when a third attempt to bring charges against the physician yielded a conviction of practising medicine without a licence. This time, the Judge levied a fifty-dollar fine and the costs of the court. This resulted in a prison term for Dr Leger, because he was unable to pay the fine. But it seemed to result that the costs to the court, once again, would be borne by the Medical Council.

Yet, the Council's efforts to make an example of Leger seemed to solve lingering problems with unlicensed doctors in the province. In 1937, the newly appointed registrar, J. M. Barry from Saint John, noted 'very little trouble with unregistered practitioners'.[51] Dr Barry told the Council that he had reports that Dr Leger, after being released, was 'confined in hospital with an incurable disease'. And so, the registrar happily reported that 'celebrated case in Northumberland County which caused [his predecessor] Dr. McDonald so much worry and the Council so much expense is, I believe, closed'.[52]

From the financial reports tabled in the minutes, the Council seemed to have expended close to $300 in the long, drawn-out process of bringing Leger to trial. Over 1934–5, legal and other fees amounted to $134.75 – the entire legal budget for three years.[53] Leger's prosecution prompted the Medical Council to review its policing practices, shifting the focus of legal attention to the local courts. The Council resolved that in future outside the City of Saint John all cases requiring prosecution would no longer go through their Saint John-based solicitor, Mr Harrison. Instead a special Laws Committee would seek out and assign a local solicitor to monitor the situation of irregular practitioners.[54] The case against Leger also prompted the Council to work more closely with the Attorney General's office and to begin political activity aimed at convincing the provincial government to take over the prosecution of such practitioners. Finally, it determined The New Brunswick Medical Act's clause for the prosecution of dealing with unregistered physicians was 'certainly not drastic enough'. The Council decided to put this problem before the Laws Committee and to step up a lobbying effort in the legislature to strengthen the wording of the Act and the penalties it outlined for this kind of offence.[55]

The Limits of Authority

The Medical Council's case against Leger highlights many limits of the power of the Medical Council in the interwar period and helps to explain their tepid attempts to regulate non-physician practitioners, such as midwives and other 'irregulars'. Even with the support of the Medical Society membership, and the legislated power to prosecute those in breach of licensing and registration regulations, the Medical Society faced at times almost insurmountable local opposition to their efforts to halt the practice of unlicensed healers. By the mid-1930s, the Council tabled serious reservations about policing physicians like Leger.[56] Apart from the expense, Registrar McDonald noted with some irritation, how on the three occasions Leger was brought to court, only once could a conviction be obtained. The Council learned that real cost lay not in the legal fees, but in the public relations fall-out that followed these trials. In Leger's case, the registrar noted with irritation how 'the culprit had the sympathy of the most important people of the County'.[57]

Letters of support had also come in from the local priest, actively involved, as many were, in the local health care. A year after Leger's conviction, he wrote on behalf of the rural Acadian population in the district to ask for the Medical Council's assistance in securing a new physician for the community. Judging from the defensive tone of the minutes, the correspondence seemed to have been couched in critical language meant to highlight the community problems emergent after the Council's prosecution and removal of the community's only doctor. In response to this, the Council made the rather unusual effort to write to Quebec's Université de Montréal and Université Laval asking them to inform their students of two openings for French-speaking practitioners in the province.[58] There is no indication of whether this resulted in a new placement, but whether through local or provincial efforts at recruitment, the community in question had a registered physician working in the area the following year.[59]

Leger's community was not the only one struggling with a problem of physician access. In Gloucester County, two Francophone communities were home to two unregistered physicians who were a 'source of worry' to the Council in the early 1930s. These physicians, like Dr Leger, were 'backed by powerful interests' in their respective communities and enjoyed local popular support. By 1934, however, the two men were gone: one doctor having been 'driven out' and the other required to take the requisite College examinations. Considering these cases in light of the costly conviction of Dr Leger, the registrar, Dr Barry, noted how powerless the Council was. He reminded his colleagues that 'it is well to remember that people in the country districts, if they need a physician, do not care if he is registered or not'.[60] The new registrar was pleased to note the Council's success managing this new situation in Gloucester, but, in both instances, he also noted how 'the Council was the subject of severe criticism'.[61]

The Council was concerned with the image of the provincial medical profession, and it wished to avoid opportunities for public criticism. In the 1920s and 1930s, the Council would occasionally write to admonish, and occasionally censure, physicians who were engaged in activities that were not deemed socially acceptable. The Council also adopted a policy – common among the provinces – of revoking the licence of any physician convicted of criminal activity.[62] However, when a priest wrote in to complain about the 'infamous conduct' of a rural physician, one Dr C, the Council members determined that 'no action be taken ... as it is not a matter [they] dealt with'.[63]

Their inaction is somewhat surprising. Not only was Dr C engaged in an open adulterous relationship, but he had also recently been arrested for driving while intoxicated. According to the report offered by the local clergyman, he was, at the time, serving a thirty-day jail sentence. While such cases were uncommon, there had been occasion in the preceding decade where the Council had stepped in to suspend the licence of physicians who had been convicted of criminal activity. One popular physician in the Fredericton area was denied a medical licence when evidence emerged that he had violated US narcotics legislation, an infraction from earlier in his career when he had held a practice in Portland, Maine.[64] In his case, the Council decided to invoke Section 38 of the New Brunswick Medical Act of 1920 and disallow his registration as a licensed practitioner.[65]

In contrast, the 'infamous conduct' of Dr C did not even result in a letter of censure, even though he was convicted of drunk driving in the province and was languishing in a jail cell. The local priest certainly had little respect for the man. One year before his conviction, Dr C had attacked the reputation of Ms F, a local nurse-midwife, who, he alleged, went about her practice in the district flouting the law and 'laughing at the Medical Profession'.[66] The priest assured the Medical Council, however, that Ms F was in fact a woman of 'good character' who provided 'great assistance nursing the poor'.[67] According to the priest, Dr C only went on calls when he 'felt like it'. This, and his questionable lifestyle, was the real reason Dr C was unable to draw and hold a practice.

The Council responded by sending a letter of warning to Ms F, but they turned a blind eye to Dr C's conduct and criminal activity. There is no record of any correspondence with Dr C, let alone a discussion about revoking his licence, among members of the Medical Council. The explanation for this inconsistent application of Section 38 might be explained by reviewing the recent history of the region where Dr C lived and worked. The community in question had been working hard to secure a local doctor before he arrived. In fact, the community where the 'infamous' Dr C had set out his shingle was the same one where local residents, a county judge and a concerned parish priest had rallied around the stubborn Leger. It would seem that Dr C was Leger's legally licensed and registered replacement.

Conclusion

The Minutes of the Council of the College of Physicians and Surgeons provide important insights into how medical elites policed practitioners in rural and remote areas of New Brunswick, Canada. Investigating rural practitioners' interactions with professional organizations reveals the nature and limits of professional authority in the twentieth-century practice of medicine. There were certainly limits on the 'monopolistic impulse' of physician organizations, and these limits seemed to have an impact on political activities and pursuits as a professional body.[68] The power of local authority, moreover, reinforces the importance of place in the history of rural medicine of the interwar period. Whether local practitioners continued to pose a challenge to the provincial Medical Council in decades to come, is a question for further research. Several scholars have argued that 'regional identities' in Canada were increasingly replaced by provincial identities on the political landscape as the twentieth century unfolded.[69] It may be that the growing importance and power of provincial governments reflects the growing power of the centralized state in local affairs of the twentieth century, including the politics of health care.[70] And provinces would, in turn, increasingly share authority with the Canadian federal government, especially after the advent of federally funded programmes of universal hospital insurance in 1957 and universal health care in 1969. For elite physicians on the Medical Council in New Brunswick, the problem of physician access fell even further into the background as they turned their attention to managing a post-war influx of immigrant and refugee physicians displaced due to the conflict. The Second World War reoriented the activities of the Council from policing medical licensing and registration within the province to the heavy task of managing physician immigration.[71]

Reviewing the Medical Council's attempts to raise and standardize the qualifications for medical practice yields three observations about the 'age of equipoise'. First, we have seen that 'irregular', traditional and 'lay' practitioners populated the rural medical marketplace of New Brunswick well into the end of the Depression era. Although marginalized as a group, some individuals persisted in viable practices, and at least some of these worked in concert and co-operation with small town and rural physicians. Judging from the responses and activities of local physicians in rural and remote areas, there was no unanimous professional opinion as to the appropriate scope of practice or medical authority for midwives, and perhaps other 'irregular' practitioners, during the interwar period. Still, midwives seemed to be common rural health-care providers, so important that their physician collaborators sometimes defended them to the College of Physicians and Surgeons. At least two physicians mentioned here supported the practice of some midwives by supplying them with drugs in service of obstetrical work.

Secondly, it seems that the strength of local authorities – operating at the county and parish level in particular – effectively challenged the Medical Council's professional power throughout the 1920s and 1930s. Geographic distance, but also religious authority and community custom (including local customary enforcement of law) in some areas of the province also played a part in challenging the legislative powers of the provincial College of Physicians and Surgeons. Although some communities, particularly northern Acadian communities, desperately needed health-care services, these communities made do with physicians like Dr C, or threw their support behind unlicensed doctors like Leger. Perhaps the local parish priest offered some medical services on the side that could act as a stopgap for community needs. Assistance would not come from the central medical licensing authority. As Linda Kealey's contribution to this volume indicates, a likely source of help in years to come would be the expanding public-health nursing system, designed for and deployed most successfully in rural nursing outposts.

A third and final conclusion is that rural health care was a critically important part of medical professionalization in New Brunswick. The Medical Council was often stymied in its policing activities because of rural communities' endemic problems accessing physician services. Inequality in the population health between north and south, rural and urban, and French- and English-speaking communities in the province, created spaces for unregulated local medical economies to operate outside the reach of elite urban-based physician organizations. Unable, or unwilling, to address the rural-urban disparity in physician services, the interwar licensing and registration policies and practices of the Medical Council of the New Brunswick College of Physicians and Surgeons weakened efforts at profession-building and consolidation. The disparities of service provision between rural and urban areas of the province ultimately proved to be the College of Physicians and Surgeons' Achilles' heel.

PART III: WOMEN, HEALTH CARE AND THE PRACTICE OF MEDICINE

Introduction

The remote regions of Europe and North America provided an environment in which women were most able to challenge and overcome many of the social and professional restrictions placed upon them. This was as true in nineteenth-century Greenland as it was in twentieth-century Canada or Finland. Mette Rønsager demonstrates that Danish authorities gave midwives tremendous responsibilities not only to bring medical care to the indigenous people of Greenland, but also to train local women to become skilled birth assistants. In this way they were instrumental to bridging the gap between Danish and Green-landic cultures and in so doing were performing many of the same duties as male explorers and bureaucrats who set out to claim and control new lands and people. Nurses in New Brunswick during the middle third of the twentieth century, who are the subject of Linda Kealey's contribution, were engaged in a particularly complex set of negotiations between local populations and the Red Cross, and between social and professional expectations and their own personal goals. The Red Cross was almost entirely responsible for providing nursing care especially in the more isolated parts of the province and relied heavily on public support for its initiatives. The nurses were charged, not only with responding to medi-cal emergencies, but also improving the health of individuals and, by extension, ensuring the health of the nation. Their medical responsibilities often brought them into conflict between the need to act even if this meant challenging the authority of some distant male physician, or waiting until a trained physician arrived even though such hesitation could result in the death of the patient. Moreover, for much of the period studied here, these women were expected to fulfil these various duties while they were still single because social mores expected married women to devote their lives to their family. Megan Davies shifts our attention away from the formally trained nurse or midwife and, using an impressive array of interviews and primary sources, vividly portrays the hardships that untrained practitioners faced when called upon to provide medical care in the remote Peace River Region of British Columbia. These women had to confront a harsh climate, rugged terrain, and a multitude of gruesome injuries. What is even more clear is the innovativeness they brought to their work. As the sole medical provider available they borrowed ideas and practices from lay, folk and academic medicine, and used whatever implements and knowledge available to care for the sick. The final paper in this section, and the collection as a whole, examines the experiences of nurses in northern Finland from approximately 1945–60. In many ways Marianne Junila's contribution addresses many of the themes addressed in this collection. The women who travelled to Lapland and took up positions as public health nurses were certainly bound by a spirit of adventure, a sincere wish to help the unfortunate, and a professional desire to use the relative autonomy they would receive to enhance their skills. They were charged with bringing medical care to an isolated part of the country and a largely unknown and previously ignored segment of the population. The state turned to these women largely because it had difficulty recruiting male physicians willing to work in northern Finland and there is no doubt that nurses were paid considerably less than doctors. However, to see this as a simple case of exploitation suggests that these women were somewhat loathe to work in Lapland and this was not the case. Many of them eagerly embraced the challenge and opportunity that working in such a harsh environment could offer.

9 THE WEST GREENLANDIC MIDWIVES 1820–1920: MEDIATORS BETWEEN THEIR COMPATRIOTS AND DANISH DOCTORS

Mette Rønsager

Introduction: The Colonial Background

Western Greenland was colonized in 1721 by the Norwegian-Danish Lutheran missionary Hans Egede. The eastern and northern parts of Greenland were colonized much later, in 1894 and 1910, and the history of these areas deviated in many respects from the history of the west coast. In this discussion, the focus will be on western Greenland only, in the period 1820–1920.

Following in the footsteps of the mission, the Danish government took over all trade along the west coast of Greenland in 1726. From the very beginning the Danes hoped to create a trade network by granting trading rights in Greenland to private Danish companies. However, Danish merchants did not succeed in establishing a profitable trade in Greenland, so in 1776 the Danish government formed the Royal Greenlandic Trade Company (RGTC). From then until 1912 the RGTC operated both as the colonial administration of Greenland as well as a trading company, and until the end of the Second World War the company maintained a trade monopoly in Greenland. During the eighteenth and early nineteenth centuries RGTC established colonies (i.e., factories) and smaller trading posts along the coast. Until the early twentieth century the company policy of the RGTC was to protect the so-called national and ancestral Greenlandic occupation of seal hunting. The protective policy was successful in spite of the fact that more and more Greenlanders found a source of income as salaried employees of the Danish Lutheran Mission in Greenland or of the RGTC itself. As a part of the trade monopoly Danes strictly controlled every trade good as well as all information entering Greenland and thereby kept Greenland closed off from the rest of the world; even Danish citizens were not allowed to enter the country without permits.[1]

A Danish Health Service in Greenland

The everyday life of the Greenlanders was dangerous. At any given time throughout the nineteenth century the majority of the Greenlandic men were hunters.
Hunting for seal and other game meant exposure to many dangers such as being
outside in all weathers, sailing in ice-filled waters and being close to wounded
animals. The Greenlanders were aware of these risks and knew both how to avoid
them and how to treat a variety of injuries, such as wounds, near death caused
by drowning or hypothermia, broken limbs, frostbite and so on. The Greenlanders also knew how to perform small operations, for instance, on cataracts. With
regards to more serious health problems, the Greenlanders believed that illness
arose from loss of the soul, too much soul or as a consequence of broken taboos.
In order to get well, the cure was either to recreate the balance of the soul or to
find the breaker of the taboo in question. The shaman was the one who restored
the balance and thereby made a person well again.[2]

In the early colonial period the Greenlandic population rarely came into
contact with European doctors. Although doctors occasionally visited the coastline on board merchant ships or whalers, they treated the European patients
only and rarely took care of the Greenlanders. The first European doctor to be
permanently stationed in the northern part of west Greenland arrived in 1793.
In 1839 another doctor was employed in the capital Godthåb (in Greenlandic:
Nuuk), followed by another in Julianehåb (Qaqortoq) in 1851. Both of these
settlements were colonies in the southern part of west Greenland. By 1916 seven
doctors worked along the coast of western Greenland.

The health service was financed and controlled by the RGTC, and the unin-
tended consequence of this arrangement was a downgrading of the importance
of the Greenlanders' state of health. This lack of concern was primarily caused by
the trade company's interest in profit, which made it reluctant to spend money
on health care. This meant that the above-mentioned handful of doctors were to
take care of the well-being of all the Greenlanders as well as the Danish colonial
officials who lived along the coast – a population of approximately 7,500 people
in 1834 (according to the first census) and approximately 15,700 in 1930, all
of whom were scattered over an approximate 2,300-km area riddled with deep
fjords. Although the population was small in number, the coastline and inland
areas were much too extensive for the few doctors to travel and were often hard
to navigate because of ice, snow and hard arctic weather conditions.[3]

In the first two decades of the nineteenth century, the RGTC acknowledged
that it was impossible to cover west Greenland sufficiently with Danish medical
staff, but did not attempt to rectify the situation. There were two important
reasons: First, it would be much too expensive to pay the salaries of all the Danish doctors and Danish midwives the area required. Secondly, a Danish medical

staff would have a hard time communicating with the Greenlanders because of language problems and other difficulties due to cultural barriers. Unlike the Danish Lutheran Mission in Greenland, the RGTC never made the effort to teach their employees how to speak Greenlandic. A majority of the Danish colonial officials learned to understand a bit of Greenlandic but seldom spoke the language themselves, even if they had been living in Greenland for several years. To a certain extent it was therefore necessary for both the Danish officials and the doctors to use Greenlandic interpreters as mediators when they addressed the Greenlandic people in matters of great importance.[4]

The Training of West Greenlandic Midwives

The need for Greenlandic-speaking medical staff and the RGTC's economic concerns were the official reasons why Greenlandic midwives with training in Danish[5] obstetrics were required in the beginning of the nineteenth century. However, there was another reason as well. The Danish surgeon Hans Lerch (1780–1855), who worked in north Greenland at the time, was appalled by the way women gave birth in the so-called traditional Greenlandic way, and he maintained that untrained birth attendants and their cruel methods were literally killing women in confinement and their infants.[6] While it is impossible to verify the truth of Lerch's statement because we lack reliable statistical information on maternal and infant mortality in Greenland in the nineteenth century,[7] we do know how Greenlandic woman gave birth: The normal posture for giving birth was kneeling or lying on one side. Two female birth attendants twined straps of sealskin around the pregnant woman's upper waist and then pulled the straps down her stomach in an effort to help the baby through the birth canal. Dr Lerch explained that if the delivery made slow progress, the procedure was to press a knee or a foot into the stomach of the pregnant woman or in some cases to call for a shaman.[8] This birthing method was regarded as primitive as well as violent by the Danish colonial officials, who considered it most imperative that Greenlandic women were taught the 'civilized' Danish ways of assisting women in labour.[9]

In 1821 the RGTC employed the first Greenlandic midwife-pupils, and from 1820 to 1920 approximately 210 midwives were trained in Greenland by doctors as well as by other Greenlandic midwives.[10] Like other women, these midwife-pupils were familiar with the so-called traditional Greenlandic ways of birth, which had been handed down from generation to generation and were deeply rooted in the believed close connexion between human beings and the surrounding natural and supernatural world. The doctors, however, discarded this knowledge entirely and trained their students in Danish technical obstetrics without any reference to the Greenlandic customs. Pupils were told over and over again not to use the old Greenlandic ways.[11]

As a part of a larger plan to improve the state of health among the Green-landers in general, the RGTC decided in 1835 to send Greenlandic midwives to the School of Midwifery at the Laying-in-Hospital (Den kongelige Fødsels- og Plejestiftelse) in Copenhagen for further training.[12] At the Laying-in-Hospital the length of the education of a Danish midwife varied over time and depended on different factors, for instance, on who was financing the education. Despite the discrepancies, it can be said that until 1843 the education of midwives took approximately half a year. In the period from 1843 to 1895 it was approximately nine months and in the period from 1895 to 1927 approximately one year. Many Greenlandic midwives stayed in Denmark for more than four years, however, often owing to difficulties arising from cultural and linguistic barriers and/or ill-ness. In the late nineteenth and early twentieth centuries the women's education often included a stay in a private Danish home in order to learn housekeeping and hygiene as well as informal nursing training in a Danish hospital.[13]

The midwife-pupils who were trained in Denmark came from the upper stra-tum of Greenlandic society. Most of them were of mixed descent and, therefore, spoke the local language fluently as well as some Danish which was needed in order to attend lectures in Copenhagen. These midwives were the first Green-landic women to be educated in Denmark, and they were indeed pioneers among their compatriots, as their numbers attest: in the century between 1820 and 1920 only thirty-three west Greenlandic women succeeded in obtaining their certificates from the Laying-in-Hospital.[14]

Remote Medicine in West Greenland

Only four Danish midwives worked in west Greenland in the period between 1820 and 1920, and they were present only because their husbands were serving as colonial officials in the area. Since the RGTC had no intention of employing Danish midwives in Greenland other than these women, the Greenlandic mid-wives became the backbone of the Danish health service in Greenland during the period in question. In most places the Danish health service was synonymous with the Greenlandic midwives. These women were able to reach the indigenous population in a way that the Danes were never able to achieve. They worked not only as midwives, but also as nurses and doctors.

Outside the colonies, the midwives worked alone in their midwifery districts as there was no doctor for many miles around. If they needed a doctor's advice in matters of life or death, they typically hired a 'kayak-man' (*kajakmand*), i.e., a local Greenlander who conveyed messages and/or medicine between doctor and midwife via kayak. In stormy, snowy weather or if the ice conditions were bad, this solution was not an option, and the midwife had to cope on her own.

In most settlements, in the absence of a doctor, a missionary or a merchant was the midwife's nearest superior, but these Danish colonial officials often lacked formal medical training and were not of much assistance. In some periods during the nineteenth century the missionaries took a very short medical course before leaving Denmark, but the merchants had no such training. Many missionaries and merchants did not know what to do; when they went on sick calls, they had to rely solely on the medical books that were at hand in every colony and trading post. The diary of the Lutheran missionary, Carl Emil Janssen (1813–84), who worked in Holsteinsborg (Sisimiut) and Godthåb (Nuuk) from 1844–9, reveals his occasional feelings of helplessness and incompetence. When Janssen had to attend a sick person, his comments on the visit were often despairing: 'Oh, I am a poor wretch; I did not know what to do at all!' He neither knew what was the matter with his patients nor how to treat them. For instance, he recorded that he often gave the small Greenlandic children a lot of molasses on gruel largely because they loved the sweet taste. Most often when a remedy was needed he simply looked at the contents of the medicine bottles and blindly chose the one that was almost full. After that, he went home and prayed for his patient's recovery.[15]

Beyond lack of training, the doctors in Greenland expressed other kinds of frustration in their annual reports to the Royal Greenlandic Trade Company and The Royal Board of Health in Copenhagen. They complained of never having enough medicine or utensils, of the few hospitals in Greenland being too small, too dirty and too outdated, and of a work-load that was too demanding.[16] Once a year they were to travel around their districts, but the districts were far too large, and often the doctors gave up before even starting and stayed at home in desperation. Furthermore, the doctors did not have their own means of transportation and had to borrow an *umiaq* (a five- to six-metre-long boat made of seal-skin) from the RGTC every time they went on sick calls. In the summertime, when the ice had broken up in the southern part of west Greenland, however, the *umiat* (pl.) were usually in use by the staff of the RGTC and unavailable to the doctors. In the north of Greenland the doctors had to travel by dog-sledges during the greater part of the year (from October to May), and the travelling was very hard. The result of these obstacles was that doctors spent most of their time in the colonies where they lived, and the sick Greenlanders had to come to them if they wanted assistance. Most of the doctors expressed powerlessness in the face of the poor health of the population. No matter how hard they worked and tried to make a difference for the well-being of the people in their districts, they felt it was never was enough.[17]

That the doctors could not possibly manage their duties without the help of the Greenlandic midwives was a fact emphasised by the doctors time and time again in their letters and reports to the RGTC. Without the midwives it would make no sense to talk about a Danish health service in west Greenland because these women covered many of the settlements that the doctors never visited. Because of the trade company's wish to bring Danish obstetrics and medicine to the Greenlanders, the RGTC decided in 1903 to employ a midwife in every settlement that had at least eighty inhabitants. The need for a high number of midwives was created by the mentioned problems of weather conditions, bad infrastructure, few doctors and bad health among the native population, as well as the fear within the RGTC that the Greenlanders wanted to use untrained birth attendants. However, the reality was that the RGTC did not want to spend the money required to employ the needed number of midwives: in 1904 the ratio was one midwife per 161 inhabitants and in 1921 one per 70 *women*.[18]

It was up to the doctors in Greenland to decide where the midwives were to be employed, and therefore the midwives often moved several times during their employment. As a general rule the midwives educated in Denmark worked in the colonies, whereas the midwives trained in Greenland were stationed in the smaller trading posts. Thus, ironically, the midwives who had the best training stayed near the doctors, where there was less need for them, and the midwives with a more rudimentary Greenlandic training often had to make do on their own without any supervisors.

But how did these two types of midwives do? Most of the time they worked as nurses or doctors tending to their sick compatriots. Usually, they had their own utensils, along with a medicine chest, which was sent to them from Denmark. Yet, it has to be stressed again that the midwives who worked in the colonies had the best conditions: their equipment was often brought with them from Denmark when they finished their training at the Laying-In-Hospital. In contrast, the midwives in the smaller settlements sometimes did not always own even a pair of scissors. In many cases these midwives relied on Greenlandic products to cure their patients, such as plants, blubber, thread made of tendon and so on.

Only a small part of the work of the midwives was actual midwifery because every year there was only a few births in the midwifery districts. Around 1900 about five to six infants were born per midwife per year – and some of the mothers even chose to give birth assisted by an untrained birth attendant instead of the trained midwife.[19] When a midwife was called to a delivery in a remote part of her midwifery district, the doctors reported that it often took several weeks before she returned. According to Dr Andersen (1878–1953) writing in 1915, the Greenlanders did not care about time and they never knew when a birth was due. So they often sent for the midwife much too early – just in case! Furthermore, depending on the time of the year, the weather often turned bad, and the midwife had to stay in the household of the woman in confinement for days on end.[20]

Between their Compatriots and Danish Doctors

The Danish colonial policy in Greenland is often described as 'a policy of protection' (*beskyttelsespolitik*), but this policy was in many respects an ambiguous and contradictory project. On the one hand, the colonial administration tried to preserve the Greenlandic hunting culture and protect it from the outside world. On the other hand, it also tried to westernize and modernize the indigenous population. This protection strategy was based upon a romantic and idealized perception of the seal-hunting population, but also upon the urge to civilize and cultivate the Greenlanders, who in many respects were regarded as primitive and childlike by the Danish politicians as well as the colonial administration.

A few of the midwives' practical obstetric and medical functions have been described above but just as crucial was their role as go-betweens in the colonial process. The Danish colonial officials in Greenland needed Greenlanders 'who stood in between' the Danish and the Greenlandic cultures to act as cultural translators and mediators. They fulfilled their roles as interpreters of the two languages but they did much more by interpreting the cultures. They provided the Danish officials with an insight into the minds of the Greenlanders, and they contributed toward bringing so-called civilization to the Greenlandic population. The policy of protection intended Greenlandic mediators to make other Greenlanders live according to Danish customs but only to a certain degree because the Greenlandic seal-hunting culture and customs had to be respected.[21] For the midwives the balance was to introduce Danish midwifery and medicine at a pace the population would accept, and this job was not always easy.

At the turn of the century 1,800 young Greenlandic men and women received western training in Denmark and in Greenland that provided them with the ability to mediate between cultures and to enlighten their compatriots by teaching them civilized ways. In the smaller settlements Greenlandic catechists taught their fellowmen Christianity and literacy. In the colonies craftsmen taught Danish crafts to other Greenlanders who then became the founders of a Greenlandic groups of artisans. During the nineteenth century this educated segment of the indigenous population, unlike the hunters, made money through full-time employment in the RGTC or in the Danish Lutheran Mission. They formed an upper Greenlandic social stratum with a high degree of social endogamy and shared habitude.[22]

Like other Greenlanders with western educations, the midwives played an important part in 'civilizing' and modernizing the Greenlandic population.

The Greenlandic midwives trained in Denmark were particularly appreciated by the doctors in Greenland for their skills as communicators of Danish values and virtues. These midwives had experienced with their own eyes and ears how Danish society worked, and they were believed to know how a cultured and well-educated woman was to behave. Most of the midwives who had been in Copenhagen were of mixed descent,[23] and they were hand-picked by the Danish doctors in Greenland to go to Denmark because of their knowledge of Danish language and culture. Some of them were used to Danish ways of living through their upbringing. Others knew of them through marriage with Danish colonial officials or with men also of mixed descent. The doctors believed that when these midwives of mixed descent were educated in Copenhagen they would be more clever and far-sighted than other midwives. In their work as well as at home, the midwives had to be aware of their status as *the* well-educated Greenlandic women, and the Danish officials expected them to set good examples for their compatriots to follow. They were told to remember that everyone's eyes were fixed upon them at any given time. In many respects the RGTC tried to put these midwives up on a pedestal: They had a higher salary than other midwives and often lived more luxuriously than their fellow-countrymen, in the sense that they had better houses and had a better access to Danish food and commodities than most other Greenlanders.[24]

The midwives' role as mediators or, in the term of anthropologist Robert Paine, 'middlemen',[25] between Danes and Greenlanders was seen in their everyday work and in everything they did. First and foremost, the midwives were interpreters of biomedicine who had to convince the Greenlanders to give up the old traditions relating to birth and medicine and choose the new Danish practices and ideas. Especially with the rise of bacteriology in Greenland in the 1880s, and with doctors' needs to disseminate the principles of good hygiene among Greenlanders, this job as 'middleman' became clear.

The midwives had to adapt their learning to the reality of their everyday work. The big gap between the Danish obstetrics and the traditional Greenlandic ways put the midwives between the Greenlandic population and the Danish colonial officials in other ways as well. The two groups put different demands on, and had different expectations of the midwives, who had to do their best to please them both. In the late nineteenth century conflicts arose time and time again particularly among the older-generation Greenlandic women who resisted the midwives' mandate to introduce good hygiene into maternity work. When, for instance, the midwife asked for water in order to wash her hands, the old women present might deny the midwife her request or give her 'a small cup filled with dirty water'. When stories like this reached the doctors, the midwives were accused of being untidy, neglecting their duties and, not least of all, of forgetting to observe the Midwifery Acts.[26] Furthermore, the doctors wondered if the midwives had forgotten everything that they have learned as midwife-pupils.[27]

Another example of the midwives' roles as middlemen and 'agents of civilization' is the Danish colonial officials' wish to teach Greenlandic women how to behave as civilized and cultured Danish housewives and loving mothers. The midwives knew about western hygiene, childcare, the importance of good nutrition and other important Danish virtues, which by the Danes in the late nineteenth and early twentieth centuries were considered necessary in order to maintain a stable home and happy family. The midwives were told by the doctors to keep their homes clean – inside as well as outside – and, just as importantly, to always welcome other Greenlandic women as their guests so that these women could see and learn how a proper home was to be kept. It also went without saying that the midwife should always think of her personal hygiene. As a role model she was to wash herself often and make sure her clothes were always clean and neat.[28]

The midwives were to be regarded by the Greenlanders as persons of authority, but the midwives sometimes chose not to adopt this status. Instead they adapted their image according to context. Despite the fact that some of them belonged to the Greenlandic elite and had some influence over their compatriots, they also wanted to take part in everyday life just like other women in their local communities. Just like these women they were often mothers, sisters, aunts and wives, and they had different obligations connected to these social roles as well. Some midwives still had to take care of their husbands' catch of seals and other animals, while others were married to wage-earners and often had little to do with hunting. Whatever their personal circumstances, the midwives were still different than other women in the settlements. They had a full-time profession, and they could not take part in long hunting trips like many other women did. Unlike any other Greenlandic woman, the midwives had to work twenty-four hours a day, seven days a week, and had a regular income.[29]

Whether the midwives themselves felt different from other women or not is hard to say. We know of no private or professional diaries kept by midwives. Furthermore, the Greenlandic midwives were obliged to send in reports to the doctors for only very short trial periods otherwise their work was only a local phenomenon, so it is all but impossible to hear 'the voices of the midwives'. In research based on diaries written by other members of the Greenlandic elite during the period in question, namely the catechists employed in the Danish Lutheran Mission in Greenland, literary historian Søren Thuesen shows how the feeling of having a calling to do their job sometimes made the well-educated male Greenlanders lonely. The catechists saw their vocation as a personal, Christian calling, as well as a calling to serve their nation and their fellow countrymen. All of this meant that the members of the Greenlandic

elite felt the obligation to reprimand their compatriots, and it was this duty
in particular that made them feel different, even from their own families and
friends.[30]

Another matter that only reinforced the loneliness, isolation and feeling of
being different among the catechists was a poor ability to hunt. In the smaller
settlements where the rest of the male population was hunters, the catechist was
often the lone member of the Greenlandic elite. In the latter nineteenth century
the majority of the Greenlandic male elite were wage-earners, and they did not
always teach their sons how to go kayaking or how to hunt. Furthermore, young
men working full-time as wage-earners would find it difficult to find the time to
become skilled hunters. This meant that catechists did not act as the majority of
Greenlanders did in the nineteenth century – but, then again, their Danish education did not necessarily make them feel that they belonged to the sphere of the
Danish colonial officials. According to Thuesen, some catechists who stood 'in
between' cultures were able to describe both Danish and Greenlandic cultures
with almost ethnographical accuracy. This was especially the case for the head
catechists.[31]

I have reason to believe that the same feeling of living a life secluded from
the sphere of their own gender can especially be applied to the situation of the
Greenlandic midwives in the smaller settlements. This suspicion is based on the
actions of the midwives and not on their words. Cases in point include midwives who left their midwife districts to go hunting with their families for several
weeks without the doctor's permission. Instances such as these might likely indicate a strong wish not to be left behind alone, but also the desire to do what any
other wife of a hunter did – follow her husband.[32]

The feeling of being different must have been emphasized by the fact that
the midwife often came as a stranger to a community, and the inhabitants did
not see a need for her advice in medical matters – they already knew how to
cope with illness and they also knew what to do during childbirth. It seems as
though the midwives in the colonies may have had more success in convincing
the Greenlanders to use the Danish ways of obstetrics and medicine than the
midwives in the smaller settlements had. Greenlanders lived in the colonies and
therefore the Danish way of living was well known to most of the inhabitants
there. It was not until the beginning of the twentieth century that the midwifery
service was increasingly acknowledged by *almost* all Greenlanders regardless of
where they lived.

With the above-mentioned problems in mind it is difficult to understand
what made the young Greenlandic women of the nineteenth century want to
become midwives. Some, as previously mentioned, were hand-picked by colonial
officials to undergo a Danish education; but these women who were to become
midwives were asked if they wanted to go. In many cases they wanted to learn

those skills because they wanted to learn Danish ways and to serve their people. Nonetheless, in the period from 1820–1920 I do not know of any Greenlandic woman who applied on her own accord for an apprenticeship. Just like in the case of the catechists, the feeling of having a calling and making a difference for their compatriots seems to have played an important role in the decision to take on the task of being a pioneer and undergo an education. This was true even if it meant that some women had to travel to another country for a couple of years or more. For these women it was a matter of the heart to bring Danish, 'civilized' manners to other Greenlanders. In other cases the education of these young girls was the result of the will of their fathers whom the girls dared not contradict. Finally, some women became midwives because their husbands asked the RGTC to finance their wives' education.[33]

In conclusion, it remains to be said that during the period 1820–1920 untrained Greenlandic birth attendants helped a fairly great proportion of women in confinement. As late as in 1914 one out of four births in the southern part of west Greenland was assisted by an untrained Greenlandic woman. In some cases this was because the Danish-trained midwives lived too far away, but in other cases it was because the woman giving birth wanted an old woman or female family members who knew the old, local ways to assist her.[34]

To summarize, the Greenlandic midwives played an important role as 'agents of civilization' and 'mediators'. The midwives were to civilize and cultivate the Greenlanders and make them live according to Danish customs. Midwives undoubtedly played an important role in the Danish civilizing project of the Greenlandic population. They were able to go where the Danish male officials could not and brought Danish customs to other female Greenlanders who conveyed it to the men, their families and to the new generations growing up. However, the civilizing process occurred only slowly and in different ways according to location, connection to Greenlandic-Danish cultures, descent and gender. The midwives' connections to both cultures were essential for the spread of Danish midwifery and medicine, and more than any of the Danish officials these women knew when and how to introduce new knowledge to the Greenlanders. If the efficiency of the midwives' role as civilizing agents is to be evaluated, it has to be considered that time worked in their favour. Over the period in question, more and more Greenlanders were receiving Danish education or coming into contact with Danish culture through trade and missionary activity. As a result Greenlanders became more likely to embrace the knowledge that midwives possessed. That said, the Greenlandic midwives as a group were committed agents of civilization despite the conflicts that arose because of their desire and dedication to help their compatriots live better lives and to see their children grow up to be healthy adults.

The west Greenlandic midwifery service was the backbone of the Greenlandic health services, and the midwives were crucial go-betweens in the colonial process. The midwives translated and introduced the Danish way of thinking among the Greenlandic population. Midwives trained in Denmark and midwives of mixed descent were particularly appreciated by doctors in Greenland for their skills as communicators. This was especially seen in the era that witnessed the rise of bacteriology and the doctors' need to disseminate the principles of good hygiene among Greenlanders. Danish officials' wish to teach Greenlandic women how to behave as 'civilized' housewives is another example of the midwives' roles as agents of civilization. The midwives were regarded as people of authority but despite the fact that most of them belonged to the Greenlandic elite and had some influence, they expected to take part in everyday life as did other women in their local communities. While this gave rise to some conflicts, by the beginning of the twentieth century the midwifery service was becoming better integrated into Greenlandic society and the work of the midwives increasingly acknowledged by Greenlanders.

10 DELIVERING HEALTH CARE IN RURAL NEW BRUNSWICK: OUTPOST NURSING IN THE TWENTIETH CENTURY

Linda Kealey

Remote and rural health-care issues have been a part of Canada's health-care challenge throughout its history. A number of voluntary groups, including the National Council of Women of Canada (NCWC), developed schemes and programmes from the late nineteenth century onwards to deal with the scarcity of health care on the prairies, in the north and in rural parts of the more settled provinces. Women's groups like the NCWC understood the great need for assistance to women who lacked access to midwives, nurses and doctors during childbirth and thus supported the creation of groups such as the Victorian Order of Nurses (VON). Similarly, in Newfoundland (which would become part of Canada in 1949), Lady Harris, wife of the Governor, brought trained midwives to the island in 1921 to serve outport and rural women and their families. The Grenfell Mission in northern Newfoundland and coastal Labrador also provided health-care services to fishermen and their families; through its office in London, England, the Mission sought nurses trained in midwifery to assist women in childbirth. Such voluntary efforts provided key assistance at a time when publicly supported health care was non-existent or minimal.[1] Of particular note is the role played by women as nurses and midwives in sustaining rural health care through both paid and volunteer labour.

As other articles in this collection underline, women's participation in health care was central in northern, rural and remote areas generally. While Megan J. Davies's research on British Columbia's Peace River region, 1920–40, emphasizes the centrality of 'mother's medicine' in the creation of female identity and in constructing a white, settler society, Marianne Junila's article on district nurses in post-Second World War Finland concentrates on the paid work of professionals serving in Lapland. These 'sisters on skis' serving in remote communities often responded positively to the notion of 'uplifting' poor Laplanders as well as the professional and independent work available. Similarly, Mette Rønsager's research on midwives in western Greenland from 1820–1920, positions the better educated and acculturated midwives who often were of mixed Danish and Greenlandic backgrounds, as 'go-betweens' or 'cultural translators' in the colonial relationship. These midwives were sometimes trained in Copenhagen and their cultural, language and medical skills were useful to Danish officials who contrasted these women's more 'modern' training with those of untrained, 'traditional' midwives who also provided nursing and medical care in these remote parts of Greenland. Thus, these examples suggest that it is crucial to understand the various ways in which women provided health care to remote areas whether as mothers, volunteers, traditional midwives or as professional nurses, midwives and doctors.

The First World War drew attention to the poor health of military recruits and by extension, to the wider population. The war brought home the great losses sustained not only on the battlefield but also from poor hygiene and preventable diseases, conditions that alarmed the emerging public health movement of the early twentieth century. In the aftermath of the war, conditions for rural health were also examined more closely. One of the most influential voluntary organizations in Canada, the Canadian Red Cross Society (CRCS), developed a peacetime plan to provide support in every province for rural health care through outpost hospitals and outpost nursing. By 1929 the CRCS had established a National Outpost Committee to advise each Provincial Division of the Red Cross. The only study of Red Cross outposts in New Brunswick, a largely rural and resource-dependent province of eastern Canada, reports that in 1929 there were a dozen facilities in four provinces: Ontario, Alberta, Manitoba and Saskatchewan.[2] Missing from this account are two small, short-lived outpost hospitals in north-western New Brunswick founded in the late 1920s and allegedly closed during the early years of the Depression. This lacuna suggests that much more research needs to be done on rural health care in New Brunswick and in particular on the important role played by outpost nursing.

This paper presents a preliminary examination of the role of Red Cross outpost nurses in New Brunswick based almost entirely on official sources, such as annual reports, Red Cross publications and files, health journals and a limited number of reminiscences. This paper argues that the CRCS and its nurses were integral to the delivery of health care in rural New Brunswick from the 1920s well into the second half of the century. A weak provincial government infrastructure depended extensively on the Red Cross to deliver rural health care. Early supporters called on patriotism and the debt owed to the men who fought in the First World War as a means of garnering donations and volunteers. In fact, the Red Cross provided monetary support for the first public health nurses in New Brunswick, thus contributing to the development of provincial health infrastructure and support for local communities. Outpost nurses working in small hospitals and nursing stations were the backbone of the system developed by the Red Cross. Although the provincial government subsidized the outpost hospitals until the late 1950s and the nursing stations into the 1970s, their contributions were relatively small until the 1960s. Thus the CRCS still played a major role in service delivery well into the 1970s.[3]

Secondly, while much remains to be discovered about New Brunswick nurses' individual experiences, those stories that have been preserved suggest that these nurses had more autonomy and more responsibility than urban hospital nurses who were more closely supervised by head nurses and doctors.[4] As Jayne Elliott's recent work on Ontario suggests, however, that autonomy was tempered by a complex set of relationships with physicians, supervisors and the community.[5] In New Brunswick's case, the official sources do not permit extensive comment on these relationships although some hints remain. Professional roles were both expanded and constrained; nurses found themselves practising beyond their training in difficult circumstances while at the same time subject to the social constraints of small communities. By and large, however, the official sources present positive statements of achievements rather than detailed commentary on problems or conflict. Thus, this paper draws attention to the opportunities and constraints faced by outpost nurses.

Thirdly, the paper follows in more detail the careers of several outpost nurses who rose through the ranks to higher administrative positions in nursing. Not surprisingly these women conformed to social expectations that careers were the purview of single women who trod a different but related path than their nineteenth-century middle- and upper-middle-class foremothers. While the latter created voluntary roles for women within a maternal welfare framework, Red Cross nurses in the post-First World War period performed nursing work for pay, though they too often shared middle-class views and aspirations as a result of their professional training.

One last point to note here is that the first half of the paper provides the context for the second. Using the extant literature and various primary sources, the paper outlines the development and decline of outpost hospitals and nursing stations in New Brunswick from the 1920s to the 1970s. The second part turns to the nurses themselves with emphasis on those who have left us with some evidence of their experiences.

Outpost Nursing: The Context

Outpost nursing has been most thoroughly studied in Ontario, which had the largest number of outpost facilities in Canada. In 1940, Ontario reached its peak of thirty-one outpost facilities with approximately 400 beds, half in small hospitals and half in nursing stations.[6] Other authors, often nurses themselves, have also reflected on outpost nursing. Muriel I. Schonberg, writing on behalf of the Committee on Public Health Nursing of the Canadian Nurses Association, began a 1947 article with this statement:

> Outpost nursing of the future will be a far cry from the grim epic of little log shacks and heroic nurses confronted with desperate emergencies and overwhelming situations ... in reality any community twenty-five miles from a medical centre, hospital or doctor is a medically unsupervised area.[7]

Her article presented an unromantic picture of the difficult task before the outpost nurse, whose duties encompassed non-nursing tasks such as writing letters, baptizing infants and conducting funeral services. Medically speaking, there were many problems stemming from poor hygiene, superstitions and local customs; Schonberg suggested that it would take about two years to instil good health practices and habits so that the outpost nurse should have to deal primarily with surgical emergencies and accidents, in addition to caring for child-bearing women and the illnesses of old age. 'Teaching by demonstration, precept and example', outpost nurses needed to embrace the idea that they were responsible for the health of the community, not just emergencies and illnesses. 'Nothing should be too trivial for the nurse, for if the people feel free to come to her for small things, she will certainly be able to influence them in matters directly pertaining to their health and welfare', Schonberg wrote.[8] In closing, the author appealed to Canadian nurses to become well prepared for outpost nursing so that they could assist in the task of nation building.[9] That task included educating the primitive and 'backward' in rural areas to middle-class standards of health.

Writing twenty years later, Ruth May, the newly appointed lecturer in outpost nursing at Dalhousie University in Halifax, Nova Scotia, accepted the fact that outpost nurses would provide services normally rendered by doctors. Furthermore she pointed out that a large number of outpost nurses were either foreign-born or foreign-educated because, unlike in Canada, schools in the United Kingdom provided midwifery training. Hence the new programme at Dalhousie would provide the necessary training for Canadians through a two-year course. The second year involved an internship, six months of which would be spent in St Anthony, Newfoundland, at the International Grenfell Association mission hospital training in midwifery. In Newfoundland and Labrador, where May had served for eight years as nurse-in-charge of the Mary's Harbour nursing station, there was plenty of experience in what was called 'outport' nursing. The Grenfell Mission, established in the 1890s, relied on small hospitals and nursing stations much like the outpost hospitals and nursing stations in Canada.[10]

Thus, historical narratives about outpost nursing tend to emphasize experiences in the north, on the western Prairie Provinces or in Ontario where the largest number of outpost facilities existed. But what about the experience in New Brunswick where a provincial Red Cross organization emerged in 1915 and the first outpost hospital was established in St Leonard, in a Francophone area along the Maine border, in November 1926? The only study of outpost nursing in the province, published by the Red Cross, designates 1941 as the date of the first outpost facility located on Grand Manan Island. While the bulk of outpost work was indeed a focus of the post-Second World War era, public health work including two outpost hospitals at St Leonard and Clair started in the post-First World War period, partly in response to the needs of returned soldiers and their families. Perhaps more significantly, the first issue of the *Canadian Red Cross* noted that the Society had given financial help to the New Brunswick Department of Health to assist five public health nurses to graduate. These nurses were placed in rural areas and small towns by the Director of Public Health Nursing, Harriet Meiklejohn, and averaged 125 home visits per month. These demonstrations of public health nursing were intended to persuade municipalities to support such a service. Infant mortality was one of the key concerns since New Brunswick had the highest rate in Canada in 1920 (134.9 per 1,000 births).[11] In September 1923 the Provincial Minister of Health, Dr William H. Roberts, acknowledged his great appreciation of the work of the Red Cross in putting into effect provincial legislation for which there were no funds. The New Brunswick Division of the Red Cross provided the initial $20,000 to set up a public health nursing service which, the Minister acknowledged, could reach more people than the government.[12] A year later the journal reported public health nurses in twenty-three communities in New Brunswick. Thus it is clear that the public sector was in its infancy in terms of health care and that the government relied on significant support from the voluntary sector, a situation that persisted well into the twentieth century.

Campbellton in the northern part of the province was one of the first towns to embrace public health nursing in winter 1922, and it illustrates the reliance of government on the voluntary sector. Interested citizens as well as the local Red Cross Society worked together to support a public health nurse with the town contributing $1,000 in 1923 to further the work. As explained in the Red Cross publication, *Despatch,* the nurse 'receiv[ed] her instructions from Miss Meiklejohn of the Health Centre at St John, N. B'. The nurse's work concentrated on school work, child welfare work, and pre-natal and maternity work. As the article noted, the public health nurse is 'constantly preaching the gospel of health'. Work among children included a well baby clinic, free milk for school children and school inspections.[13] By 1925 the Red Cross money had run out but a number of communities had benefited from a public health nurse for at least part of the year.[14] The Annual Report of the New Brunswick Division for 1924 reported financing the salaries in whole or part for twenty-seven public health nurses while the infant mortality rate had dropped from 134.9 to 103.2 'and we believe it is now even less'. The annual report for 1927 bemoaned the fact that the 'Red Cross does not get the credit which is its due, for the establishment and maintenance of those who are known as Public Health nurses in various parts of the Province'. This same report noted that the Red Cross had granted the Department of Health $60,000 in total to be spent on this work.[15] Clearly the CRCS provided the much needed infrastructure for public health in New Brunswick. By contrast, in these early years the province paid Red Cross nurses a mere $100 per annum to examine school children. As historian Sharon Myers demonstrates the provincial government 'would not put its money where its mouth was; as elsewhere, given limited resources and material inequality, a more conservative education campaign took the place of material reorganization and fundamental social change'.[16]

St Leonard (on the border with the State of Maine) was the first New Brunswick community to feature an outpost hospital. Sibella Barrington, the Red Cross's Dominion Organizer for Home Nursing, was instrumental in establishing this outpost hospital in 1926, along with one at Clair, bordering on Quebec. Reporting on St Leonard, she announced that the trial period had been a success and that all costs had been borne by the Home Nursing Grant given by the Central Council of the CRCS, not by the Provincial Division. Appealing to the central body's sense of Christian charity and patriotism, Barrington praised the work of francophone registered nurse Olida Daigle and commented that 'Red Cross work is God's work'. She urged the province to support more outpost hospitals, more home nursing classes and more Red Cross workers, noting that 'Outpost hospitals caring for children ... are part of the ideals those men died for', referring to the soldiers of the First World War.[17] The five-bed hospital established above Dr A. B. Violette's shop in St Leonard soon proved its worth during a typhoid epidemic in 1927; that same year the hospital moved to larger quarters featuring an operating room and a dozen beds. A second facility was noted in Clair in 1928 when both hospitals were reported as self-sustaining.[18] Three years later, however, both had closed for lack of funds, according to the annual report.[19]

Not until 1941 did another outpost hospital emerge in New Brunswick. During the Depression, financial support for outpost hospitals and nursing stations was difficult to come by in the province though requests were made to the Red Cross for more of these facilities. Canada-wide, however, there were sixty-four outpost facilities in 1935,[20] up from forty-eight reported in 1931. Despite major threats of typhoid, whooping cough, scarlet fever, diphtheria and epidemics of measles (1934–6) and polio (1937–8), all of them particular threats to

New Brunswick children, it was difficult for the Province to take charge, with few exceptions. The 1940s also saw repeated outbreaks of polio and diphtheria while tuberculosis was a major cause of death among the young. Thus, the appearance of a new hospital must have been welcome. Grand Manan's outpost hospital opened its doors in October 1941, in co-operation with the locally established Hospital Board for a term of one year; the Red Cross provided the operating funds and the arrangement was so successful that the agreement was renewed. In the meantime the Board worked at reducing the debt and persuading more residents to subscribe to the hospital scheme.[21]

The successes at Grand Manan convinced the provincial office of the Red Cross to expand its hospital work. Between 1941 and 1959, the Red Cross operated six small hospitals.[22] Because of a shortage of nurses, the first matrons often were the only professionally trained staff on duty; they relied on Red Cross volunteers to cook, clean and do laundry as well as sew curtains and linens and fundraise for the hospital. Local Red Cross groups also subsidized the cost of X-rays and several branches supplied milk and cod liver oil to schools; a few gave relief to the poor. According to the 1942 annual report, nursing received a shot in the arm as more and more women joined the Emergency Nursing Reserve to learn first aid while volunteers with more intensive training worked in hospitals.[23]

Community support and co-operation were key to the establishment of these hospitals because the Red Cross required significant community participation before a hospital opened. Administration was shared between the provincial Red Cross officials and local supporters. The Red Cross supplied the operating costs and the staff while the community had to find a suitable building and equip it to the society's standards. The local area was also responsible for forming a Red Cross branch and a hospital board. In general the local group had to raise funds and provide volunteers where needed. Each hospital needed a minimum of ten beds, and separate areas for delivery, operating and nursery. Elective surgery was limited to the removal of tonsils and adenoids, though emergency surgery depended on circumstances and the decision of the physician. By 1951, the Grand Manan hospital became independent of the Red Cross though the latter continued to donate supplies. The island's Hospital Auxiliary helped to maintain the hospital, and in 1970 a new facility opened to house the patients since the original building had been condemned.[24]

Nurses in these hospitals worked long hours until 1950 when the Red Cross, facing recruiting problems, mandated six eight-hour days with a month's holidays for $100 per month ($150 for matrons), plus room and board. The annual report noted that a substantial increase 'was necessary to prevent a complete breakdown of the whole program on account of shortage of staff and over-fatigue'. Subsequently, staff turnover was reportedly reduced, and by 1964 the Red Cross's Nursing Committee recommended that nurses' salaries conform to the level recommended by the New Brunswick Association of Registered Nurses.[25]

Due to legislative changes in health care in the late 1950s, the government began to assume some responsibility for medical facilities and the outpost hospitals ceased to be run by the Red Cross in New Brunswick and in most other provinces, except Ontario. As a result, nursing stations in New Brunswick became more important in providing residents with medical help in isolated areas.[26] In 1956, Dr J. P. McInerney, chair of the Outpost Hospitals and Nursing Stations Standing Committee, had expressed his hopes that more nursing stations would be established when the hospitals became the responsibility of the provincial government. By 1959, only Ontario continued to run outpost hospitals, peaking at eighteen in 1961, with six nursing stations. In New Brunswick, however, only seven nursing stations remained in 1959, decreasing to a half dozen throughout the 1960s and early 1970s, dropping to four in the period up to 1975.[27] In his 1960 report, Dr McInerney raised questions about the financial role of the government, pointing out that in 'most other provinces where Red Cross operates Outpost Hospitals and Nursing Stations, generous subsidies are provided by the provincial government concerned'. Although New Brunswick subsidized public health services such as those carried out by outpost nurses in St Stephen/Milltown, subsidies to nursing stations, for example, remained small and patients' fees were often impossible to collect.[28]

By the mid-1960s, statistics in the annual reports demonstrated a reduction in the number of home and office visits, a trend reinforced in subsequent reports. As a result, nurses gradually took on more public health work and the contributions made by the provincial government increased from a few hundred dollars to about $6,000 per station. In 1963, for example, the government spent a total of $33,000 on six nursing stations while the Red Cross's contribution amounted to $26,000. Previously the Red Cross had supplied the bulk of the funding supplemented by local fundraising and patient fees.[29] In the late sixties fees were increased several times, though the 'Nursing Stations Report' for 1967 admitted there were many patients who could not afford even part of the fee since they subsisted on government welfare. A year later the annual report noted a sliding fee scale and that the government paid the fees for those on welfare, thus alleviating the budget deficit.[30]

When the CRCS recommended in the late 1960s that the government take over responsibility for the costs of the nursing stations across Canada, a detailed study of the role of nursing stations followed in 1967–8. The study found that in the previous ten years there had been numerous changes: such as increases in the number of doctors, nurses and hospitals as well as improved transportation services and a diversification of public health services. The financing of the stations varied from treating them like hospitals, to maintenance grants from provincial health departments to fee-for-service payments. The final recommendation of the study reinforced the need for negotiation with provincial authorities for an arrangement that would finance these facilities from public funds or insurance benefits. Although the number of Red Cross nursing stations across Canada had diminished to twenty-one in 1968, the study emphasized that those stations that remained filled 'a need which would not otherwise be met and it seems likely that our expanding frontiers will continue to create small centres of population where this facility will be required'. Similarly, in New Brunswick, the Nursing Stations report for 1969 emphasized the important, round-the-clock service they provided, despite a decline in the number of users. In the early sixties, around 11,000 patient visits were recorded, but by the latter part of that decade the numbers had dropped to under 7,000 per year.[31] By 1970 with the imminent participation of New Brunswick in Medicare and the reorganizations carried out by the government of the day, decisions had to be made about the role of nursing stations.[32] Two were closed and the four remaining expanded their public health and home nursing roles and by 1974 the provincial government approved additional funding for the nursing stations 'until such time as the service is replaced by the Department of Health'. The next year the four remaining stations were transferred to government and by 1978 only two – Miscou Island and Juniper – survived.[33]

Outpost Nurses: Who Were They?

What do we know about the nurses who staffed these hospitals and stations in New Brunswick? Very few recorded their experiences first-hand, though the few reminiscences we have show both the opportunities and constraints these women faced. Most were single in the pre-Second World War era and a number of them developed ties to their communities, sometimes through marriage. Most found themselves at least occasionally performing duties normally assigned to physicians, thus stretching the boundaries of the profession.

In 1973, Kathleen G. DeMarsh published her account of 'Red Cross Outpost Nursing in New Brunswick' in the *Canadian Nurse*, and the Red Cross's *Despatch* captured DeMarsh in photographs and stories in 1946–7. Trained at the Saskatoon City Hospital, DeMarsh attributed her attraction to remote nursing to the stories of a Saskatchewan outpost nurse and to her brother who had been assigned to Miscou Island as a summer theology student. He had been in touch with the New Brunswick Red Cross and found that they needed a nurse. DeMarsh accepted the assignment even though the prospects were daunting – two channels of water had to be crossed to reach Miscou, with a population of 1,300 mostly French-speaking residents. Access was restricted during some weeks of the fall and spring because of ice conditions; there was no electricity and only two phones on the island. The nearest doctor and hospital were on the mainland. As with many of these accounts, the emphasis is on pioneering and obstacles overcome – for DeMarsh, the need to learn French and win over the islanders. One month after her arrival, DeMarsh received the gift of a horse and the residents worked together to build a barn, an indication to her that she had achieved a measure of acceptance. The horse, 'Nellie Rothesay', was the gift of the Rothesay branch of the Red Cross and the nurse used it for her rounds on the island.[34] According to the *Despatch*, Nurse DeMarsh 'made 158 home visits, cared for 16 patients and delivered five babies' in her first six weeks on the job.[35] Perhaps the most telling evidence of the community's support for the out-post nurse came in March 1947 when DeMarsh brought two branch members from the island to the annual meeting of the New Brunswick Red Cross Society. Helen G. McArthur, National Director of Nursing Services (1946–71) for the CRCS wrote: '[I]t was the two branch members from the Islands that accompa-nied her who could really speak with feeling of the need that was being met and of their desire to work tirelessly for the advancement of their Outpost'.[36]

DeMarsh's memoir celebrates the adventure she found on the island but also underlines how nurses faced situations beyond their training. DeMarsh notes that in many situations 'I had to proceed according to my own judgment ... and then report to the doctor after the fact ... In many instances I found myself making judgments and taking action that in normal situations I would not have dared to make or take!' In the case of a shooting accident DeMarsh recalls sutur-ing the man's hand using drugs and chloroform 'all without a doctor's order. But after all, this was an emergency!' Indeed she challenged the doctor's authority by objecting to his advice that a finger needed to be removed. Instead she per-suaded the patient to submit to massage and exercise, thus saving his finger. Her experiences led her to question 'whether or not society as a whole is prepared to allow the nurse to function at her full capacity ... Is there a lesson here that could be learned in relation to the proposed community health clinics?' she asked.[37] These early experiences prepared DeMarsh for her promotion later on to the CRCS's Assistant National Director of Nursing Services and Vice-President (Nursing), Health Sciences Centre in Winnipeg.

A few excerpts of outpost nurses' memories were captured by McIntyre in her brief history of New Brunswick outposts. Typically, these stories focus on transportation difficulties in getting to patients or getting them to hospitals. The dangerous nature of woods work appears in Jean Sweet's memories of two cases of severed limbs in the Juniper area. Her brother-in-law severed his hand in a logging accident and days later another man had his leg amputated in a mill accident, both incidents requiring trips to the hospital twenty-five miles away. Genevieve Eaton of Campobello Island recalled many adventures including the rescue of a haemorrhaging lighthouse keeper as the tide came in. Edith Pinet, local nurse and midwife in Paquetville, remembered a terrible snowstorm that forced her to keep an injured patient at the station for three days warmed by her gas stove. Dorothy Ward's stories of Miscou Island also focused on storms and on deliveries without the assistance of a doctor using the back of a truck as delivery room. The *Despatch* ran a similar story in autumn of 1951 relating the birth of a baby in a Red Cross truck aboard a ferry scow between Miscou Island and Shippagan. Nurses Lorna Russell and Jean Lapointe had been summoned by the wife of a fisherman expecting her sixth child. When complications arose the nurses decided to take her to Shippagan after failing to find the nearest doctor on the mainland. The baby delivered in mid-channel and mother and child were taken to the hospital. According to the article it was all in a day's routine for outpost nurses.[38]

As Jayne Elliott's most recent article suggests, there were complex relationships with the community that nurses negotiated. DeMarsh's account takes a bemused tone when she recalls her first year on Miscou Island; visits to patients' homes attracted neighbours who wanted to get a look at the new nurse and the local store furnished much gossip about the nurse who came to buy supplies for the station. As DeMarsh remembers, news of her successes and failures spread rapidly over the island so that when she had some success using the fairly new drug, penicillin, patients would flock to her hoping to relieve diverse complaints.[39] Clearly it was difficult for outpost nurses in these small communities to maintain a private life. Nevertheless, romantic attachments are recorded in the official documents. While some communities were concerned about such liaisons, Grand Manan's 1944 Annual Report coyly warned about sabotage,

> with Cupid aiding and abetting the saboteur, who was none other than one of the Hospital Board Members, who contributed to the shortage of nurses, by marrying the nurse in charge and during the same season, another staff nurse was married to one of the Islanders.

Once married, nurses tended to withdraw from paid labour, though some continued to work part time as far as their family commitments allowed. The 1950 annual report noted that 'Miss Mary Daly followed out the tradition of matrons at Grand Manan and married after being with us a year. She is the fifth of seven matrons to marry during the last eight years', the report stated. Furthermore the report noted that six staff had left during the year on account of marriage while five others went to positions in other provinces or countries. While Grand Manan may have been an extreme example, turnover was a serious problem for isolated locations.[40] Even the much-loved DeMarsh and her colleague Therese Arseneau resigned in autumn of 1948 to take up other positions.[41]

Although Grand Manan assumed control over its hospital from the Red Cross in 1951, the experiences of Bessie Bass, a graduate of the Saint John General Hospital, is of interest as one of very few personal reminiscences of outpost nurses. The eldest of eight children, she taught school before becoming a nurse. Arriving in Grand Manan in April 1951 for what began as a summer job, Bass quickly became the matron of the hospital, a position she retained until she married in 1954. She recalled working alone on 1 January 1957 when she had to call for help in the delivery of twins. After marriage she worked only occasionally until her children were older, returning to full-time work in 1965 and once again becoming matron from 1975 until 1985 when she retired. Her narrative demonstrates the constraints that married nurses lived under but also illustrates the increasing presence of married nurses in the post-war period.[42]

Paquetville, an economically depressed francophone community dependent on lumbering, farming and construction, enjoyed the services provided by Mrs Edith Pinet who became a Red Cross nurse when the nursing station opened in 1951. A 1960 report penned by the Director of Maternal and Child Health in the province noted Pinet's varied services to communities within a ten-mile range. Since doctors rarely visited the area, patients had to travel fourteen to thirty-five miles to find medical care; thus Pinet's presence was highly valued. She not only delivered babies but also gave injections on the doctor's advice and described patients' symptoms over the telephone. Pinet's duties also included home visits and health education, and she 'made her own vegetable garden in order to set an example to other people', many of whom suffered from malnutrition. As her daughter remembered, tuberculosis was common because of the poverty and lack of good nutrition. Daughter Elizabeth Cripps also became a nurse and she reminisced about her mother's practice. She remembered the ox cart that often took her mother to deliveries day or night. As the mother of eleven children, Pinet had to have the assistance of maids to keep the household running. Paquetville's nurse continued to provide care into the 1970s as the area remained isolated and impoverished.[43]

One of the women whose career demonstrates considerable job mobility is that of Lorna Russell who began her stint on Miscou Island in 1949 after graduating from the Miramichi Hospital School of Nursing and working there as a staff nurse. In 1952 she won a bursary to study public health nursing at Dalhousie and returned briefly to the Fredericton Junction outpost hospital in 1953 before becoming the Director of Outpost Hospitals and Nursing Stations that same year. She replaced Margaret Pringle who had been the director since 1946. Russell's appointment brought the hospitals and nursing stations under one department head responsible for central purchasing, finances, staff and liaison with hospitals. The following year the Commissioner's report on the four hospitals and eight nursing stations remarked of the twenty-six outpost nurses: 'These girls deserve the highest possible praise'. Lorna Russell's 1954 report, co-signed by Dr J. P. McInerney, chair of the Outpost Hospital and Nursing Station Committee, indicated that the Miscou station had to close temporarily from April to September because of the illness of one of the nurses just as ice prevented passage to the island and an unspecified epidemic broke out among the children. Russell reported that the military had provided plane and helicopter assistance to land two nurses on the island to help with the outbreak. From these reports it is apparent that finding nursing personnel was not always easy and Russell reported temporary closures of stations and occasional new ones throughout the 1950s. Her 1954 report also noted that Kathleen DeMarsh, formerly in charge of Miscou station, had assumed the position of acting Director of Nursing Services and had paid a visit to the New Brunswick provincial office to see old friends. As noted previously, DeMarsh moved on to higher posts.[44]

In 1955 Russell reported that the difficulty of obtaining nurses and associated costs meant that Miscou would be reduced to one nurse instead of two for a trial period. In her capacity as Director of Outpost Hospitals and Nursing Stations, Russell also assumed other duties such as assessing the possibility of opening new stations or moving them. In April she had visited the Escuminac and Bay du Vin areas to assess the feasibility of moving the station from Bay du Vin to Escuminac since the former was not serving enough people to warrant keeping it open; however, she reported little interest from Escuminac. Similarly she visited Canterbury to assess a request for a new station there which eventually opened in spring 1956 just after Bay du Vin closed.[45]

By the late 1950s, as the last of the outpost hospitals were turned over to the government, Lorna Russell found herself working with the hospital boards and staff teaching them the basics of hospital administration. In autumn 1957 Russell spent a few months at Harvey and Fredericton Junction in anticipation of the hospital hand over in early 1958; later that year she provided the same guidance to the board and staff at the Rexton hospital, the last Red Cross outpost hospital in New Brunswick. That same year she assumed the role of Director of Nursing Services in addition to Director of Outpost Hospitals and Nursing Stations. Nursing stations closed at Harcourt and Deer Island while a new but short-lived one opened at Tabusintac. Russell remained in her post until 1965 when she resigned to take up a position with a local company as an industrial nurse. In 1977 she was named as Provincial Director of Red Cross Nursing Services.[46]

Nursing stations remained important in New Brunswick, however. Isolated places such as Campobello Island and Miscou Island maintained nursing stations into the late 1970s after most of the others had been closed. Mrs Genevieve Eaton, a native of Campobello Island, opened the station in 1950 and ran it for the next twenty-eight years until it closed. In addition to bedside care and obstetrics she faced emergency cases related to the fishing industry. Prior to 1962, emergency cases had to be taken by ferry or boat to the mainland for hospitalization either in Maine or to St Stephen, sixty miles away. Eaton ran nursing services from her home and was on call twenty-four hours a day. From 1970 onwards, she ran a public health nursing programme, in which child health clinics and visits to schools were the prime focus.[47]

Miscou Island, initially served by Kathleen DeMarsh, Therese Arserneau, Lorna Russell and Jean LaPointe, was under the care of Mrs Dorothy Ward from 1957 into the seventies. Isolation was not as severe for Ward because a causeway had been built to connect Lameque and Shippagan islands with the mainland and larger treatment centres in Tracadie and Caraquet. By the 1960s there were fewer calls for nurse's services except in bad weather and thus Ward, like other outpost nurses, was recruited to assist with public health nursing in the schools and well-baby clinics. As the annual report of the New Brunswick Division noted in 1961, the nursing stations were 'very useful adjuncts to the Medical Services and the Department of Health in the areas in which they are located'.[48]

Moving up in the Red Cross hierarchy as Kathleen DeMarsh and Lorna Russell did was not an opportunity for most outpost nurses, a number of whom were married and closely tied to specific communities. In theory, according to Elliott's work on Ontario outpost nurses, supervisors expected nurses to move when reassigned. Evidence is lacking in the New Brunswick case about such reassignments but there is ample proof that outpost nurses were well connected to their division nursing supervisor and the National Supervisor of Nursing Services, Helen McArthur. In the case of New Brunswick's nursing supervisors, outpost nurses had frequent contacts with them, sometimes through her visits to their stations and annually when all the outpost nurses attended a spring meeting to discuss problems and developments in their area.[49]

On numerous occasions annual reports reflect the presence of the National Supervisor of Nursing Services at the annual conferences. Helen McArthur made her career as national supervisor from 1946 until her retirement in 1971. From Edmonton, she had experience as a public health nurse in Alberta and had studied at Columbia University. She served both as director of the University of Alberta's school of nursing and as director of the Alberta Public Health Nursing Division. While working with the Red Cross she also served in a variety of voluntary roles, including president of the Canadian Nurses Association. Despite the extent of these activities McArthur visited New Brunswick often; for example, she spent a week visiting hospitals and nursing stations 'offering many constructive suggestions' in July 1948. In June 1951 she was the principal speaker at the annual conference of nursing staff from the hospitals and nursing stations and offered helpful policy advice. The timing of 1952's conference was changed so that McArthur could attend and her 1953 visit in the autumn included a meeting of hospital matrons in Saint John. The following year DeMarsh became Acting Nursing Director when McArthur was seconded as the Coordinator for the League of Red Cross Societies in Korea. Upon her return from Korea, McArthur resumed her position as National Director visiting New Brunswick many times before her 1971 retirement. In some ways her exit signalled the beginning of the end of an era in rural health care as the need for outpost facilities declined in the 1970s. With the phasing out of nursing stations, the last four nurses retired, each of them with at least twenty-five years of Red Cross service.[50]

Conclusion

Outpost nursing, whether in small hospitals or nursing stations, provided essential health care to rural residents in New Brunswick as elsewhere. As a voluntary organization, the CRCS gave vital assistance to the government by funding the first public health nurses as well as hospitals and nursing stations. As Mariana Valverde argues in *The Age of Light, Soap and Water* about the late nineteenth and early twentieth centuries, the voluntary sector maintained its key role in providing assistance to governments for social reform and welfare activities.[51] In the New Brunswick case such interdependence lasted well into the second half of the twentieth century and can be said to have aided in state-building functions in health care. Key to these developments was the role of women who performed the health-care labour needed to build the infrastructure. While this paper has focused on nurses, women from the elite class also played a role in providing voluntary leadership and services through the Red Cross. This latter activity was shared with male leaders – politicians, professionals, religious leaders and the occasional military man. Strikingly, however, the official reports say little about the medical men of New Brunswick; instead they focus on the outpost nurses who established the links between isolated rural populations and medical assistance.

While there is limited data about the lives of individual nurses, there is evidence that nurses often became part of the communities they served, most clearly by marriage. Annual reports noted marriages and commented on married nurses 'helping out' in times of need, thus underlining the normative expectation that these women would be single, at least until the post-war period when married nurses became more common. Clearly in the incidences of upward mobility within the Red Cross and beyond, the three examples discussed – Kathleen DeMarsh, Lorna Russell and Helen McArthur – were single women who made lifelong careers in nursing.[52]

Outpost nurses generally had to negotiate their roles not only within their communities but also as professionals. As some of the evidence indicates, professional independence could be a source of pride but also presented a challenge to the scripted roles of nurses who were not supposed to encroach on the roles of medical men. In emergencies nurses had to take action and make decisions that normally would be taken by physicians. In the case of childbirth, where no doctor was available and where nurses had limited training in midwifery, they had to rely on their training and sometimes each other for a successful delivery. In short, New Brunswick's outpost nurses were part of a long tradition that stemmed back to the late nineteenth century and the VON. Their work was integral to community- and state-building in Canada; they 'helped lay the foundation for formal government involvement in health and medical care, aiding in the construction of a major component of the social welfare state'.[53]

11 MOTHER'S MEDICINE: WOMEN, HOME AND HEALTH IN THE PEACE RIVER REGION OF BRITISH COLUMBIA, CANADA, 1920–40[1]

Megan J. Davies

In the mid-1920s young Eden Robinson was hand-logging on Philip and Emily Tompkins' farm at Halfway, a remote Peace River community at the midpoint between Fort St John and Hudson's Hope, when a tree came down on his head. The force of the impact pushed Robinson downward onto a sharp snag which entered his mouth from below. This was a bad bush accident, leaving Robinson with a nasty scalp injury and serious jaw damage. With the nearest doctor and hospital in Pouce Coupe 100 miles away, transportation to medical assistance was out of the question. Alice Summer (née Tompkins), then a child, remembers the young man being carried into the house, placed on the dining-room table, and given hard liquor to dull the pain. Working in consultation with Dr Archibald Watson of Pouce Coupe over the telegraph, Alice's mother, Emily Tompkins, sterilized a moccasin needle with boiled snow, and stitched up the head wound with silk thread. Turning to Robinson's other injuries, Emily used tweezers to remove the wood chips embedded in the roof of his mouth while her husband Philip walked over to the Robinson home for adhesive tape to bind Robinson's lower jaw.[2]

This dramatic story, which has survived well in folk memories of the region, spotlights the healing talents of one lay woman, Emily Tompkins, a war bride who had worked in a greeting-card factory in Bristol, England, before immigrating to a new life on the Canadian frontier. Despite her lack of formal medical training Tompkins clearly had the temperament, and the sewing skills, to stitch up a nasty head wound. When Dr Archibald Watson arrived one week after the accident he told Emily that she had done an excellent job.[3] Remembered by her daughter as a woman who 'when need arose could find whatever it took to cope', Emily Tompkins managed the family's health using mustard plasters and 'sniffs' – mixtures of camphor and eucalyptus oils – to clear chest colds and advised her children to run scratches and bumps under cold water. She served on occasion as a lay midwife in

Halfway, BC, delivering Martha 'Pat' Bazely's son Ted in the 1930s and a premature baby girl in 1941. Tompkins's life in Halfway also underscored the hazards of
coping with health concerns in remote regions: two of her own children died, one
at birth from an umbilical cord cut too short and another when, suffering from
pneumonia, he was transported too late to hospital.[4]

While Emily Tompkins's dining-room-table surgery demonstrates the dramatic potential of health and healing in remote regions in British Columbia's
past, taken as a whole her work as a healer was not exceptional. Indeed, the life
history of Tompkins is a fine illustration of the diverse historical roles which
lay women have played in the provision of health care in pioneer settlements.[5]
In this paper I present these activities as a key facet of 'motherwork', whereby
women employed a range of different health knowledge systems (Aboriginal,
folk, common sense and biomedical) in places where access to health professionals and health institutions was uncertain.[6] More than just a set of skills and a
response to human need, the 'health' labour of women like Tompkins also needs
to be understood and appreciated as central both to the maternalist creation
of Euro-Canadian settler society and to the construction of female identity in
a remote rural setting.[7] The locales of home and local community in the Peace
were spaces where non-native women were engaged in the collective project of
building 'white' rural British Columbia.[8] Mothers incorporated rural feminine
norms of caring, coping and curing into their identity as frontier women and
utilized them as a base of female authority and power.[9] As scholars across the
disciplines have noted, understandings of colonial power relations and gendered
identities require an appreciation for material conditions, everyday 'life-world'
experiences, and the ways in which the body serves as a canvas for the creation
of civic society.[10]

This article side-steps the historical establishment of hospitals, public-health
units, women's institutes and hospital auxiliaries, and the roles of the pioneer
doctor and the district nurse – all of which are important elements of the history
of health care in the Peace. Instead, I use oral and local histories as sources to
explore understandings of health and healing and health strategies in the context
of the local and the everyday.[11] The relatively late period of Euro-Canadian family settlement in the region, which primarily took place in the 1920s and 1930s,
allowed me to access the memories of women who went to the Peace as girls and
young women. This process served two happy ends: reclaiming the life work of a
generation of women and opening wide my intellectual appreciation of women's
health work done in the context of home and family. I would also like to note
the key role of local histories, community-produced narratives of family and
place, compiled by women and men of the Peace over the 1970s and 1980s in
my research. These invaluable volumes – each the size of a big-city telephone
directory – have been my most select bedside reading for the past few years, and

the source of tales of snowy trips to the hospital, tragic farming accidents, summer berry picking and social fundraisers for school dental care.[12]

The Peace River of this pioneer period is best understood as a 'belated frontier'.[13] Pamela Banting uses this phrase to describe the experience of growing up in an area where white settlement was a recent phenomenon of only a few decades.[14] Like Banting, the people of the Peace existed simultaneously in two historical moments – the first Euro-Canadian woman at Cecil Lake, for example, gave birth on a bed constructed from a piece of deer or moose hide tacked on a wooden frame in an era where women in urban Canadian hospitals were being given preparations to induce labour and anaesthesia to ease pain of childbirth, and having episiotomies and forceps employed in the final stages of birth.[15] Women's approaches to health and healing on the Peace River frontier reflects this dualism: their collective action through the women's institutes demonstrates an awareness of contemporary concerns about the health of children, while geographic distance and lack of ready cash often limited access to modern medicine.

These women operated within a 'contact zone' where health knowledge was informed by a range of cosmologies – folk, humoral, biomedical and indigenous.[16] John Crellin's term 'home medicine' is most useful in describing this kind of popular medicine which crosses the boundaries of Aboriginal, traditional, folk and biomedical systems.[17] Pioneering women of the Peace employed methods of treatment and understandings of disease causation which 'travelled' with them from Europe and other regions of North America.[18] Biomedical expertise was certainly privileged within their range of therapeutics, but when it was not available women would call on other strategies for dealing with fever, infectious disease and injury. Indigenous and folk healing modalities were used, alongside older Galenic holistic understandings of the humoral body, where healing involved restoring balance of body humours through food, drink and medicine. The 'belated frontier' might also explain a relative openness to Aboriginal peoples and Aboriginal healing modalities. My sources suggest that women employed a pragmatic, pluralistic approach to therapeutics, using materials available to them in a remote frontier setting. The kitchen, the barn and the Eaton's catalogue were all sources for items in an eclectic non-prescription *materia medica*.

This paper begins by providing a brief history of Aboriginal and Euro-Canadian settlement in the Peace River region of British Columbia (BC), paying attention to the creation of transportation and communication infrastructures and medical institutions, and tracing the history of medical professionals in the area. I then move to a discussion of childbirth, midwifery and the seasonal regulation of white bodies, highlighting the role played by women in these processes. The final section of the piece considers the management of illness within the context of home and community.

Locating the Peace River Region

The communities that these women were involved in creating were located in the Peace River lowlands, an area which transverses the northern boundaries of the provinces of Alberta and BC and includes some twelve-million hectares on the BC side.[19] Wide plateaus of parkland and boreal shrub forest are bisected by the river known locally as 'The Peace', a waterway that has carved its way deeply into the land, creating bench lands and terraces beneath the flat plateau area at the top.[20] Summer days are long and warm, while temperatures can drop as low as minus 40–50 °C in the winter months.

By the late 1920s, BC's Peace River Block (the official designation before the land was turned over to BC), in anticipation of the transfer of some 500,000 acres from the Federal Government of Canada, had become the country's 'Last Best West' for agricultural settlement by non-natives.[21] Earlier white involvement in the region had been primarily linked to trapping and involved mostly transient single men, but migration in the 1920s and 1930s was family-based and agricultural in intent. Between 1921 and 1931 the population of the Peace River increased from 2,144 to 7,013.[22] Treaty Number 8, signed in 1899 between representatives of the Canadian Government and the Dene-thah First Nations Peoples, included BC's Peace River region and effectively cleared the region for white settlement.[23] With new strains of hardy, early-maturing wheat and the expansion of the railway to Dawson Creek in 1930, hopeful farming families flocked to the region – many fleeing drought and ruined prairie homesteads.

Medical resources followed the pattern of settlement on the BC side of the Peace River region with Dr Archibald Watson setting up a practice in Pouce Coupe in 1921, the same year that the Red Cross established an outpost hospital there.[24] Another outpost hospital, staffed by one nurse and a housekeeper, opened in Grandhaven in 1930, and moved to Cecil Lake five years later. The Catholic Sisters of Providence opened hospitals in Dawson Creek in 1931 and in Fort St John in 1932. By 1930 roads linked the communities of Pouce Coupe, Dawson Creek, Rolla, Rolla Landing and Fort St John and a telegraph line had been strung west to Hudson's Hope. However, transport was slow at any time and particularly difficult in the spring when the ice broke up on the river and the roads turned to 'gumbo' mud.[25]

Incoming physicians and district nurses broadened the sphere of medical influence. Dr Hubert Brown arrived in Fort St John in 1930 and by 1932 there were two other doctors, Dr Beckwith and Dr McKee, practising in the South Peace region. In 1934 Dr Brown took on the post of Indian Agent and turned over much of his practice to Dr Garnet Kearney.[26] Dr Edward Hollies came to practise in Pouce Coupe in 1936 following the death of Dr Watson.[27] The first step toward a network of public-health nurses, the result of pressure from local

Women's Institute groups, began in 1931 when Nurse Nancy Dunn was posted to Sunset Prairie, funded jointly by the Red Cross and the Provincial Board of Health.[28] The 1935 establishment of a Provincial Health Unit in the government centre of Pouce Coupe solidified public health in the Peace with a full-time doctor and cadre of district nurses.[29]

Although by 1935 elements of a biomedical presence in the Peace had been put into place, this was still a 'belated frontier'. The vast distances which comprised the region, the short period of time which had elapsed since the beginning of white familial settlement and the challenges posed by seasonal weather and limited transportation and communication systems, all served to limit the impact of modern medicine and foster a range of alternative healing modalities.

Creating, Nurturing and Sustaining White Bodies

The health 'motherwork' done by women served practical purposes, but also worked to foster community links in a new settler society and a frontier female identity that integrated reproduction, care-giving, knowledge and capability.[30] Frontier women of the Peace were thus intimately connected with white bodies, particularly when they lived in communities that did not have ready access to hospitals, doctors and nurses. Acting together as lay midwives, women pooled knowledge and skill to deliver children in remote regions. As mothers, they strove to create a healthy home where children could be raised with strong bodies ready to resist the extremes of northern winter weather and the dangers of infectious disease. In both instances the home functioned as the primary 'field of care'.[31]

Although settler women who had the money or lived close to physicians, nurses or hospitals might use these resources when they gave birth, there also existed a network of community-based, female-centred supports for birthing women. These were not organized structures like the Women's Institutes that dotted the region by the mid-1930s, but rather a set of local understandings and systems of expertise. Oral and local histories tell of a number of trusted and well-used 'community' midwives, lay women who took on this work in lieu of a local physician or nurse, but likely did not identify themselves as 'midwives'.[32] Additionally, local women with nursing training, many of whom are recalled as unique and important community individuals, delivered many babies in remote areas of the Peace.

Lay midwifery in the Peace was a joint enterprise in a youthful settlement that was linked to both the creation and the continuance of community and supports Lesley Bigg's understanding of this kind of midwifery as taking form in response to the particular historical moment of settlement.[33] Local and oral histories demonstrate that some women were known and used in a region as women skilled at helping with births, supporting Wendy Mitchinson's argument that midwives did not disappear during the period.[34] Early midwives of the Peace did not necessarily claim the title of 'midwife', nor were they known as such, but their skill was acknowledged and appreciated nevertheless. These patterns of informal settler midwifery echo the ties of womanhood and the crossover of women between public and private spheres demonstrated in Laura Thatcher Ulrich's classic *A Midwife's Tale*.[35] Ada Herald, whose family homesteaded at Fish Creek in the 1920s, recalled, 'Mom rode miles, to deliver babies'.[36] In the Rolla district there were at least three women acting as midwives in first fifteen years of settlement, and '[r]egardless of night or day, Mrs Miller [Mary Lois Miller, née Fey] delivered many, many babies in those early years'.[37] Ada Cadona came to the aid of Luella Fredrickson (in 1928) and Veta Latimer (in the early 1930s) when snow and cold kept the women from getting medical attention.[38] Known for serving 'many mothers in distress',[39] Kate or 'Ma' Edwards, who settled south-east of Rolla, delivered Ellen Coons' children in 1916, 1918 and 1921, as well as Klara Johnson's fourth baby in August 1916 in their dirt-floored cabin and Pearl Taylor's child in July 1917.[40]

Glena Southwick, who settled at Charlie Lake around 1920, followed a pattern of exchanging service, helping neighbouring women give birth at home in the area over the 1920s and receiving help when she was in labour herself. She was midwife for several of Walter 'Red' and Evelyn Powell's children, and also at the birth of Tommy McMartin, child of Blanch Dopp Hipkiss.[41] Evelyn Powell in turn assisted when the Southwick children who were born through the 1920s; as the chronicler of the Southwick family history noted, 'Mrs Powell and my mother were midwives for one another, some times their babies were quite close together, but they made out some how'.[42]

As Glena Southwick and Evelyn Powell demonstrate, birth was a collective female event and lay midwifery was framed in the context of female friendship and being a good neighbour.[43] Edith Freer, who homesteaded in Taylor Flats from 1915 to 1923, had a neighbour woman come from twenty miles distant to assist when her three children were born.[44] This may have been Charlotte Taylor, a First Nations woman and a known midwife in the region.[45] Pearl Smirl of North Pine recalled,

> The first winter we were on the homestead Mr and Mrs Alex Thompson came to see if Ruby might stay with me as her second baby was already overdue. The summer before we had come to be very good friends with much visiting back and forth.[46]

Such a request for help could not be ignored. Martha Tower, born at home on a 'chinooky day' in 1934 at Sweetwater, north of Dawson Creek, described Mrs Trail, her midwife, as a neighbour and a good friend of her mother.[47]

It is not clear why particular women would take on the role of lay 'midwife' in a community. Some of my informants suggest it was because they had a talent for, or some experience of, nursing. Others noted that the women in question had worked with birthing animals, and indeed Kate Edwards of the Rolla district was known for her work with both people and livestock. A further explanation was that women like Kate Edwards, Mrs Trail at Sweetwater, and Mary Lois Miller, all middle-aged when they worked as midwives, had themselves given birth and were at a stage of life where their temporary absence from the household could be managed.[48] Where did Emily Tompkins of Halfway acquire her midwifery skills? Her daughter noted that as the oldest of ten children, the youngest of whom was fifteen years her junior, and as woman who had given birth to eight children, 'she knew the routine' – and local people knew that she had the ability.[49]

In some instances need dictated action. Though she had no medical training, Frances Kemp came immediately when her husband called in to say there was a woman 'down the way' in labour in the autumn of 1930.[50] Kemp continued to act as midwife at Cecil Lake during the first years of white settlement in the area, apparently stopping when the outpost hospital was opened there in 1935. She assisted with the birth of George Maginnis Jr in May 1931 and of Fay Bonnell a few weeks later.[51] Elizabeth Spence, her friend and neighbour, helped her out, calling on the nursing training which she had received before her marriage to successfully knead a woman's abdomen when the afterbirth did not appear. With fourteen-year-old daughter Dorthea running the family home, Frances Kemp was able to stay on and help for five days.[52]

As might be expected, any Peace River women with nursing training were understood to be competent at childbirth. Katherine Mixer, a Belgium nurse who lived in Kilkerran, delivered babies.[53] Coming to the area to settle in 1924, Ethel Holgate used her nursing training to help deliver 'quite a number of babies in the area'.[54] Kathleen Peck (née Sheppard) and Gertie Lucas (née Gaylor) helped women in childbirth in Hudson Hope. Gertie Lucas of Hudson Hope, who trained as a nurse in Calgary before marrying and coming to the Peace, wrote: 'I helped at any nursing that was needed in the area, and delivered six babies for neighbours who couldn't get to Fort St. John, the nearest hospital, some 70 miles away'.[55] As local histories recount, a trip to the hospital from Hudson Hope was expensive during the Depression years and involved a three-day overland trip in winter or a ride in a boat followed by a wagon or car trip in the summer. Considering the risks involved in transportation, some who opted to stay close at home contributed to local mythologies of pioneering childbirth:

> Gertie and Reg [Lucas] were known to have been awakened in the middle of the night and obliged to give up their bed to a mother in labour. Gertie quickly stripped the bed and remade it, climbed up through a trap door into the attic and brought

down a box containing her obstetric requirements, scrubbed and soon was in business.[56]

While the midwifery exploits of Gertie Lucas in Hudson Hope are certainly memorable, the most legendary settler midwife was Anne Young (née Roberts). A Welsh woman and registered nurse and midwife who accepted a post at the Grandhaven Red Cross Hospital in 1930, Anne continued to work as a community midwife after she married – a job for which she was paid fifteen dollars per birth by the provincial government. She is said to have delivered between 300 and 400 births in all, continuing her practice well beyond the time when other women had ceased acting as midwives. A memorial quilt made for Anne, famous for venturing out on her horse when it was two a.m. and forty below zero with blowing snow, hangs in the Fort St John Museum, each of the ninety-nine squares embroidered with the name of a baby that she caught on its way into the world, an eloquent testimony to a woman cherished by the community.[57] The quilt demonstrates both the time spanned by Young's midwifery practice and the geographical parameters of her work. Between 1930 and 1951 she initially delivered babies around Grandhaven, west of Fort St John: later her practice was centred around Rose Prairie, where her husband ran the post office, covering Rose Prairie, Monteney, North Pine, Doig River and Stoddart Creek.

Like childbirth, regulating and maintaining healthy bodies was women's work. Mothers monitored the well-being of their children and sometimes of the farm hands and farm animals as well. 'Mother kept track', Alice Summer recalled, 'and sensed when somebody wasn't feeling well. Never my father.'[58] Other interviewees echoed this perspective. 'Mothers did the most of it', stated Ellen Dewetter (née McDonnell). 'They were more in the house.'[59] From the perspective of the women of the Peace, good diet, suitable clothing and keeping bodies strong in the face of cold, heat and infectious disease were tasks that they performed as part of their motherwork.

Understandings of seasonal health remedies were brought to the Peace and adapted to the local environment. For the English settlers in the region, spring tonics were a yearly ritual of purification and part of creating and maintaining a healthy child's body. Rooted in Galenic understandings of body functions, but also linked to an early-twentieth-century medical concept of 'autointoxication', the spring tonic was meant to purge the body of impurities built up over the cold, dark winter months.[60] It is not surprising that this task of cleansing the internal body was done by mothers, as their roles in cleaning both the outside of the body and the home were clear.[61] A mixture of molasses and yellow powdered sulphur, the spring tonic was hated by children: from Sunset Prairie, where Winnie Williams reported that the school atmosphere turned blue with the stench of children passing air after receiving their tonics, to Hudson's Hope, where the Beattie children downed their seasonal dose.[62] Girlie Powell (née Beattie) reported on the spring tonic: 'Terrible. We had to have a big spoonful of that. And I always say that the cure was worse than the disease'.[63]

District nurses like Nancy Dunn of Sunset Prairie taught 'nutrition' through the Women's Institutes, but oral and local histories demonstrate that many settler women already had a good empirical understanding of diet that incorporated both local produce and culturally familiar food to ensure a balanced diet throughout the year. I suggest that this combination of the familiar (that 'travelled' with women to the frontier) and the new (that was the result of 'shared' knowledge on the frontier) was another element of the construction of female identity in the Peace River. Emily Tompkins, living in Halfway in the 1930s, canned saskatoon berries native to the region, and rhubarb and vegetables in the summer so the family could have fruit and vegetables year-round.[64] The Tompkins's diet demonstrates the pluralistic nature of food strategies in a remote frontier settlement: local saskatoon berries had been traditionally used by First Nations People and rhubarb, typical English fare, would have been familiar to Emily from her English childhood.[65] Similarly, at Cecil Lake scurvy was avoided by eating preserved rhubarb in the winter and gathering the first spring greens – lamb's quarters or 'pigweed' as it was known locally – which grew copiously on the farmyard manure pile.[66] John Crellin's work on home medicine in Newfoundland suggests that the spring consumption of pigweed might have been both a health and a seasonal ritual.[67]

The construction of settler community and the frontier mother was deeply connected with the way in which the women of the Peace undertook the 'motherwork' of bearing, regulating and maintaining white bodies. This process involved utilizing both the culturally familiar and the new, as women drew from a range of healing cosmologies to feed, nurture and sustain their children and families. An informal system of midwifery, folded into the daily world of home and local community operated when geography and weather meant access to hospital, nurse and doctor was not possible. The health work of women in this remote region thus needs to be understood as part of the creation of community and a set of skills developed in response to challenging conditions – both aspects of their 'motherwork' were keys to the creation of a regional female identity.

Tending the Body: Sickness, Accidents and Home Nursing

Accidents and illnesses punctuated the front pages of the weekly *Peace River Block News*, as well as the local and oral histories which I draw upon in my work. While tending illness was centred on the female world of the home, serious accidents and disease transcended the boundaries of home to encompass the workplace, the doctor's office and the hospital. Peace River pioneers employed a 'hierarchy of resort' in dealing with health issues, moving from self-help, to consultation with others, to professional medicine as a health concern was assessed and acted upon. However, the uncertainties of obtaining medical assistance meant that women also lived in what I call 'a state of preparedness', having on hand the necessary knowledge, tools and preparations and ready to take action on illness when necessary. Women kept a family 'doctor's book', homemade salves, patent medicines and bandages on hand, alongside the ingredients ready to concoct home remedies. They purposefully gathered knowledge from a plurality of healing systems – biomedical, folk and Aboriginal. They called on the services of local health 'experts' when it was deemed necessary. When a cold or fever arrived, when children scalded themselves or men became injured dealing with farm equipment, mothers used a variety of strategies to order the process of disorder created by illness or accident.

Most settlers had a 'doctor's book', a good medical reference book.[68] The family history of the Westergaards of Charlie Lake makes reference to a 'well-thumbed doctor book'.[69] Dorthea Smith of Cecil Lake told me that her mother had a good doctor's book which she brought from Saskatchewan. Did she use it? 'You bet she did! That doctor book was always ready to go and sterilized items that she might need'.[70] Florence Barrington, a pioneer who came to Sunset Prairie in the early 1920s, had a book called *Doctor's Home Advice*, brought with her when she immigrated from England. And she used it as well, for her daughter Winnie told me that Florence used to study the book.[71]

Tales of 'doctor's books' reveal patterns in lay health knowledge and indicate a first step in the hierarchy of resort (a strategy whereby the person seeking medical assistance begins with self-medication, then moves to consultation with peers and to professional assistance.) Interviewed at Pouce Coupe in 2005, Elizabeth Gibbon noted that the books served as a substitute for the expert voice of the absent physician: 'There wasn't a doctor helping like today, so when anything went wrong we would look at it'.[72] The book owned by Elizabeth's mother covered both humans and livestock, indicating both the importance of cultivated animals in a farming community and a fluid female 'curing' role that might encompass both house and barn.[73] In 1933, when Amy Smith came north from Saanichton on southern Vancouver Island to get married, her mother gave her the family medical book. This meant that Amy drew on the same knowledge system that her mother used as a young mother and shopkeeper in the Yukon and later as a mother and berry farmer on Vancouver Island. 'I went by that book a good deal', Amy told me. 'I used it a lot. So did my mother'.[74]

Without a physician nearby and only a doctor's book in hand, women sought out other knowledge systems in their search for healing. Here, hierarchies of resort might include a range of healing modalities. In the early days of white settlement, and in areas where contact between First Nations peoples and white settlers persisted, women like Florence Barrington learnt about health care from Aboriginals who lived nearby.[75] Similarly, the Starnes family, who moved to Moberly Lake in 1913, were taught about medicinal properties in the buds of certain trees and in the pitch of the spruce and pine from local Cree, Saulteaux and Dunneza peoples.[76]

Women coming west from the prairies may have brought with them First Nations remedies that had been shared with an earlier generation of female healers. 'Mother Rose' Sowden's black poplar salve, made from the sticky spring buds of the tree and used for burns, sores and chapped hands, suggests a contact between Plains peoples and her mother.[77] When the young Margaret Sowden fell against a cross-cut saw, her brother was sent on horseback to buy chewing tobacco, a remedy also reported by Bertha Lentendre (née Gauthier), a First Nations woman from Moberly Lake.[78] Mixed with water to soften it, the tobacco was then wrapped in a cotton cloth, sterilized in the oven, and put on Margaret's leg. The pain was so great that Margaret passed out.[79]

In the 'country of home-mades', as one public-health nurse described the Peace River, women exchanged information about remedies which could be made and kept on hand for a range of complaints.[80] The Women's Institute was one forum for this activity, sometimes formalizing the creation of collective knowledge. In March 1933 Mrs Hollingsworth Jr of the Sunset Prairie Women's Institute gave a talk on home treatment for burns.[81] Three months later the west Saskatoon Women's Institute answered roll call with remedies for a cold, burn or poison.[82] Similarly, at the September 1934 meeting of Cecil Lake's Nor' Pioneer Women's Institute members answered the roll call with 'home remedies'.[83] Frances Kemp, one of Cecil Lake's first pioneers, was likely at the Institute gathering that day, sharing the remedies that her daughter remembered her making.[84]

Women also drew on folkloric knowledge systems of health which may have come from the 'Old Country' or from a blend of Aboriginal and European understandings of healing, demonstrating the flexibility of medical systems in frontier communities distant from scientific medicine. Forbes Grout, a Metis living in the Sunset Prairie region during the first years of white family settlement, showed Florence Barrington how to extract poison from a foot injury by binding it with an old copper penny.[85] In Pouce Coupe Catherine McDonell used her gold wedding ring to stop the spread of eczema on the face and in the early 1940s instructed her daughter to dig strawberry root so that she could treat diarrhoea with a tincture made from the plant.[86]

Home remedies used by the mothers of the Peace were linked to an older or Galenic understanding of the body as a humoral system that became ill when a healthy balance of hot and cold had been disturbed. Warming a body which had been compromised by the chill northern climate could restore an individual to a healthy state.[87] Hot poultices were made by women in their kitchens and placed on the patient's chest were standard practice for respiratory illness.[88] Like many other women, Florence Barrington employed mustard plasters with bacon fat for severe cold or chest infection or fever.[89] Called to aid a young baby suffering from respiratory problems, neighbour Mrs Doonan advised the application of a mixture of ground onions and warm goose oil.[90] Rosie Westergaard at Upper Halfway used hot, wet towels, coal oil, brown sugar and prayer for childhood croup attacks and hot compresses for pneumonia.[91]

Interestingly, notions of the humoral body persisted in places where access to biomedical assistance was readily available. When little Verner Ulrich of Sunrise went into convulsions the night after the district nurse vaccinated him in 1943, mother Elly 'never lost her nerve', giving him a warm bath.[92] Catherine McDonnel of Pouce Coupe, with ready access to doctor and hospital, also used mustard plasters, indicating that the earlier association of this healing modality with physicians survived the rise of scientific medicine.[93] Her daughter Ellen Dewetter described the process: 'Got hotter than Hades ... liquid that came through would burn like a son of a gun. Sometimes the cure was worse than the problem.'[94]

Some remedies used in the Peace River region demonstrate a pragmatic reworking of older folk therapeutics to incorporate products readily available in frontier homestead kitchens and barns. Dorthea Smith's mother-in-law used baking soda for everything – and always on a burn.[95] Sisters Toulie Hamilton and Girlie Powell (née Beattie) both remembered their mother treating boils with daily application of poultices of milk, sugar and cooked onion.[96] Florence Barrington would place a bread and soap poultice over a sliver, swelling or infection to 'soak the poison out' and the practice of staunching the flow of blood from a bad cut by sealing the limb inside a bag filled with flour.[97]

The medicinal uses of kerosene and sheep or stock dip – a disinfectant wash used to prevent vermin in sheep – all readily available on a farm, suggest another thread of antiquated medical belief known as counter-irritant theory. It was believed that the burning, astringent qualities of these substances would serve to draw out noxious humours that were the cause of the infection.[98] Nurse Rita Mahon of the Peace River Health Unit reported in 1937 that many residents placed a boiling tin of Lysol or kerosene solution on the stove as means of warding off scarlet fever infection.[99] Elizabeth Beattie used kerosene and sugar for cold and sore throats.[100] Arriving with her family, the second white family in the region, at Cecil Lake in 1930, Elizabeth Spence used diluted stock dip for cuts and sores, soaking the affected limb in sheep dip or using it as a poultice.[101] What is interesting, and indicative of the fluid boundaries between folk and scientific medicine in remote settler communities, is the fact that Elizabeth Spence had received some nursing training before she married and came west to the Peace.[102]

Organization and planning were keys to being prepared for dealing with an accident or illness in a remote setting and another way of ordering ill health. Elizabeth Beattie had a small cabinet specifically for medicines at their farm outside of Hudson Hope. She also washed flour bags and made bandages from the fabric.[103] Several women told me that their mothers created medical 'kits' for dealing with injuries, so they could simply grab a kit and run if their services were needed.[104] Amy Smith's mother would post lemons from Victoria for her daughter and North Pine neighbours to have on hand for colds and sore throats.[105]

Patent medicines were kept on hand, purchased through the Eaton's catalogue, from one of the travelling salesmen active in the district or at drugstores in Pouce Coupe, Dawson Creek or Fort St John. Though there was concern about the overuse of patent medicines in Newfoundland and the Scottish Highlands and Islands during the early twentieth century, my rather impressionistic conclusion is their use was not widespread in the Peace.[106] Particularly in the early years of the Depression, this was a cash-poor economy where purchases were generally limited to essential items. Elizabeth Beattie bought medicinal supplies through the Eaton's catalogue or at the Hudson Hope Hudson's Bay Shop: liquorice sticks for coughs, Minard's Linament for bruises, rheumatism and sprains, Vaseline for cuts, rough hands and cracked lips, Epson salts to be taken in coffee for constipation, and Castoria for the same complaint among small children.[107] The 'Rawleigh Man' or the 'Watkins Man', usually local farmers trying to earn extra money during the Depression, visited farms in the Rolla region of the South Peace two or three times a year selling castor oil, epson salts and cough remedies along with spices and Bird's Eye Custard Powder.[108]

Mothers living distant from physicians and hospitals opted to use self-help, administering first aid and then leaving an injury deemed less serious to heal. Home treatment utilized materials on hand. Alice Summer's (née Tompkins) mother Emily never made a fuss of scratches and bumps; her children were told to run the injured limb under cold water.[109] Ellen Dewetter's mother treated bee stings by covering them with mud.[110] This *laissez-faire* mode was used by the Beattie family when they were out on their farm, thirty miles outside Hudson Hope. When she was seven years old Girlie Beattie cut herself on the face with a double-bitted axe. The wound was at least an inch in length, but her mother just bandaged it up and left it to heal.[111] Mrs D. Cuthill of Hudson Hope gave Henry Stege three stitches in his left hand when he cut it slicing meat.[112]

Acute illnesses were 'read' by the mother who might then decide to seek professional help. Nurse Pauline Yaholnitsky was a rookie district nurse stationed in Progress in 1936 when called out by a mother to see a sick boy. With the child's father away at work, the two women worked as a team. Nurse Yaholnitsky observed a rapid pulse, high temperature and sore right side and diagnosed possible appendicitis. Together, the women decided to rush the boy to the doctor, taking him over thirty-five miles of snowy and icy roads. En route to the hospital, they worked together to replace a flat tire. The tone of the tale, written up by Yaholnitsky for the provincial *Public Health Nurses' Bulletin*, is one of collegiality rather than of a professional and lay person.[113]

In her memoir of life in the Sunrise area during the 1930s, Lily Dingman noted that settlers shared expertise to fill in gaps in the professional sector: 'We all helped each other. Every district seemed to have someone skilled in different trades, a barber, a carpenter, a nurse and veterinarians, etc'.[114] Lay health 'experts' were female in the Peace River, and stories of these women in the first decades of white settlement demonstrate that in the absence of medical credentials lay 'expertise' was predicated on practical ability, and these individuals were widely acknowledged as valuable members of the community. Thus, as in systems of folk medicine elsewhere, authority and creditability did not emanate from an institution located outside the Peace, but related instead to the pragmatic and everyday world of the local.[115] Taylor Flats postmistress Charlotte Taylor (née Ankenam), a convent-educated Aboriginal woman married to Hudson's Bay Company trader Herbie Taylor, was known north of the Peace River for her extensive knowledge of medicinal herbs.[116] Amy Smith remembers Charlotte Taylor as, 'a well-respected member of the community because she helped people'.[117]

'Aunt Kate' Edwards served as nurse, vet, dentist and healer to the people of Rolla and district throughout the 1910s and 1920s, when there were no health professionals in the area. Travelling west from Georgetown, Ontario, with her brother Jack Coutts in 1912, Edwards characteristically wore men's bib overalls and smoked 'roll yer own' cigarettes. Her niece recalled

> stories of how she would ride or drive horses day or night to help the sick or needy ... In 1915, when dysentery swept through this area she was credited with saving many lives. It didn't matter if it was an animal or human being in need of medical or dental help; she would do her best.[118]

In 1947 Edwards, who had abandoned male clothing and solitary cattle-ranching and had moved to Dawson Creek, was awarded an Honorary Canadian Citizenship Award.[119]

Local histories present a string of women who brought nursing training to the remote communities of the Peace and were remembered and appreciated for their ability to deal with a range of health conditions. Doctor's wife Rosa Watson, who had St John's Ambulance training and had worked for the Red Cross during the First World War, tended to minor cuts and diseases and helped deliver babies in the Pouce Coupe area.[120] May Birley, an Australian-born nurse who had also served in France during the war, came to Fort St John in 1920 with her brother Ken and sister Nina. Famous for her English garden, tennis court and garden parties, 'May was always ready to give a hand when someone was hurt, or to help nurse someone back to health'.[121] Kathleen Peck (née Sheppard) of Hudson Hope, an English nurse, came to Hudson Hope in 1923 with her trapper husband Victor and four boys.[122] Toulie Hamilton (née Beattie) described this local healer in action,

> She was 'Pecky' to everyone that knew her. A lovely person. Good hearted. They would go to her and she would go to their houses too when they were sick. She would do everything, eh, that she could except cut you open or whatever ... She could stitch you up, bandage you, put splints on. That sort of thing.[123]

Peck also looked after First Nations peoples in the region.[124]

Conclusion

On a summer evening in July 2002 I drove our rental car up the zigzagging curves of Beatton Hill on the road from Fort St John to Cecil Lake. It was snowing lightly. I wanted to hear more from the women waiting to speak with me about the 'life-world' of healing, which had been the subject of a group interview at the Dawson Creek Museum the night before. Asked about their mothers' involvement in the Women's Institute and their memories of the pioneering provincial health unit in Pouce Coupe, the women of the Peace told me instead about local midwives, husbands away at work, mustard plasters, medical 'kits' and getting to the hospital in wintertime.

My Cecil Lake interviews, and a subsequent set which took place in Fort St John the following day, added to my understanding of heath care as an important element of women's work in the frontier home. I heard about women making home remedies, adopting Aboriginal healing practices, cleaning wounds with diluted sheep dip and kerosene, eating rhubarb and pigweed to avoid scurvy, and calling on the services of community healers. As this paper makes clear, I have come to see this female sphere of health care as a flexible, pragmatic system that drew on a range of healing cosmologies. Belief systems and health-care practices were as eclectic as their *materia medica*, drawn from the kitchen, the barn and the Eaton's catalogue.

What makes this story particular to a remote, rural setting? This was a healing system that often operated in the physical absence of biomedicine, deeply rooted instead in the local, the female, the everyday and in an understanding of community as a place where 'you helped your neighbour where and when you could'.[125] It was also a healing system that had to be ready to adapt to the vagaries of seasonal weather and the vast geography of the region. The life stories and local histories which the people of the Peace generously shared with me allowed me a unique entry into this 'belated frontier', a place where biomedicine co-existed with local networks of lay midwives, home remedies and Aboriginal healing modalities, and facilitated my exploration of how the health work of women served to construct both frontier female identities and Euro-Canadian settler society.

Historical studies of post-Second World War rural BC are still too limited to speak with certainty about how health arrangements were altered by improved transportation and increased access to mainstream medical care. But it is certain that the spatial and economic elements of health care shifted for British Columbians in remote rural locations: hospitals and doctors became easier to reach and more affordable, no matter what the season. Thus, in a practical sense, there must have been much less reliance on the motherwork and community systems that I have explored in this paper. There were likely attitudinal changes as well that undermined the use of traditional home cures: one of my respondents recalled being offended when her daughter-in-law referred to the use of a damp wool sock around the neck for a cold as an 'old wives' tale. This was a remedy that had been passed on by her own mother, but it had become suspect by the 1940s.[126] The story of the scorned wool sock suggests an important transitional moment, the demise of lay and place-related rural health systems centred around home and community and the expansion of health professionalism and the biomedical state.

12 CALL OF THE WILD: PUBLIC HEALTH NURSING IN POST-WAR LAPLAND

Marianne Junila

In Finland, the public health care system started to develop gradually just before the Second World War. The basic units for arranging health care were municipalities that concentrated mainly on the medical treatment of communicable diseases, especially tuberculosis. Tuberculosis was prevalent and maternal and child mortality was high, especially among the poor social classes.

After the war, municipalities started to build up the public health care system by contracting general practitioners, midwives and public health nurses and by building maternity and childcare centres. The midwives and public nurses were salaried, but the general practitioner's income came primarily from payments by patients. For the physicians, working in the remote, poor or sparsely populated areas meant lower income than in other parts of the country, and this led to a constant lack of physicians in the northern parts of Finland, especially in the Province of Lapland. Because of this the public health nurses here had to work more alone and more independently than their colleagues in more urban municipalities.

Although the activity for public health and welfare had wide-ranging support in Finnish society since the late 1920s, rural health-care services commonly suffered from a shortage of trained personnel. In Finland, this problem was accentuated in the eastern and northern provinces, which included the most sparsely populated and the poorest regions of the country. The differences in availability of the health services remained strikingly large until the late 1960s.

Working in these 'remote areas' (*syrjäseutu* as they are called in Finnish) required different professional skills and personal qualities, as well as a different attitude, than working in more densely populated regions with higher standards of living and better infrastructure. As the chief public health nurse of Lapland put it in 1951: 'Lapland has its pros and cons. And there will always be nurses who are willing to sacrifice their best years to it'.[1] In this article, I will discuss these pros and cons. I will ask what made public health nurses seek employment in Lapland, the northernmost province of Finland. What were the qualities that public health work in this environment required? And how did public health nurses cope with the challenges presented by the local conditions?

I will approach the activities of the public health nurses who worked in post-war Lapland from three points of view. First, official sources, most importantly the reports written by the chief medical officers and chief public health nurses of the province,[2] will show how public health agencies and society at large regarded the public health nurses' work. Secondly, oral history sources and autobiographical accounts by the nurses themselves will shed light on their personal experiences and their means of coping. Thirdly, the local people of Lapland[3] also had their own views on public health nurses. Their voices can be heard in some extensive oral history collections about health-care work.[4]

During the Lapland War, which constituted the last phase of the Second World War in Finland, the province of Lapland was almost burned to the ground. Unsanitary temporary lodgings, poor diet and ubiquitous landmines threatened the health of the population. Among the gravest problems that the public health services faced in the north were maternal and infant mortality, which were many times higher than elsewhere in the country, and tuberculosis, previously rare but now rampant.[5] The post-war period of reconstruction coincided with a major health care initiative, *viz.* the institution of an extensive network of local maternity and children's health centres (*neuvola*). Trained health-care workers were in great demand all over the country, and there was reason to fear that the shortage would be particularly acute in Lapland. The state could no longer simply order the workforce around, as it had been doing during the war. In medical services, wartime practices lingered for a relatively long time; as late as spring 1945 the National Board of Health (*Lääkintöhallitus*) posted some district nurses to Lapland.[6]

Before the Second World War, when Finnish public health services were mostly in their infancy, private charitable organizations such as the Mannerheim League for Child Welfare (*Mannerheimin lastensuojeluliitto*) and the Finnish Red Cross were major players.[7] Between 1926 and 1935, the Finnish Red Cross had contributed significantly to public health by founding a series of cottage hospitals, one of which was located in the Province of Lapland. A district nurse resided at the hospital, treating patients, giving health advice and visiting schools and homes. The Red Cross also ran some mobile health clinics from 1945 to the 1950s. A mobile clinic was staffed by a physician and a nurse. They visited those parts of the province where roads were accessible by car (between spring and autumn) and the road less regions on skies (in April) or on foot (during the summer). In May, when the melting snow flooded the roads, travelling came to a halt.[8] Thanks to such activities, the notion of community nursing was known even before the Act on municipal public health nurses was passed.

Answering the Call

Could not young nurses sacrifice a few years [of their lives] for work in the wilderness, for the benefit of people in difficult straits?[9]

The year 1944 saw the passing of important pieces of legislation that proved pivotal for the development of public health services in Finland. Of most importance were those that addressed municipal public health nurses and midwives, and the provision of municipal child health and maternity centres. The new legislation obliged all municipalities to open maternity and children's health centres and to employ midwives and district nurses, and it also defined the number of public health nurses and midwives per municipality. Fortunately for the sparsely populated Lapland, local circumstances were taken into account when the ratio of public health nurses and midwives per inhabitant was fixed.[10] Lapland thus received a fair number of public health nurses' posts. The trick was to find qualified occupants for these posts.

By 1946 pessimists were already predicting that the municipalities of the northern provinces would not be able to recruit qualified health-care workers to the new posts. Trained public health nurses were in short supply, and there was reason to fear that they would opt for towns or for wealthy rural municipalities which could secure them adequate facilities and accommodation, thus leaving remote rural areas without trained personnel. Health education was sorely needed in Lapland, but would southerners be able to deal with 'the loneliness, the cold and the barrenness' of Lapland?[11] One could not count on Lapland-born nurses easing the shortage because there were so few of them among the newly graduated public health nurses. The region clearly needed marketing.

One way to attract especially young public health nurses to Lapland was to appeal to their sense of duty and professional ambition. Public health nurses shared the ethos of the voluntary welfare organizations: they believed that the privileged women of the educated middle classes had a duty to help the disadvantaged (women) of the rural north. Such voluntary aid work also entailed the possibility of exerting the power that came with the privileged position. People engaged in public health services were called upon to improve both the quality and the quantity of the population.[12] Lapland was, for several reasons, particularly well suited for acting upon this creed.

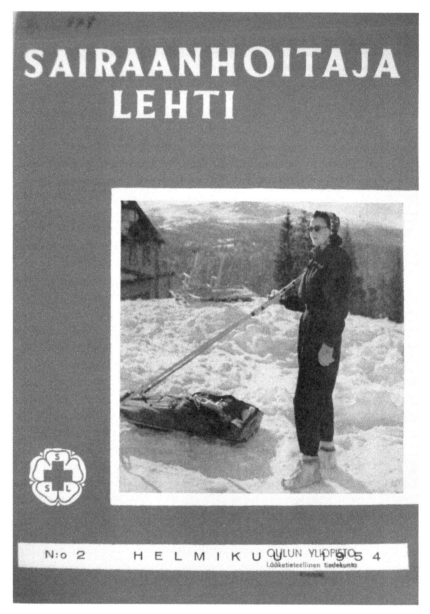

Figure 12.1: The cover of *Sairaanhoitaja-lehti* (Finnish Journal of Nursing), 2 (1954); reprinted by permission of the journal. Several special issues were distributed for Lapland in the 1940s and 1950s. Such attention was not paid to any other province in Finland.

Nursing journals such as *Sairaanhoitajalehti* (Finnish Journal of Nursing) (see Figure 12.1) and *Kätilölehti* (Finnish Journal of Midwifery) rallied for the Lappish cause. While stressing that no one would be expected to spend all their active years in Lapland, *Sairaanhoitajalehti* assured young nurses that public health work would give 'the energetic and intelligent' an opportunity to 'raise the Lappish people from their sorry state by hard work and sound advice, and [thus] to accomplish something of great and lasting value'.[13] Lapland was the place to be for those who really saw public health nursing as a vocation. The gratitude of the Lappish people would be a lasting source of satisfaction. *Kätilölehti* warned that it might take some time for the local people to learn to appreciate the nurses' efforts. At first, they might even be suspicious of the nurses' attempts to raise them from their 'sorry state'.[14] For an ambitious nurse, however, this was merely an added challenge.

Public health nurses who came to Lapland from other parts of the country remember being animated by a pronounced frontier spirit. They were full of enthusiasm, and they firmly believed in their own ability and that of public health services' ability to improve the health of the northern population, especially the health of children.[15] The realities they faced when they arrived at their posts, which could lie 150 km away from the nearest physician or a colleague, could feel crushing at first:

> I am responsible for the therapeutic and preventive care of six hundred people who live scattered [throughout a vast region]. They would first turn to me, whatever the emergency. – I am 24 years old, newly graduated, and about to start in my first job as a public health nurse.[16]

The public health nurse was recognized by her uniform: a blue dress with white collar, occasionally covered by a white apron. On her travels she naturally dressed according to the weather and the season. Before public health nurses entered the scene, local people had relied on deaconesses and midwives for help, and for some time to come they would find it easier to approach these more familiar figures. While the deaconess, in particular, was associated in people's minds with strong personal vocation, even self-denial, the public health nurse was seen rather as a professional on official business. On the other hand, one did not dress up in one's Sunday best for seeing a public health nurse, like one did for seeing the doctor.[17] The public health nurse was a novelty, someone whose status and exact job description were not familiar to the local people. She was, therefore, treated with some caution at first.

The Lure of Lapland

Summer there was short, and the sun was shining all night and all day, turning it into a paradise.[18]

The unique nature of Lapland was an asset in the recruitment of public health nurses. Although it was obvious that visiting Lapland differed greatly from living there, holiday experiences sometimes proved decisive: 'I had fallen in love with northern Lapland during my yearly hiking trips. I had grown fond of its people and its landscapes.'[19]

Lapland held a particular attraction for those nurses who enjoyed winter sports and outdoor life. Skiing from one village to another on the glimmering spring snow, they were able to combine business with pleasure. Spring and summer in particular could be breathtakingly beautiful in Lapland – an experience not to be missed.[20] 'We often went for our rounds [on skis] on beautiful, sunny spring days. With weather like that, travelling was a great pleasure. We admired the bright spring snow, the sunshine, and the days getting longer and longer.'[21]

Lapland was recommended by fellow students, or perhaps by a spouse. A public health nurse who had been working in Petsamo by the Arctic Ocean reminisced fondly about the tight-knit community of 'southerners' that was formed there.[22] Social life in Lapland was characterized by community spirit and a supportive, family-like atmosphere, something which constituted an experience in itself. Travellers came to Lapland in the autumn to see trees and bushes glow in red, yellow and brown, or in the winter to see the northern lights. For a resident, however, the natural environment was a less constant source of delight. It could also present a formidable challenge, for instance at the times when it was so cold that water and electricity became unavailable. Few public health nurses planned to spend their whole career in Lapland. Most of them had their craving for the exotic fully satisfied by a short term as a surrogate nurse in the summer, or by a spell with a mobile clinic in late spring.

There was plenty of peace and quiet in Lapland. One had to learn to endure, or even to enjoy solitude, and to soften it with little things like needlework and listening to the radio.[23] A public health nurse who disliked her own company could not work in Lapland for very long.

Some nurses found Lapland attractive *because* life there was rough. Hissu Kamila had trained as a public health nurse and worked in a field hospital during the war. After the war, she had gone to work in a small rural community in central Finland, but had found her work there frustrating. A job as a public health nurse in the vast northern municipality of Enontekiö fully satisfied her yearning for both new challenges and for greater professional autonomy. The few public health nurses who originated in Lapland were particularly strongly committed to the welfare of the local people and often stayed their whole career in the same community.[24]

Some parts of Lapland were more attractive than others. What was true of the country as a whole also applied to the Province of Lapland: professionals and the trained work force favoured the most densely populated locations, and they often preferred to stay in or close to the area where they had been educated. Thus, the few towns of southern Lapland and the rural municipalities immediately adjacent to them had no difficulty in recruiting qualified public health nurses. Surprisingly, the municipalities that experienced the greatest trouble in finding public health nurses were not the most sparsely populated municipalities located in the very far north. In the early 1950s, the municipalities of Enontekiö and Utsjoki both employed a qualified public health nurse who remained for more than ten years. In contrast, their southern neighbours, the municipalities of Muonio and Sodankylä, kept losing their public health nurses. In Salla, too, the turnover was high.[25]

The fact that Enontekiö, Inari and Utsjoki were regarded as the most exotic and the most genuine parts of Lapland may have added to their appeal.[26] Luck perhaps also played a role. Given that there was only one public health nurse's post in each of these municipalities, one dedicated public health nurse was enough to solve the recruitment problem there for a long time. Sodankylä and Salla had far more inhabitants and also several extensive nursing districts, with tens of both permanent and ambulant maternity and child health centres.[27] Although both municipalities employed several public health nurses, each nurse still had a considerable patch to cover.

Until the early 1950s, public health nurses were in short supply all over the country. In fact, the shortage hit many other regions, Kainuu for instance, worse than Lapland. Every seventh post remained vacant in Lapland, while the figure for the country as a whole was one in four. With its vast patches of uninhabited wilderness, Kainuu was not unlike Lapland. However, the Kainuu region suffered a far more serious shortage of public health nurses despite the fact that they were educated in the nearby town of Oulu since 1945. Thanks to increased investments in public health nurses' training, their shortage eased both in Lapland and in the country as a whole in the 1950s.[28]

The beauties of nature drew some public health nurses to Lapland. Another motivating factor was the collective compassion that the destruction of Lapland had aroused, and the desire to help the people of the devastated province. Additionally, for some years after the war, public health nurses working in Lapland were also paid extra.[29]

Another factor that spoke in favour of working in Lapland was the Children's Hospital of Lapland, founded in Rovaniemi in 1952. The hospital was a progressive and modern specialist unit, which also functioned as a training hospital.

Public health nurses from all over country attended the further training courses offered by the hospital. The medical staff of the hospital took active part in the training, and the cooperation between the hospital and the health care workers on the field was successful in other respects. The presence of a high-quality hospital in the province, even if it were hundreds of kilometres away from the public health nurse's home base, was an asset.

Autonomy and Responsibility

I was far too inexperienced to work independently in an unfamiliar environment, but perhaps my enthusiasm compensated for my shortcomings. I made mistakes, but I'm sure I also did a lot of good.[30]

The US and Britain led the way in the development of preventive health care. The first Finnish public health nurses were trained in Britain at the Bedford Nursing College which offered a graduate training course in public health nursing. Between 1920 and 1930, sixteen Finnish nurses took this course. The first Finnish training courses for nurses were organized by the Mannerheim League of Child Welfare in the mid-1920s. At the end of the decade, the state assumed the responsibility for training nurses for preventive health services. The State Nursing Institute (*Valtion terveydenhuolto-opisto*) was founded in 1930. It provided a graduate course in public health nursing and remained the sole educator of public health nurses until 1945. However, because the output of public health nurses failed to meet the demand, their work was sometimes done by deaconesses, tuberculosis nurses and district nurses.[31]

According to law, the public health nurse assisted the physician at the maternity and child health centre, carried out home visits, and fought contagious disease. Her primary duty was to guide and advise the members of the community on matters of health, with special emphasis on the health of children, from infants to school children. If the municipality was unable to provide home nursing in any other way, the public health nurse might also be assigned some acute care nursing, but this was supposed to be in exceptional cases only.[32]

In the day-to-day work of the public health nurse these legal obligations intertwined with many other tasks. Physicians seldom had time to work actively at maternity health centres, so the centres were run by public health nurses. Home nursing was supposed to be the province of district nurses, but because they could not be recruited to Lapland in sufficient numbers, public health nurses provided some therapeutic care at home as well. Because the hospitals of Lapland had been destroyed by the war, public health nurses also treated acute cases. They managed small health care units by themselves. The public health nurse of Utsjoki even cooked for the patients of the cottage hospital.[33]

The responsibilities of the public health nurse covered highly varied tasks at irregular hours. She was never truly off duty, because she always had to be prepared to leave for a home call.[34]

> There were no working hours. A call could come night or day, on a Sunday or on a weekday. If no one answered at the local health centre, there would always be someone to tell [the caller] where I was headed. Then they would try and reach me by phone, calling house after house, although telephones were rare.[35]

Physicians were few and far between, and they made home calls only exceptionally. In the countryside, public health nurses treated patients at their homes and carried out procedures which, in urban areas, were left for the doctor. The public health nurses of the rural municipalities of Lapland and Oulu often – more often than colleagues elsewhere – faced situations that would have called for medical training. A home call required solid professional skills and self-confidence. The great distances characteristic of Lapland also complicated things. By the time that the public health nurse got to the patient, the latter's condition might have changed drastically from what it had been when the nurse had first been called, thus presenting new and unexpected problems. There was rarely a phone for calling the doctor for instructions or advice.[36]

It was often the public health nurse who decided whether the expensive and laborious trip to the nearest physician was worth taking. Physicians were usually posted in the major villages, the closest of which might be 100 km away. Driving the whole way was seldom an option. People relied on whatever transportation was available: horse, reindeer, boat or bike, or they simply walked. If the weather or the road conditions were poor enough, there was no way of getting medical care.[37]

Public health nurses belonged to the elite of the nursing occupation, and local authorities were eager to make use of their skills and expertise. They often sat on the municipal social, health and child protection boards, or worked for the boards as social and child welfare inspectors.[38] They were free from the harsh discipline that, for example, hospital nurses, especially those housed at the hospital, were subjected to. Resident hospital nurses had little privacy, and they were under the control of the sister even when they were off duty. Midwives and public health nurses, however, enjoyed exceptional autonomy both in their work and in their private lives.[39]

Nurses who came to Lapland from the other parts of the country found the local conditions professionally and personally demanding. It was commonly believed that the loneliness and the isolation of the wilderness could unsettle even healthy, well-balanced people and make them lose their critical capacities.[40] Some public health nurses had their social contacts mainly restricted to their patients, with few opportunities to talk to colleagues. The combination of large workload, loneliness and lack of diversion could indeed be depressing.[41]

Work in the remote corners of the country provided an enthusiastic and self-confident public health nurse with a fine opportunity to work independently and to make full use of her professional skills. The public health nurse's job was about quick decisions, responsibility and freedom.

Ultima Thule

Our province has offered its public health nurses lots of work and many hardships, and few diversions and modern comforts.[42]

The Province of Lapland covered almost one third of the whole area of the country, and there were villages in all its municipalities that could only be reached on foot. In the 1950s, there were approximately 500 maternity and child health centres in the country. One tenth of these were permanent 'central centres' and nine out of ten were temporary, which functioned in schools or larger houses at certain times.[43] Whether the purpose was to nurse the sick or to provide health instruction, it was the nurse, and not her clients, who travelled. She might start her journey by bus, if there was a connection, and then change into a horse-and-carriage or a reindeer-drawn sleigh, and perhaps walk the rest of the way. Not even footpaths led to the remotest Lappish villages. The public health nurse skied in the winter, and cycled or walked in the summer.[44] When she travelled to set up a roving clinic, she usually had to carry all her equipment with her. She would also take a piece of dry birch bark and matches with her, in order to start the fire quickly in case a bear strolled uncomfortably close. Her rounds of home visits typically lasted for several days. Since there was no way to reserve accommodations beforehand, they had to be improvised as the journey went on.[45] Figure 12.2 shows a public health nurse and midwife travelling together.

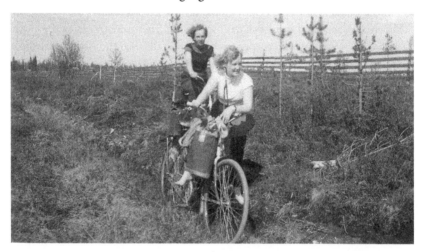

Figure 12.2: Public health nurse Marja Aikio with midwife Lea Kuivila, on their way to a home call; held within the Aikio Family Collections and reprinted by permission of the Aiko family.

In conditions such as these, transportation was a major issue. The combination of vast districts and poor transportation was one of the things that exhausted public health nurses and made them leave Lapland. While the distance between an ambulant clinic and the major centre was approximately 15 km in most rural municipalities, it was about 25 km in Lapland. There were, on average, six ambulant clinics per public health nurse in Lapland and three per nurse in the other parts of the country. Matters were made worse by the reluctance of local authorities to provide public health nurses with cars, or with fuel. The public health nurse of Savukoski was willing to buy a car with her own funds, but gave up the idea when municipal authorities refused to cover the cost of the fuel. Cars were not particularly reliable in the harsh northern conditions, where very low temperatures and poor roads were hard on them. Both the driver and the client became familiar with problems such as frozen brake fluid and broken car parts. Alternative means of motor transportation were sometimes considered. For example, there was a Jawa moped on display at the annual public health nurses' meeting in 1957.[46] Economically minded local authorities were more likely to equip a nurse with a moped than with a car.

Public health care services were based in local welfare centres (*terveystalot*), which were designed to meet the new legal requirements: there were consultation rooms for the medical officer, the midwife and the district nurse, plus apartments for the latter two (see Figure 12.3). Some welfare centres also included a small cottage hospital with a few beds. Lapland had foreign donations to thank for many of its local welfare centres. The United Nations Relief and Rehabilitation Administration (UNRRA) financed the local health centres of Rovaniemi and Sodankylä, and the furnishings of the welfare-centre-cum-cottage-hospital of Utsjoki were received as a gift from Sweden. These new houses of health were practical enough, but they tended to be cold in the winter.[47]

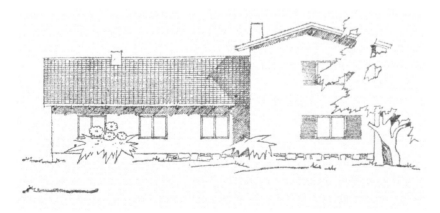

Figure 12.3: Sketch of a newly planned local health centre; reprinted by permission of The Finnish Medical Society Duodecim. Source: *Terveydenhoitolehti*, 4 (1948).

Many public health nurses had come to Lapland because they wanted to work in a region in which inhabitants had suffered particularly hard during the war, and they knew that the conditions would be poor. Nonetheless, their modest expectations were sometimes set too high:

> Of course I would have a centre and up-to-date accommodation under the same roof. Of course I would have all modern conveniences. [But] there was no centre; what I got was a bag, an old bicycle and a bus that ran once a day.[48]

Even if the newly employed public health nurse had had the foresight to ask in advance whether the centre was equipped with running water and electricity and been answered in affirmative, still she might be disappointed: 'Once I got there it turned out that the water had to be pumped by hand and electricity was available only at certain hours'.[49] Bleak and crammed housing was a post-war reality, particularly in Lapland. Dwellings were so small 'that not even the soul fits in'.[50]

Life in a far-away village was very different from life in town. One newly arrived public health nurse first did things by the book. She dressed up in her uniform in the morning and waited at the centre for the customers to come, and visited homes in the afternoon. She got a seemingly chilly reception: no one came to the centre, and she was not welcome in the homes either. She got over her disappointment once she realized that the locals fished all through the sunny summer nights and slept through the nurse's office hours.[51] After this, she learned to adapt herself to local conditions.

Travelling in the far north was best done in company. A natural companion for the public health nurse was the municipal midwife. Sometimes local officials – the priest, the policeman and public health nurse – travelled to the farthest villages together.[52] Society thus came to the citizens, bringing sacraments, justice and vaccinations. A public health nurse who visited remote households was sometimes expected to take care of all the official business by herself. One public health nurse, coming to vaccinate a baby, was taken to a table with a white sheet and a book of hymns. The mother wanted her to baptize the baby before vaccinating it and felt that a priest could well sanction the act later.[53] More patient mothers waited for the joint home call of the local servants of the state and the church to have their babies baptized and vaccinated.[54]

The People of the North

In the bus I thought about my destination. I was going to treat the children of Lapland.[55]

In Finnish public health-care nursing, the well-being of the children of Lapland was of a primary concern. They were the poorest among the poor people of Lapland. The nursing staff who for the most originated from other parts of Finland did not usually make clear distinctions between the two groups of Lappish people: Finns and Sami. Although the Sami were identified as a special ethnic group, as patients they did not differ much from the rest of inhabitants: they were not educated and they came from poor social classes, usually from big families with low income.

Poverty made people ill. Malnutrition and unsanitary housing resulted in less resistance to disease, and Lappish people of all ages were in poorer health than other Finns. Children's health, in particular, was a matter of great concern. Children born in Lapland were much less likely to survive their first year than children born elsewhere in Finland.[56]

Some children bore visible marks of deprivation on their bodies. They were pale and thin, sometimes with legs deformed by rickets. Their milk teeth were often brown and decayed thanks to the local habit of soothing a baby by giving it a piece of gauze soaked in honey to suck.[57] The high morbidity and mortality of children in Lapland were largely due to deficiencies in infant care.[58] There was thus a lot to gain by health education and infant-care advice.

Working among the poor, public health nurses could see first-hand how poverty bred illness. The poor could not have their illnesses medically treated, because they could afford neither the doctor's fee and expenses nor the long trip to the local health centre – which also entailed loss of income. The public health nurse, on the other hand, would make a home call for free and charge only for medications.[59]

Preventive measures could also be beyond the means of the poor. Health advice was free, but vaccinations, for instance, were not. One of the central aims of the public health administration was to have the Finns vaccinated against the most common and the most dangerous communicable diseases. Full immunization against some of these diseases required a series of multiple vaccinations. A poor family that could not afford a full series of vaccinations for all its members had to choose whether to vaccinate everyone incompletely or have some of them fully protected.[60]

Health education was not unimportant, however. The public health nurse was supposed to learn the ways and beliefs of the local people and, whenever she detected something inimical to health in them, 'to make an improvement'. A home visit gave the public health nurse an opportunity to teach the family how to deal with health risks, and her jurisdiction also extended to workplaces (see Figure 12.4).[61] Lappish people were regarded by outsiders as easy-going and unspoiled, but also oddly primitive. Northern people were in many respects still one with nature, and some of their habits were obsolete and downright superstitious. Public health nurses were sometimes astonished by the persistence of 'old folk beliefs' in Lapland. It was not easy to implant new, healthier ways of life in a region where the most narrow-minded fathers did not allow their daughters to take part in school physical education on the grounds that it was indecent.[62]

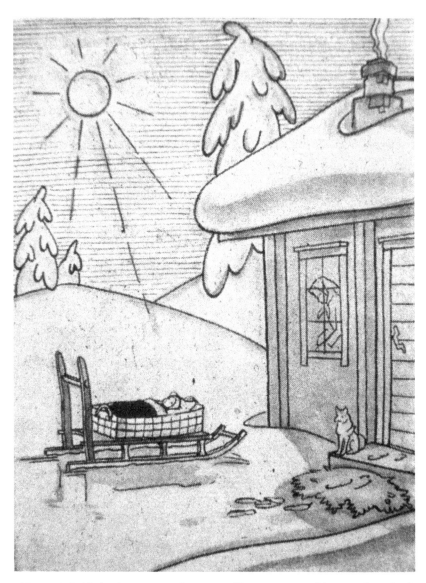

Figure 12.4: A baby sleeping outside; reprinted by permission of the Finnish Medical Society Duodecim. Source: *Terveydenhoitolehti*, 2 (1945). Sleeping outside, regardless of weather, was considered very important for the health of infants. Both public health nurses and paediatricians campaigned forcefully for this habit.

Lappish people could be fatalistic about disease, and particularly about children's diseases and deaths. They saw little sense in fighting the inevitable. If the parents regarded their child's illness as a divine punishment, the public health nurse would have to work extra hard to persuade them to have the child medically treated. Rumours about children whom not even the expensive trip to the hospital had saved further undermined the trust of the local people in official medicine.[63] The idea of visiting a health centre *before* falling ill was initially completely alien to the local people, and public health nurses had to train them to bring their children to the centre for the vaccinations.[64]

The primary target of the health instruction given by public health nurses were the local women. The idea was that the women who received up-to-date knowledge on healthier habits would gradually pass it on to the community as a whole. It was therefore important for the public health nurses to reach all mothers and children. Not all mothers were able to visit the maternity and child health centres, however. The women who lived in remote parts of the district and took care of the children, the household and the cattle all by themselves, with the men of the household out herding reindeer or logging, could not leave for the centre, not even in case of illness. Longer journeys in the winter might also be out of the question because the children lacked warm clothes.[65] The public nurse's visit could be the only adult contact in a long time for the lonely women of the isolated houses, and the visit was thus important not only for their physical but also for their mental well-being.[66] Public health nursing brought women together, although not necessarily on equal footing, given the nurse's often middle-class background, her education and the paternalistic nature of her duties.[67]

Local people had great faith in the public health nurses, district nurses and deaconesses. Both children and adults crowded to the child health centres to get their complaints seen to. Only two-thirds of the customers of these centres were children, while one-third were adults seeking help and advice. The public health nurse measured blood pressure, tested blood, removed ear wax, treated wounds, and she transported children and old people to hospital.[68] She took interest in the health of the whole family. During home visits, she wanted to know not only how the mother and the children were doing, but also how the old people were taken care of and what the family did to support the 'municipal poor'. Sometimes people even took their sick animals to see the public health nurse.[69]

Public health nurses' training was designed to be wide-ranging. The name 'welfare sisters' (*huoltosisaret*) was suggested for the new class of nurses, to indicate that their expertise covered not only matters of health and disease but also other problems arising at different stages of life.[70] A public health nurse working in a sparsely inhabited remote region had to be particularly versatile. She filled in application forms, contacted various official agencies, ordered medications, and even organized property registrations and estate inventories for her clients.

When the mail office could not decipher the address on an envelope, the letter would end up on the public health nurse's desk.[71] After all, she knew everybody.

In towns, public health nurses' work description was less varied. They primarily worked at the maternity and child health centres, making fewer home calls than their rural colleagues. Townspeople sometimes regarded a visit from a public health nurse as an embarrassment, as an unwelcome indication that the health of the family or the sanity conditions of the household were poor enough to call for official intervention.[72] Because townspeople had medical help – doctors and hospitals – readily available, the public health nurse's position in the community was not as prominent as it was in rural communities.

Rural people sometimes had greater faith in the public health nurse's expertise, judgement and practical experience than in those of a physician. The latter was too high up the social hierarchy and too expensive to be consulted about minor complaints. Some of the physicians who ended up working in the north were also so eccentric that local people avoided them and rather relied on the public health nurse. The public health nurse was regarded as an expert, and some patients would not follow the doctor's orders before she had sanctioned them. The trust shown by the local people heightened the public health nurse's sense of obligation.[73] A newly graduated public health nurse could not always share her clients' trust in her own abilities:

> I was oh so afraid, but nevertheless tried to seem as if I knew what I was doing. – People had lots of trust and great expectations, and the nurse couldn't show how little she knew or how insecure she felt inside.[74]

Public health nurses had to shoulder a great responsibility for the scattered population of the remote areas. It was no wonder, then, that they became trusted confidants whose opinion was carefully heeded.

Many public health nurses had been warned in advance that the locals might be cool towards 'southerners', but in fact they found working in Lapland more rewarding and the people more receptive and grateful than elsewhere. Their professional expertise was greatly appreciated, and the locals were friendly and warm, if perhaps a little shy, rather than rejecting.[75] It was empowering for the public health nurse to know that a correct diagnosis or a successful procedure might prove decisive for a patient's course of life.[76]

The chairwoman of the Nurses' Union, based in southern Finland, wondered how her colleagues managed among the rough people of Lapland, with no civilized company. But public health nurses were not the only educated women working in the north. Primary school teachers, like public health nurses, were often young, and the representatives of the two occupational groups got to meet and to know each other during school health inspections.[77] Her work brought the public health nurse in contact with many different people, and some of these encounters led to firm friendships which outlasted the nurse's years in the north.[78] The public health nurses who had been working in the north for a longer period of time usually adopted local ways of dressing and travelling, which made it easier for them to function in the northern conditions. A public health nurse who wore shoes made of reindeer skin and insulated with dried hay, like the local people did, would feel comfortably warm when she made her rounds in a reindeer-drawn sleigh.[79]

Municipalities Drag their Feet

The post-war period of reconstruction put northern municipalities in financial straits, a situation which hampered the implementation of the new public health legislation. Despite state subsidies for local health care, many municipalities could afford only the bare necessities. When the state allocated health care subsidies it did not take local circumstances or special needs into account (as it did with education subsidies). Health-care provision therefore put greater economic strain on the Lappish municipalities than on more populous municipalities.

Money was short, but the attitude of local authorities also left much to be desired. They showed little enthusiasm in implementing health-care legislation, and failed to found municipal boards of health, or to hire health-care personnel and to provide them with adequate facilities.[80] Local authorities were surprisingly reluctant to listen to public health nurses' proposals for improvement. Apparently, some of the authorities in the rural municipalities failed to see the significance of preventive health care altogether, and the most conservative of them thought that any investment in the health of women and children was a sheer waste of money.[81] This attitude is also reflected in the salaries of trained midwives, which was considerably lower in rural Finland than elsewhere in the Nordic countries.[82]

The law obliged the municipality to provide its public health nurses with lodgings that comprised at least a room and a kitchen and included free lighting and electricity.[83] However, in post-war Finland, and particularly in post-war Lapland, a single woman could rarely expect to have this much living space at her disposal. The public health nurse had to settle with the prevalent standard of housing and often lodged in shop attics or twin rooms in hostels, and many of them worked in cold and draughty temporary huts.[84] Public health nurses and municipal midwifes understood how poor the municipalities were and they did not immediately demand what was theirs by law. However, they did get annoyed because they always seemed to be the ones asked to economize.[85]

Some public health nurses felt that the stinginess of the local authorities had a detrimental impact on their work. Parsimonious municipalities even complained about the cost of the needles and syringes needed for vaccinations. The law obliged the public health nurse to interfere whenever she saw health hazards or shortcomings in health care, but it was not easy to make significant improvements in municipalities where mere vaccination equipment was a bone of contention.[86]

Facilities, too, were often grossly inadequate. When the number of local health centre buildings grew, maternity and child centres increasingly found homes in them. Prior to that, however, much depended on the resourcefulness and negotiation skills of public health nurses. Firm action was needed, for instance, when a municipality that had been donated money for setting up a local health centre kept postponing its construction, or when a municipality tried to appropriate the finished building for other uses. In one case, work on the local health centre building got under way only after successful lobbying by the midwife and the public health nurse, who personally visited every member of the municipal council.[87] When population increase became the top priority of state population policies, the state put more pressure on the municipalities. Local maternity and child health centres played a key role in the new pro-natalist population policies. By the 1950s, more than 500 local health centres had been constructed, thirty-three of which were in the Province of Lapland.[88] Thanks to this building spree, the quality and quantity of the maternity and child health centres was reaching acceptable levels.[89]

The public health nurse could use a taxi on her rounds only when accompanied by a medical officer. When she travelled alone, she had to use cheaper forms of transportation. Increasingly, public health nurses learned to drive and bought cars for themselves. To begin with, public health nurses who drove their own cars on duty had to cover all the expenses themselves, with no help from the municipality. As one local authority put it, 'public health nurses have always cycled'. When driving became more common among public health nurses, municipalities only reimbursed them for a limited number of kilometres. The on-duty driving of, say, the municipal constructor was not limited in this way, because, went the reasoning, he needed to be able to look after communal property effectively. The municipality gave the public health nurse a home phone but regarded it as taxable income. No wonder, then, that public health nurses could be very frustrated by the attitude of local authorities.[90]

At the beginning of the 1960s, there were roughly seventy public health nurses in Lapland. Sixteen of them owned a car. The majority still relied on public transportation or on their own feet.[91] At the end of the decade, some municipalities still allowed the public health nurse to use a car in emergencies only. State agencies sometimes took action against municipalities that systematically neglected the public health nurse's needs, her living and working conditions.[92] The National Board of Health reprimanded some municipalities for underpaying fully qualified public health nurses.[93]

The mobility of the public health nurse mattered for the community. Public health nurses working in remote areas regarded the long and difficult journeys as one of the greatest hindrances that they faced in their work. A considerable part – as much as one third – of their working hours was spent on the road.[94] Their time and expertise would have been better spent if they had been allowed to use a car whenever the road conditions allowed.

Public health nurses looked towards the local boards of health for understanding and support. Unfortunately, they were often disappointed in this respect. Some local boards of health took no interest whatsoever in their work. In other municipalities, not even the admonitions coming from state agencies could convince local authorities to set up a board of health.[95] These municipalities feared the extra expense, and they were no doubt right in believing that a health board with active and committed members would have demanded added resources for health care.

As Sirpa Wrede expresses, local authorities had to be made to see the value of women professionals.[96] Getting their work the appreciation it deserved was not only a matter of money, it was also a matter of perceptions relating to gender. Local authorities needed to learn to set greater value on both female health-care workers and on the health of the women and children who primarily benefited from their efforts.

The Brisk Pioneers of Welfare Work

One must wonder at the dedication, faith and fitness of the staff that stays on in such extreme conditions.[97]

To work in Lapland presented a dream and a challenge for many public health nurses. Those who were attracted to Lapland primarily by the unique, untouched nature were sometimes disappointed – the natural environment did not necessarily prove such a constant source of delight at close range – but those who came looking for challenges and responsibilities were not. Lapland was the right place to be for a public health nurse with a strong sense of vocation (see Figure 12.5).

Health-care work in post-war Lapland called for enthusiasm, initiative and independence, as well as good physical and mental health. Courage was a plus. The public health nurses who came to Lapland in the aftermath of the war no doubt possessed the same sort of boldness and frontier spirit that today makes people undertake relief work in developing countries.

Public health nurses did not leave Lapland because of the harsh environment but rather because they were frustrated by their inability to harmonize their professional ideals with the everyday realities of their work. Their time was often taken up by the treatment of acute complaints rather than by the preventive nursing that they had been trained for and employed to do.[98] Eventually, their calling would desert them.

> After having driven 100 kilometres a day in hail and storm for twelve years, I realized that I would not be able to take this until retirement.[99]

The turnover among public health nurses was great, which surprised neither the local people nor the health care agencies. Rather, there were reasons to wonder why the shortage in the work force was no greater than it was. Public health nurses were paid relatively little, the cost of living was higher in Lapland than elsewhere in the country, the quality of housing was lower, and the great distances made the work harder and more strenuous and also entailed extra expenses (for the accommodation, meals and clothing needed on the road). However, the most common reason that public health nurses named for leaving Lapland was the dissatisfaction that they felt with their job description and with the results of their work.[100]

The period characterized by major public investments in the public health services of remote rural areas did not prove to be very long. It started right after the war, and twenty years later the work was all but done. Starting from the mid-1960s, mass emigration to towns and to Sweden emptied rural Lapland, leaving behind few people to be treated. The health-care work of state provincial governments was now focused on solving the problems caused by urban over-crowding.[101]

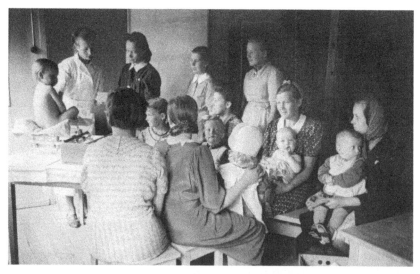

Figure 12.5: A public health nurse at the local health centre of Sodankylä; held at the Collections of Rovaniemi Local Heritage Society Totto and reprinted by permission of Kotiseutuyhdistys Rovaniemen Totto ry.

However, a solid basis had been built for welfare society during those twenty years. Growth in production and income are necessary but not sufficient conditions for increased welfare. Nor can simple economic indicators measure the level of social welfare. The level of social welfare crucially depends on the availability of such things as public health services, educational opportunities, sanitary housing, clean water and good nutrition. Economic growth is not enough to guarantee these. In contrast, British economist Dudley Seers maintains that the best indicators for measuring the level of social welfare are infant mortality, life expectancy and literacy. A society that fares well does not display abject poverty or gross inequality in educational possibilities or in the accessibility of health care.[102] Welfare is attainable only if resources are distributed in a way that makes a good life possible for everyone. Whether economic growth becomes transformed into welfare depends on social values and political will.

During the war and the mass evacuation, infant mortality in Lapland was almost twice as high as in the country as a whole. In the worst years, more than one child in ten died before the age of one. In the mid-1940s, only one child in ten was being monitored by a public health nurse. At the beginning of the 1960s, however, more than nine out of ten children regularly saw a public health nurse. By that time, infant mortality in Lapland was on the same level as in the rest of the country.[103] There was a marked improvement in children's health, which was largely due to the development of the network of local maternity and child health centres and to the health instruction delivered by public health nurses.

The Finns made a value-laden choice in the aftermath of the war: they decided that a return to the pre-war society with its many inequalities was unacceptable. Public welfare was promoted by hard work and for the benefit of all. Some of the problems that post-war health care services faced in the remote areas of the north – long distances, social and economic problems, shaky municipal economies and lack of trained personnel and hospital beds – still existed in the 1960s.[104] However, thanks to many years of hard work, the gravest problems had been solved. The professional skill and competence of public health nurses had been a key factor in the success of this endeavour.

NOTES

Curtis, 'Introduction'

1. See http://www.ipy.org/development/themes.htm [accessed 1 January 2011].
2. See, M. Mörner, 'The Colonization of Norrland by Settlers during the Nineteenth Century in a Broader Perspective', *Scandinavian Journal of History*, 7 (1982), pp. 315–38. The concept of frontier has come under considerable criticism in recent years largely because of the problem of defining it, and the social and cultural assumptions it makes about those living on either side of it. For a useful summary of this debate see, for example, E. Furniss, 'Imagining the Frontier: Comparative Perspectives from Canada and Australia', in D. Bird Rose and R. Davis (eds), *Dislocating the Frontier: Essaying the mystique of the outback* (Canberra: Australian National University, 2005), pp. 23-46.
3. Many current studies of medical provision in areas similar to those studied here demonstrate that governments must be prepared to listen to the sick and respect their traditions rather than simply try to impose a particular type of medical care upon them. See, for example, J. O'Neil, J. Bartlett and J. Mignone, *Best Practices in Intercultural Health: Report* (Winnipeg: Centre for Aboriginal Health Research, 2005); K. Hooper, Y. Thomas and M. Clarke, 'Health Professional Partnerships and their Impact on Aboriginal Health: An Occupational Therapist's and Aboriginal Health Worker's Perspective', *Australian Journal of Rural Health*, 15 (2007), pp. 46–51.
4. See, for example, Y. Berhane, *Women's Health and Reproductive Outcome in Rural Ethiopia* (Umeå: Umeå University, 2000), p. 43. In 1999, G. Walraven and A. Weeks pointed out the necessity of paying heed to the strength of local cultures: 'Cultural sensitivity and the ability to have one's help sought and advice followed may be just as important as technical skill in making an impact on maternal health'. G. Walraven and A. Weeks, 'The Role of (Traditional) Birth Attendants with Midwifery Skills in the Reduction of Maternal Mortality', *Tropical Medicine and International Health*, 4 (1999), pp. 527–9, on p. 527.
5. Among these are M. Grey, *New Deal Medicine: The Rural Health Programs of the Farm Security Administration* (Baltimore, MD: Johns Hopkins University Press, 1999); S. Lee Barney, *Authorized to Heal: Gender, Class, and the Transformation of Medicine in Appalachia, 1880–1930* (Chapel Hill, NC: University of North Carolina, 2000); and S. Stowe, *Doctoring the South: Southern Physicians and Everyday Medicine in the Mid-Nineteenth Century* (Chapel Hill, NC: University of North Carolina, 2004).
6. R. Bowman and J. Kulig suggest that thinking in terms of rural versus urban is probably more useful when studying modern societies than those of the past. R. Bowman and J. Kulig, 'The North American Section of Rural and Remote Health: The Time has Come', *Rural and Remote Health*, 8 (2008), at http://www.rrh.org.au/publishedarticles/article_print_1016.pdf [accessed 1 January 2011].

7. Recent historical studies underscore the growing interest in rural health care although there remains much more work to be done in this area. A fine example is J. L. Barona and S. Cherry, *Health and Medicine in Rural Europe, 1850–1945* (València: University of València, 2005). This collection, a result of the relationship between sponsoring European academic institutions, quite reasonably emphasizes rural health activities in Spain and England but also contains a couple of insightful essays addressing rural medicine in Norway and in Russia.

8. European Association for the History of Medicine and Health. Heidelberg, 3–6 September 2009.

9. See for example, I. Wallerstein, *The Modern World System: Capitalist Agriculture and the Origins of the European World-Economy in the Sixteenth Century* (New York: Academic Press, 1974).

10. H. Vuorinen, 'Core-Periphery Differences in Infant Mortality', *Social Science and Medicine*, 24 (1987), pp. 659–67, on p. 661. See also D. Seers, B. Schaffer and M-L Kiljunen (eds), *Underdeveloped Europe* (Hassocks, Sussex: Harvester Press, 1979), pp. 3–62. Although this collection of essays primarily examines the economic characteristics of cores and peripheries, they also touch upon the social consequences of this unequal relationship. Johan Galtung's work also belongs to this brief summary of the emergence of core/periphery models in the last decades of the twentieth century. He also perpetuated the image of a strong, decision-making core able to exert its will over what is often perceived as a weak, passive or even indifferent periphery. J. Galtung, 'Sosial posisjon og sosial avferd', in *Periferi og Sentrum i historien* (Studier i Historisk Metode X, Universitetsforlaget, Oslo, 1975), p. 9, cited in C. Smout, 'Centre and Periphery in History; with some Thoughts on Scotland as a Case Study', *Journal of Common Market Studies*, 18 (1980), pp. 256–71, on p. 257.

11. Christopher Smout wrote more than two decades ago that there are different hierarchies in this core-periphery relationship that are revealed at the level of parish, province, country, continent or even international region. Smout, 'Centre and Periphery in History', p. 263.

12. Much of the motivation for a re-examination of the nature of the relationship between cores and peripheries, and particularly the alleged passivity of the latter, can be attributed to the new postcolonial histories that emerged first in the late 1970s. Considering the histories of these countries in their own right often reveals a dynamism we would not otherwise expect had we envisioned them solely as mere pawns controlled by others. Mark Harrison argues that when it came to the introduction of new medicines in the colonies even as late as the early twentieth century there was a good deal of reciprocal borrowing between western doctors and local medical practitioners. M. Harrison, 'Science and the British Empire', *Isis*, 96 (2005), pp. 56–63, on pp. 58, 61. David Baranov makes a similar case that we must examine more closely the process of negotiation that enabled western medicine to make inroads in Africa. D. Baranov, *The African Transformation of Western Medicine and the Dynamics of Global Cultural Exchange* (Philadelphia, PA: Temple University Press, 2008).

13. S. Mayhew, 'The Impact of Decentralisation on Sexual and Reproductive Health Services in Ghana', *Reproductive Health Matters*, 11 (2003), pp. 74–87.

14. A. Simões, A. Carneiro and M. P. Diogo (eds), *Travels of Learning: A Geography of Science in Europe* (Dordrecht, Boston, MA, and London: Kluwer Academic Publishers, 2003). The contributors are well aware of the limitations of thinking about cores and peripheries as distinct entities and emphasize the importance of cultural negotiation that occurs between them.

15. T. Hägerstrand, *Innovation Diffusion as a Spatial Process*, trans. A. Pred (Chicago, IL: University of Chicago, 1967).

16. See, for example, N. Skillnäs, 'Modified Innovation Diffusion – A Way to Explain the Diffusion of Cholera in Linköping in 1866? A Study in Methods', *Geografiska Annaler*, series B. 81 (1999), pp. 243–60; R. Ormrod, 'Local Context and Innovation Diffusion in a Well-Connected World', *Economic Geography*, 66 (1990), pp. 109–22.

17. E. Moscardi and A. de Janvry, 'Attitudes toward Risk among Peasants: An Econometric Approach', *American Journal of Agricultural Economics*, 59 (1977), pp. 710–16.

18. R. Ormrod, 'Local Context and Innovation Diffusion in a Well-Connected World', *Economic Geography*, 66 (1990), pp. 109–22. See also L. Fitzgerald, E. Ferlie, M. Wood and C. Hawkins, 'Interlocking Interactions, the Diffusion of Innovations in Health Care', *Human Relations*, 55 (2002), pp. 1429–49; I. Aaraas and E. Swensen, 'Policy Report, National Centre of Rural Medicine in Norway: A Bridge from Rural Practice to the Academy', *Rural and Remote Health*, 8 (2008), at http://www.rrh.org.au/publishedar-ticles/article_print_948.pdf [accessed 1 January 2011]. They write: 'In rural practice, narratives related to illness, family, culture, context and life history often contain information crucial to appropriate patient-centred understanding and decision-making'.

19. T. Valente, 'Social Network Thresholds in the Diffusion of Innovations', *Social Networks*, 18 (1996), pp. 69–89.

20. Barbara Duden's magisterial work illustrates how a careful reading of journals kept by an eighteenth-century German physician can be used to illuminate popular ideas about the workings of the body. See B. Duden, *The Woman Beneath the Skin: A Doctors' Patients in Eighteenth-Century Germany* (Cambridge, MA: Harvard University Press, 1991). Unfortunately, such detailed sources are very rarely found.

1 Cherry and King, 'Medical Services in a Northern Russian Province'

1. Respectively, Reader and Research Fellow in the School of History, University of East Anglia, Norwich, UK.

2. Prof. M. I. Kapustin, a former *zemstvo* doctor, quoted in E. A. Osipov, I. V. Popov and P. I. Kurkin, *Russkaya Zemskaya Meditsina* (Moscow: Izd. Pravleniem Obshchestva russkikh vrachei pri sodeistvii Moskovskoi gubernskoi zemskoi upravy, 1899), p. 96.

3. See also F. King, 'Rural Health Care in Russia: A Northern Case Study', in J. Barona and S. Cherry (eds), *Health and Medicine in Rural Europe c.1850–1945* (Valencia: Scientia Veterum, 2005), pp. 83–102; S. Cherry, 'Rural Health Care in Zemstvo Russia c. 1864–1917', in A. Andresen, T. Gronlie and T. Ryymin (eds), *Science, Culture and Politics: European Perspectives on Medicine, Sickness and Health*, report 4 (Bergen: *Rokkansenteret Report*, 2006), pp. 155–72.

4. See N. Frieden, *Russian Physicians in an Era of Reform and Revolution 1856–1905* (New Jersey: Princeton University Press, 1981), p. 239.

5. The National Library of the Republic of Karelia provides extensive online primary sources concerning Olonets *guberniya*. See http://elibrary.karelia.ru/.

6. See S. C. Ramer, 'The Zemstvo and Public Health', in T. Emmons and W. S. Vucinich, *The Zemstvo in Russia: An Experiment in Local Self-Government* (Cambridge: Cambridge University Press, 1982), pp. 279–314. A contrasting study is P. F. Krug, 'The Debate over the Delivery of Health Care in Rural Russia: The Moscow Zemstvo, 1864–1878', *Bulletin History of Medicine*, 50:2 (1976), pp. 226–41.

7. See, for example, the 1775 Statute on the Provinces. See M. Raeff, *The Well-Ordered Police State: Social and Institutional Change through Law in the Germanies and Russia, 1600–1800* (New Haven, CT: Yale University Press, 1983), pp. 192, 199, 236, 243.

8. H. Seton-Watson, *The Russian Empire 1801–1917* (Oxford: Clarendon Press, 1967), p. 97.

9. Frieden, *Russian Physicians*, p. 80.

10. Ibid., pp. 85–6; Ramer, 'The Zemstvo and Public Health', p. 283. Almost half of the peasantry were on privately owned estates, depending upon landlords or their own efforts for health care.

11. Frieden, *Russian Physicians*, pp. 85–6. There were 414 village pharmacies in 1827 and 749 by 1852: see Seton-Watson, *The Russian Empire 1801–1917*, p. 213.

12. D. T. Orlovsky, *The Limits of Reform: The Ministry of Internal Affairs in Imperial Russia 1802–1881* (Cambridge, MA: Harvard University Press, 1981), pp. 124, 152–3.

13. *Russkaia Starina*, 6 (1913), p. 543, cited in Krug, 'The Debate over the Delivery of Health Care', p. 227.

14. Ramer, 'The Zemstvo and Public Health', pp. 279–80.

15. 'Zemskaia Meditsina', *Entsiklopedicheskii slovar*, 12a (1894), pp. 482–91, cited in B. Veselovsky, *Istoriya zemstva za sorok let*, 4 vols (St Petersburg, 1909), vol. 1, p. 325.

16. Boris Veselovsky (1880–1954) a historian of local government produced between 1909 and 1911 a massive four-volume study reviewing the history of the *zemstvo* over its first forty years. Veselovsky, *Istoriya zemstva*, vol.1, pp. 301–2, 312–13.

17. In 1859 just 4 per cent of the population were serfs, living in the more productive, southerly *uezds* of Lodeynoe Pole and Vytegra. See A. Troinitskii, *The Serf Population in Russia According to the 10th National Census* (Newtonville, MA: Oriental Research Partners, 1982), pp. 43, 61–3.

18. I. Blagoveshchensky, 'Zemledelie', in I. Blagoveshchensky (comp.), *Olonetskiy sbornik, vyp. 4* (Petrozavodsk, 1902), pp. 3, 7, 10.

19. *Pamyatnaya knizhka Olonetskoy gubernii za 1868–69 god* (Petrozavodsk, 1869), pp. 145, 152, 164; *Olonetskaya guberniya: Statisticheskiy spravnochnik* (Petrozavodsk, 1913), pp. 1, 23, 31, 343.

20. *Olonetskaya guberniya*, pp. 29, 30.

21. *Sbornik postanovleniy olonetskikh gubernskikh zemskikh sobraniy s 1867 po 1897 g. (vklyuchitel'no)* (Petrozavodsk, 1898), p. 1. All translations are by the authors unless otherwise indicated.

22. *Zhurnaly vtorogo Olonetskogo gubernskogo zemskogo sobraniya 1867 goda* (Petrozavodsk, 1867), p. 21. In this period 20,000 roubles were worth about £2,000.

23. Ibid pp. 4–5. V. Badanov, 'Zemskaya meditsina na severe Rossii', *Sever*, 11 (1998), p. 129.

24. Ibid, pp. 15–22.

25. Ibid, p. 22.

26. I. A. Shif, 'Kratkiy ocherk razvitiya zemskoy meditsiny v Olonetskoy gubernii', in *Vrachebno-sanitarnyy obzor Olonetskoy gubernii* (Petrozavodsk, 1912), no. 1, p. 41.

27. *Zhurnaly ... 1867*, p. 17; Badanov, 'Zemskaya meditsina', p. 129.

28. *Zhurnaly ... 1867*, p. 35; Shif, 'Kratkiy ocherk', pp. 38–9.

29. Shif, 'Kratkiy ocherk', p. 40.

30. *Zhurnaly Olonetskogo gubernskogo ocherednogo zemskogo sobraniya* (Petrozavodsk, 1872), p. 107.

31. *Zhurnaly* (1872), p. 100.

32. Ibid., p. 101.
33. National Archive of the Republic of Karelia (NARK), f. 10, op. 1, d. 15/5, l. 6; *Zhurnaly* (1872), p. 105.
34. *Zhurnaly ... 1867*, p. 19.
35. Osipov et al., *Russkaya zemskaya meditsina*, p. 74.
36. Veselovsky, *Istoriya zemstva*, vol. 1, pp. 332, 337.
37. Krug, 'The Debate over the Delivery of Health Care', p. 231.
38. Ibid., pp. 233–4.
39. Veselovsky, *Istoriya zemstva*, vol. 1, pp. 310, 354.
40. Osipov et al., *Russkaya zemskaya meditsina*, p. 75.
41. Ramer, 'The Zemstvo and Public Health', p. 292. There were 2,620 independent feldsher points in 1910.
42. *Svedeniya o sovremennom sostoyanii Zemsko-Meditsinskogo dela v Olonetskoy gubernii za 1891 god* (Petrozavodsk, 1892), p. 9; *Protokoly zasedaniy II s"ezda zemskikh vrachey Olonetskoy gubernii* (Petrozavodsk, 1897), p. 70; Blagoveshchensky (comp.), *Pamyatnaya knizhka Olonetskoy gubernii na 1903 god* (Petrozavodsk, 1903), pp. 212–15.
43. *Protokoly II* (1897), Dr Isserson, p. 72.
44. Blagoveshchensky, *Pamyatnaya knizhka*, p. 260.
45. Ibid., pp. 212–15; Report No. 154, Olonets guberniya zemstvo assembly (27 November 1906), p. 5.
46. See *Otchet Obshchestva vzaimopomoshchi fel'dsherov, fel'dsherits i akusherok Olonetskoy gubernii za vremya s 23 marta po 31 dekabrya 1914 g.* (Petrozavodsk, 1915), p. 13.
47. Frieden, *Russian Physicians*, p. 323.
48. Ibid., p. 323; Ramer, 'The Zemstvo and Public Health', p. 292.
49. This table is based on statistics provided in Frieden, *Russian Physicians*, pp. 358, 360; Veselovsky, *Istoriya zemstva*, vol.1, p.703.
50. Veselovsky, *Istoriya zemstva*, vol. 1, pp. 699, 702.
51. Ibid., vol. 1, p. 366.
52. Ibid., vol. 1, pp. 703, 360, 363.
53. Shif, 'Kratkiy ocherk', p. 41.
54. *Zhurnaly* (1872), p. 21.
55. *Protokoly I* (1887), Dr Isserson, p. 31.
56. *Protokoly II* (1897), Dr Isserson, p. 28.
57. Ibid., p. 29.
58. Dr Shif, *Kratikiy ochark*, p. 43.
59. *Vrachebno-sanitarnyy obzor*, no. 1, p. 129.
60. Veselovsky, *Istoria zemstva*, vol.1, p. 386. Prikaz hospitals could be very poor: that in Samara was grossly overcrowded and 'the majority of cases ... regarded the necessity of going in to hospital as a punishment from God', according to P. B. Alabin, *Dvadtsatipya-tiletie Samary, kak gubernskago goroda* [The Twenty-Fifth Anniversary of Samara as a Guberniya town] (Gubernskaya tipografiya Samara, 1877), p. 14.
61. Veselovsky, *Istoria zemstva*, vol. 1, p. 388. Data on 1,054 of the 1,440 hospitals identified suggests that nearly 60 per cent of these had fifteen beds or less.
62. Ibid., vol. 1, pp. 388–91.
63. *Protokoly I* (1887), p. 72. The 761 patients in 1886 included just 165 women and 22 children, with 11 babies delivered. Muscular rheumatism, syphilis and ulcer cases featured prominently.
64. Ibid., p. 48.

65. Ibid., p. 62; *Svedeniya o sovremennom*, p. 8.
66. *Protokoly I* (1887), p. 28, pp. 96–7.
67. Blagoveshchensky, *Pamyatnaya knizhka*, pp. 208–12.
68. *Sbornik postanovleniy ... 1867 po 1897*, p. 16.
69. S. Cherry, 'Medicine and Rural Health Care in 19th Century Europe', in Barona and Cherry (eds), *Health and Medicine in Rural Europe*, pp. 19–62, on pp. 26–38.
70. The infant mortality rate averaged 243 per 1,000 births in 1867 and still 237 per 1,000 in 1911. B. R. Mitchell, *International Historical Statistics: Europe 1750–1988* (Basingstoke: Macmillan, 1992), pp. 138–41. Roughly half of those born died by the age of five years.
71. V. Veresaeff (V. Smidovitch), *The Confessions of a Physician*, trans. S. Linden (London: Grant Richards, 1904), p. 281.
72. D. I-va, 'Russkaia mysl', 12 (1884), p.78, cited in Veselovsky, *Istoriya zemstva*, vol.1, p. 289.
73. Frieden, *Russian Physicians*, p. 239.
74. R. L. Glickman, 'The Peasant Woman as Healer', in E. B. Clements, E. A. Engel and C. W. Worobec (eds), *Russia's Women: Accommodation, Resistance, Transformation* (Berkeley, CA: University of California Press, 1991), vol. 1, pp. 148–62, 154.
75. N. Frieden, 'Child Care: Medical Reform in a Traditionalist Culture', in D. L. Ransel (ed.), *The Family in Imperial Russia* (Chicago, IL: University of Illinois Press, 1978), pp. 220–45, on p. 240.
76. O. Tian-Shanskaia, *Village Life in Late Tsarist Russia* (*c*.1891), trans. D. Ransel (Bloomington, IN: Indiana University Press, 1993), respectively pp. 24–5, 13, 19.
77. '[T]hus Praskoyva Korotchenkova left her hospitalized baby son, suffering from pneumonia, to tend a cow about to calve, because "the cow ... feeds everyone ... How was I going to manage without the cow? What was I going to feed the children?"', cited in D. Ransel, *Village Mothers: Three Generations of Change in Russia and Tataria* (Bloomington, IN: Indiana University Press, 2003), p. 186.
78. Frieden, 'Child Care', p. 240.
79. State Archive of Samara Oblast (GASO), f. 4, o. 4, d. 214 1.47.
80. Veresaeff, *The Confessions of a Physician*, p. 230.
81. Veselovsky, *Istoria zemstva*, vol. 1, pp. 309–10.
82. NARK, f. 14, op.1, d. 19/18, ll. 34–5. Letter, 23 April 1874.
83. See J. K. Pratt, 'The Free Economic Society and the Battle against Smallpox', *The Russian Review*, 61 (October 2002), pp. 560–78, 566, 573. The Society promoted calf lymph supplies and *teliatniki*, vaccine supply units.
84. *Protokoly I* (1887), Dr Isserson (Lodeynoe Pole), pp. 36, 37.
85. *Doklady Olonetskoy gubernskoy zemskoy upravy gubernskomu zemskomu sobraniyu sessiy chrezvychaynoy 31 maya i 1 iyunya 1901 goda i XXXV–y ocherednoy s 29 noyabrya po 15 dekabrya 1901 goda* (Petrozavodsk, 1902), p. 390.
86. *Protokoly II* (1897), Dr Isserson (Lodeynoe Pole), p. 31.
87. Ibid., p. 14.
88. Ibid., pp. 14–15.
89. Ibid.
90. See *Protokoly II*, (1897), p. 32.
91. *Zhurnaly* (1872), p. 103; *Sbornik postanovleniy ... 1867 po 1897*, p. 38.
92. *Protokoly II* (1897), p. 32.
93. See *Vrachebno-sanitarnyy obzor*, no. 1, pp. 70, 83.

94. Osipov et al., *Russkaya zemskaya meditsina*, pp. 28–9. The comparable average for England and Wales was 152.
95. *Zhurnaly ... 1867*, pp. 17–18.
96. *Protokoly II* (1897), Dr Isserson (Lodeynoe Pole), pp. 108, 103.
97. Ibid., Dr Shepilevsky (Olonets), p. 14.
98. Ibid., Dr Ol'gsky (Kargopol'), p. 22.
99. Ibid., p. 107.
100. Ramer, 'The Zemstvo and Public Health', p. 220.
101. *Sbornik postanovleniy ...1867 po 1897*, p. 2.
102. Reports appended to *Protokoly I* (1887), pp. 2–3, 7–9.
103. NARK, f. 10, op. 1, d. 80/52. 'On Organizing a Congress of Doctors in Olonets guberniya', ll.1–2ob. Letter dated 6 November 1885 from Kargopol' uezd zemstvo uprava to Olonets guberniya zemstvo uprava.
104. Ibid., Letter dated 6 November 1885.
105. *Protokoly I* (1887), appendix, p. 11; *Protokoly II* (1897), p. 121.
106. A. A. Tsvetaev, *O vvedenii sanitarnoy organizatsii v Olonetskoy gubernii i smetnykh soobrazheniyakh na 1913 g.* (Petrozavodsk, 1912).
107. *Protokoly II* (1897), p. 119 (reporting on the 1896 Olonets Doctors' Congress).
108. Krug, 'The Debate over the Delivery of Health Care', p. 236.
109. See E. Fee and D. Porter, 'Public Health, Preventive Medicine and Professionalization: England and America in the Nineteenth Century', in A. Wear (ed.), *Medicine in Society: Historical Essays* (Cambridge: Cambridge University Press, 1992), pp. 265–75, on pp. 250–1.
110. Our comparator study of Samara province quotes an Alekseevka doctor: '[T]here is never complete trust (but) ... the injection of diphtheria serum, which represents such a great step forward ... does enjoy a certain authority; it is very rare that the injection is refused'. GASO, f. 4, op. 4, d. 214 l.47 11.6. Similarly in Buguruslan: '[O]ne only needs to remove a cataract ... and almost all the sick there will turn up requesting the "knife"'. GASO, f. 4, op. 4, d. 214 l.47 11.4. See S. Cherry, 'Rural Health Care in Zemstvo Russia', *International Journal of Regional and Local Studies*, 2:2 (2006), pp. 72–91, p. 86.
111. Glickman cites a study of 125 herbs used by *znakharki*, who also used mercury toxins in the treatment of pox, for example. Glickman, 'Peasant Woman as Healer', p. 155.
112. This was the experience of an eighteen-year-old dropsy sufferer in September 1910. NARK, f. 236, op.1, d. 10/90, pp. 58–60.
113. In *zemstvo* areas 34 per 1,000 population were registered sick compared with 14 per 1,000 in non-*zemstvo* areas, with 68 per cent attended by a qualified doctor (c.f. 53 per cent) and 4 per cent securing hospital treatment (c.f. 3 per cent). Veselovsky, *Istoria zemstva*, vol. 1, pp. 421–3.
114. Ibid., p. 430. *Zemstvo* medical spending per head was 56 kopeks in 1904, compared with 22 in non-*zemstvo* European Russia, 44 in the Don, 33 in Siberia, 32 in the Caucasus and just 9 in Central Asia, although 66 in the Baltic.
115. J. F. Hutchinson, *Politics and the Public Health in Revolutionary Russia, 1890–1918* (Baltimore, MD: Johns Hopkins University Press, 1990), pp. 470–2; J. F. Hutchinson, 'Death of Zemstvo Medicine', in S. G. Soloman and J. F. Hutchinson (eds), *Health and Society in Revolutionary Russia* (Bloomington, IN: Indiana University Press, 1990), pp. 1–15, 13.
116. Veselovsky, *Istoriya zemstva*, vol. 4, p. 277, p. 429.
117. Badanov, 'Zemskaya meditsina', p. 132.

118. Veselovsky, *Istoriya zemstva*, vol. 1, p. 712; for his overall assessment of Olonets *guberniya*, see vol. 4, pp. 622–31.
119. Shif, 'Kratkiy ocherk', p. 40.
120. Veselovsky, *Istoriya zemstva*, vol. 1, pp. 684–5.
121. Ibid., vol. 1, pp. 698–9, 703.
122. Ibid., vol. 1, p. 133.

2 Ryymin, 'Changing Minority Culture'

1. Between 1920 and 1945, the eastern national border in Finnmark was with Finland, which had gained access to the Arctic Ocean through the so-called Petsjenga (Petsamo) corridor in the aftermath of the First World War. Finland ceded this territory to Russia after the Second World War.
2. Statistisk sentralbyrå/Statistics Norway, Befolkning, table 3.2., Hjemmehørende folkemengde etter fylke/Resident population by county, at http://www.ssb.no/histstat/tabeller/3-3-2t.txt [accessed 31 January 2011].
3. See Norwegian official report (NOU) number 18, *NOU 1984:18 Om samenes rettsstilling* (Oslo: Universitetsforlaget, 1984), p. 83, table 3.1.
4. The standard reference work on these issues is K. E. Eriksen and E. Niemi, *Den finske fare. Sikkerhetsproblemer og minoritetspolitikk i nord 1860–1940* (Oslo: Universitetsforlaget, 1981).
5. See T. Ryymin, 'Civilizing the "Uncivilized": The Fight against Tuberculosis in Northern Norway at the Beginning of the Twentieth Century', *Acta Borealia*, 24:2 (2007), pp. 143–61, on, pp. 144–6.
6. See, for example, C. Gierløff, *Gjennem Finmarken med renskyss* (Kristiania: H. Aschehoug & Co. (W. Nygaard), 1918), p. 45, where he describes the Sami as 'et folk viet til undergang'. See J. Raftery, *Not Part of the Public. Non-Indigenous Policies and the Health of Indigenous South Australians 1836–1973* (Kent Town: Wakefield Press, 2006), pp. 159–64 for a discussion of a similar 'doomed race' discourse in an Australian context.
7. For a telling example, see A. Helland, *Topografisk-statistisk beskrivelse over Finmarkens amt. Anden del. Befolkning og historie*, Norges Land og Folk topografisk-statistisk beskrevet, 20 vols (Kristiania: H. Aschehoug & Co., 1906), vol. 20, p. 425: see also Eriksen and Niemi, *Den finske fare*, p. 37.
8. *NOS. Beretning om Sunnhetstilstanden og Medicinalforholdene i Norge 1900*, 4:55 (Kristiania: Direktøren for det Civile Medicinalvæsen, 1902), pp. 271–82 (Finmarkens amt), table on p. 271.
9. I. Elstand and T. Hamran, *Sykdom. Nord-Norge før 1940* (Bergen: Fagbokforlaget, 2006), pp. 121–3.
10. *Om sykehusforholdene i Finnmark og planene for gjenoppbygging av de permanente sykehus*, St.meld., nr.19 (1948), p. 1; *Medisinalmelding for Finnmark 2001*, Fylkeslegen i Finnmark 2002, p. 5, at: http://www.helsetilsynet.no/upload/Helsetilsynet%20i%20 fylkene/finnmark/finnmark_medisinalmelding2001.pdf [accessed 26 May 2010].
11. On the role of voluntary associations in the provision of health services in Northern Norway, see Elstand and Hamran, *Sykdom, passim*.
12. J. Vea, 'To ulike kriser, to ulike svar. Fiskerbondesamfunnet i Nordland 1896–1940', *Heimen*, 38 (2000), pp. 3–14, on p. 4.

13. '"Fællesgammerne" og det Liv, som der leves, antagelig danner Lavmaalet af menneskelig Tilværelse i Europa'. District medical officer in Kistrand, N. Christoffersen, in *NOS. Beretning om Sunnhetstilstanden og Medicinalforholdene i Norge 1903* (Finmarkens amt), p. 283. All translations by Teemu Ryymin.

14. J. Backer, *Trend of Mortality and Causes of Death in Norway 1856–1955* (Oslo: Central Bureau of Statistics of Norway, 1961), pp. 208–9, table 138.

15. Helland, Topografisk-statistisk beskrivelse, p. 48.

16. This table is based on statistics provided in *Sunnhetstilstanden og medisinalforholdene* (1933), p. 13; (1935), p. 23; (1940), p. 25.

17. A. Steen, *Finnemisjonen 75 år. 1888 – 28. februar – 1963* (Trondheim: Norges Finnemisjonsselskap, 1963), pp. 9–15.

18. For an overview of the debates on Læstadianism, see E. A. Drivenes and E. Niemi, 'Også av denne verden? Etnisitet, geografi og læstadianisme mellom tradisjon og modernitet', in Ø. Norderval and S. Nesset (eds), *Vekkelse og vitenskap: Lars Levi Læstadius 200 år* (Tromsø: Universitetsbiblioteket i Tromsø, 2000), pp. 157–87.

19. Steen, *Finnemisjonen*, p. 19.

20. 'Det er i det hele taget utrolig, hvor mange syge og vanføre, halte, blinde og døve i alle Aldre, der findes blandt Finnerne. Paa enkelte Steder kan man rent forfærdes over deres Mængde og over den navnløse Elendighed, de maa leve i. Jeg tror, jeg trygt tør sige, at der ikke er et Sted i Landet, der en saadan Rigdom paa afsidesliggende Steder, hvorhen Presten aldrig har Anledning til at komme, og en saadan sørgelig Overflod paa Krøblinge, der aldrig kan komme til Herrens Bord, som Finmarken'. Statsarkivet i Tromsø, Privatarkiv 69 Norges Sememisjon (hereafter SiTØ PA 69), 128 Årsberetninger, G. Tandberg in *Norges Finne-mission 1896*, p. 24.

21. J. Lye, 'Samemisjonens utvikling 1888–1925' (MSc dissertation (hovedoppgave), University of Tromsø, 1999), p. 34; H.-J. Wallin Weihe, *'Social Work' and Missionary Work as Part of the Power Game. A Discussion through Two examples: Hans Egede Missionary in Greenland 1721–1736 and The Norwegian Saami Mission in Finnmark: The Period of Establishing Missions and Social Services 1888–1900* (Lund: Socialhögskolan, 1999), pp. 187–9.

22. Wallin-Weihe, *'Social Work' and Missionary Work*, p. 223.

23. See A. B. Wessel, 'Bidrag til Finnmark fylkes medisinalhistorie', in *Tidsskrift for Den norske lægeforening* 49 (1929), pp. 992–1006, 1047–62, 1094–1110, 1149–65. Three of the thirty-nine institutions were not yet built in 1929.

24. I. Tjelle, *Omsorg og overgrep: Møter med barnehjemsbarn* (Alta: Nordnorsk forlag, 2005), p. 18.

25. Elstad and Hamran, *Sykdom*, pp. 242–5, 258–63, 359–64, 377–97, 420–2, 480–6.

26. See *Finnmark Fylkestings forhandlinger* (hereafter *FF*), 93 (1931), p. 379; *FF* 56 (1932), p. 293.

27. Elstand and Hamran, *Sykdom*, pp. 362–4.

28. O. Ugland, *Der Herren bereder vei* (Oslo: Hellstrøm & Nordahls Boktrykkeri A.s., 1948), p. 27.

29. B. Evjen, *Et sammensatt fellesskap. Tysfjord kommune 1869–1950* (Bodø: Tysfjord kommune, 1998), pp. 137–8; K. T. Andersen, 'Læstadianismen i Tysfjord fra 1850 til andre verdenskrig' (unpublished manuscript, 1995), pp. 35–6, available at http://ask.bibsys. no/ask/action/show?cmd=alle&pid=061274925&kid=biblio [accessed 1 January 2011].

30. See Elstand and Hamran, *Sykdom*, pp. 486–7.
31. See A. Andresen, 'Perspectives on the Interaction of Medicine and Rural Cultures: Spain, Norway and European Russia 1860s–1910s', in J. L. Barona and S. Cherry (eds), *Health and Medicine in Rural Europe (1850–1945)* (València: Seminari d'estudis sobre la ciència, 2005), p. 160.
32. See Steen, *Finnemisjonen*, pp. 29–30, 34–6, 88–91, 109–113.
33. 'Samenes eget mål blir å benyttes i den utstrekning som ansees fornøden, så lenge samene selv ønsker det samiske språk benyttet'. Articles of association for Norsk Finnemisjons-selskap, 1926, cited in Tjelle, *Omsorg og overgrep*, p. 77.
34. Tjelle, *Omsorg og overgrep*, p. 77.
35. See SiTØ PA 69 number 123, Årsberetning 1925; number 128, Årsberetning 1923–4, p. 6; number 123, 'Hovedstyre til J. Børrezen', 14 March 1941; Elstand and Hamran, *Sykdom*, pp. 483–4.
36. 'Det Norsk-Luth. Finnemissionsforbund 1910–12.juli-1920', in *Det Norsk-Lutherske Finnemissionsforbund 1910–1920* (Stavanger: Dreyers, 1921), pp. 11, 29.
37. Ibid., p. 10.
38. Ibid., p. 11.
39. 'Heve deres (samenes) kulturelle nivå ved å bibringe dem vår norske kulturs fordeler'. G. Tandberg in *Lappernes Ven*, 19 (1911), cited in B. A. Devik, *Sameskolen i Havika 1910–1951. Et tidskifte i sørsamenes kulturreising* (Tromsø: Tromsø Museum, 1980), p. 42).
40. 'har længe nok været foragtet, de har længe nok faat bo i jordhuler, de har længe nok været skubbet tilside fra de bedste pladser, deres aandsevner har længe nok været forkrøb-let av fornorskningen, de har længe nok faat høre at de ikke duet til noget stort, men at det var bra om de kunne bli norske mænds tjenere. Litt efter litt vil dette forandres under Guds naadessol', *Det Norsk-Lutherske Finnemissionsforbund 1910–1920* (Stavanger: Dreyers, 1921), pp. 29–30.
41. *Norsk Finnemisjons Blad*, (1918), p. 122.
42. K. Brevik, 'Vårt kristelig-sociale arbeide', in *Norsk Finnemisjonsselskaps Årbok 1931–33* (Trondheim: Finnemisjonsselskapet, 1935), p. 46; 'Ordentlig husliv', cited in Wallin-Weihe, *'Social Work' and Missionary Work*, p. 175, n. 117; see also p. 253.
43. '[D]e gamle beredes til den siste reis inn i evighetens verden', *Norsk Finnemisjonsselskaps Årbok 1938–1944* (Trondheim: Finnemisjonsselskapet, 1945), p. 22.
44. See Steen, *Finnemisjonen*, pp. 95–6, 118, 172–8; B. Regeland, 'Fra Øytun ungdomsskole', in *Det Norsk-Lutherske Finnemissionsforbund 1910–1920* (Stavanger: Dreyers, 1921), p. 48 and p. 49; Devik, *Sameskolen, passim*; *Utgreiing av skoledirektøren i Finnmark om: Særlige tiltak vedkommende opplæringa i de språkblandede distrikt*, in *Tilråding om Samiske skole- og opplæringsspørsmål* (Oslo: Samordningsnemnda for skoleverket, 1948), appendix 2, p. 21.
45. '[A]v stor vigtighet er det jo ogsaa at faa sat barnet paa ret kjøl mens det er saa litet. Derved kan man ha haap om at faa fjernet de medfødte tilbøieligheter og kanter, som vel er mere merkbare blandt et naturfolk som lapperne end blandt de folk som gjennem aarrækker har været under kultur. Årsberetning for Haviken hjem og skole for lappebarn, 1917–1918', *Norsk Finnemisjons Blad*, 1918, p. 141.
46. Devik, *Sameskolen*, p. 35; Steen, *Finnemisjonen*, p. 176.
47. 'Det Norsk-Luth. Finnemissionsforbund 1910–12.juli-1920', p. 26; J. Otterbech, 'Vort arbeidsfelt', in *Det Norsk-Lutherske Finnemissionsforbund 1910–1920* (Stavanger: Drey-ers, 1921,) pp. 52–3.
48. The following discussion is based on Ryymin, 'Civilizing the "Uncivilized"'.

49. 'Men ved siden av herav gjælder det om at være opmerksom paa og støtte alt, som bidrar til ellers at utvikle landsdelen i økonomisk, kulturel og hygienisk henseende'. *Tuberkulosen i Finmarken og dens bekjæmpelse. Indstilling fra den av Den norske nationalforening mot tuberkulosen nedsatte komite* (Bergen: Nationalforeningen, 1914), hereafter *TiF* (1914), p. 16.

50. R. Dubos, *The White Plague: Tuberculosis, Man and Society* (1952; New Brunswick: Rutgers University Press, 1996), pp. 197–207.

51. *TiF* (1914), pp. 14–15, 18.

52. Ibid., pp. 11–12, 36–41.

53. Ibid., p. 41.

54. T. Ryymin, *Smitte, språk og kultur. Tuberkulosearbeidet i Finnmark* (Oslo: Scandinavian Academic Press, 2009).

55. See T. Ryymin, '"Tuberculosis-Threatened Children": The Rise and Fall of a Medical Concept in Norway, c.1900–1960', *Medical History*, 52 (2008), pp. 347–64.

56. Odelstingsproposisjon (Ot.prp.), 10 (1914), *Om utferdigelse av Lov om smaabruk- og boliglaan m.v.*, pp. 74–7 (§ 83); *Lov om smaabruk- og boliglaan m.v. 23. juli 1915* (§ 83).

57. *Forhandlinger i Stortinget*, 19:5 (1915), pp. 789, 793.

58. Ryymin, 'Civilizing the "Uncivilized"', p. 150.

59. Ryymin, '"Tuberculosis-Threatened Children"', p. 356.

60. '[A]t støtte alt det, som har til formaal at øke befolkningens almindelige oplysningstilstand', *TiF* (1914), pp. 111–12.

61. L. Lind Meløy, *Internatliv i Finnmark. Skolepolitikk 1900–1940* (Oslo: Det Norske Samlaget, 1980); Eriksen and Niemi, *Den finske fare*, pp. 59–61.

62. 'I hygienisk henseende kan deres betydning neppe overvurderes. Ved siden av undervisning i de almindelige skolefag lærer barnene ogsaa at klæ av sig, at ligge ordentlig i seng, istedetfor som ofte i hjemmene at ligge fuldt paaklædt paa gulvet, at ordne denne, naar de staar op og lufte sine sengklær, at vaske sig, samt at holde sit rum i orden. Videre lærer de at sitte ordentlig til bords, at spise med kniv og gaffel, og at ha hver sine kopper m.v. under maaltiderne'. *TiF* (1914), pp. 116–17.

63. See *TiF* (1914), pp. 115–17, 118–19.

64. Ryymin, 'Civilizing the "Uncivilized"', pp. 149–150; T. Ryymin, 'Formaningens former i et flerspråklig område. Opplysningsarbeid mot tuberkulose i Finnmark', in K. Malterud, K. T. Elvbakken and P. Solvand (eds), *Sunnhet og sykdom i kulturelt perspektiv* (Bergen: Rokkansenteret, 2005), pp. 90–4.

65. Eriksen and Niemi, *Den finske fare*, pp. 122, 141, 160.

66. 'Finmarkens beliggenhet er saa utsat, dens befolkning saa opblandet med fremmede elementer, at ethvert arbeide, selv det mindste, for at knytte denne landsdel til det øvrige land, ogsaa blir et nationalt arbeide av betydning. Det øker fædrelandsfølelsen og styrker samfølelsen og de dager kan komme, da begge skal staa sin prøve', *TiF* (1914), p. 18.

67. Ryymin, 'Civilizing the "Uncivilized"', pp. 152–5.

68. Ibid., pp. 155–6.

69. See the annual reports of activity of the Finnmark County Tuberculosis Board in the 1930s in *FF*; see also Elstad and Hamran, *Sykdom*, pp. 423–4.

70. '[D]erfor blir det tidlig diagnose av nye tilfeller, oppsporing av mulige smittekilder av nyere og eldre dato, og behandling og helst uskadeliggjøring av alle oppdagede tilfeller som blir det viktigste for oss', *FF* (1939), Sak 24.1939, p. 84.

71. Ryymin, 'Civilizing the "Uncivilized"', pp. 156–7.

72. Ryymin, '"Tuberculosis-Threatened Children"', p. 359.

73. K. Evang, 'Noen aktuelle oppgaver ved gjenreisningen av den norske folkehelsen og det norske helsevesen', *Tidsskrift for Den norske lægeforening*, 65 (1945), pp. 266–71; K. Evang, *Gjenreisning av folkehelsa i Norge* (Oslo: Fabritius & Sønners forlag, 1947).

74. Evang, *Gjenreisning*, p. 97.

75. See R. Slagstad, *De nasjonale strateger* (Oslo: Pax Forlag, 1998), p. 210.

76. National Archives, PA-1245 Nasjonalforeningen for folkehelsen. Af Sentralstyret, 2, Sentralstyret 1952–1954, 'Til sentralstyrets medlemmer', 15 November 1952; Minutes from a meeting of the National Association central board, 18 November 1952. The brochure can be found in National Archives, S-1285, Sosialdepartementet, Helsedirektoratet, D, 70, 'Brosjyrer vedrørende BCG-vaksinasjon'.

77. 'Til fylkesmannen i Finnmark. Dekning av utgifter til trykning av brosjyrer på samisk i forbindelse med skjermbildefotograferingen i Finnmark i 1954', 17 February 1954, National Archives, S-1285, Sosialdepartementet, Helsedirektoratet, D, 61, jnr 774/54.

78. 'Fylkeslegen i Finnmark til Helsedirektoratet, tuberkulosekontoret', 26 January 1954, National Archives, S-1285 Sosialdepartementet, Helsedirektoratet, D, 61.

79. See brochures in Sami for 1958 and 1960 in National Archives, S-1285 Sosialdepartementet, Helsedirektoratet, D, 103; for newspaper notifications, National Archives, S-1285 Sosialdepartementet, Helsedirektoratet, D, 61.

80. In 1952, 284 Finnish citizens were screen examined in the Tana Valley. This number increased in 1956 to 365. National Archives, S-1285 Sosialdepartementet, Helsedirektoratet, D, 102, Finnmark county medical officer Jonassen to *länsläkare* Hirvonen, 'Tuberkuloseundersøkelsen i Tanadalen 24.mars-17.april 1952', 28 April 1952; Finnmark county medical officer Jonassen to Helsedirektoratet, Tuberkulosekontoret, 'Skjermbildefotograferingen i Finnmark 1958 – den finske grensebefolkning', 12 November 1957.

81. 'Fylkeslegen i Finnmark til Helsedirektoratet, tb.kontoret', 16 March 1951 National Archives, S-1285 Sosialdepartementet, Helsedirektoratet, D, 102; 'S.D.jnr. 3470/51 H.dir.3. *P.M. Skjermbildefotograferingen i Finnmark 1952*', 6 August 1951.

82. 'Samene er et livskraftig folk, kulturelt tilpasset det circumpolare miljø ... Det som er truet av utdøen, er den samiske kultur som er utsatt for et voldsomt press i forbindelse med de senere års industrialisering og mekanisering av livet i bygdene'. J. Torgersen, 'Noen populasjonsgenetiske data fra samene', *Tidsskrift for Den norske lægeforening*, 76 (1956), p. 810.

83. Torgersen, 'Noen populasjonsgenetiske data', p. 810.

84. 'Flyttsamene har bare sparsomt fått del i den materielle og kulturelle fremgang i tiden. Hittil er det aldri blitt utdannet en samisk lege, en samisk ingeniør eller tannlege. Samene har ikke høve til å få almenkunnskaper på sitt morsmål. De er henvist til å erverve dem via norsk i løpet av en kort folkeskole, hvor norsk først må læres ... Lægene bør når det gjelder helseopplysningsarbeidet bruke det samiske språk der det lar seg gjøre'. Ø. Jonassen, 'Sosiale og hygieniske forhold i flyttsamenes basisområde', *Tidsskrift for Den norske lægeforening*, 79 (1959), p. 118.

85. '[H]elsestellet ... bør forsøke å bygge mest mulig på det verdifulle i samenes egen livsførsel fra gammelt av. Vondt kan ellers bli verre', Jonassen, 'Sosiale og hygieniske forhold', p. 118.

3 Andresen, 'The Sami, Sami-ness and the Staffing of Health Services in Northern Norway'

1. Senter for samisk helseforskning, at http://uit.no/medsamisk/2011/?colapsemenu=col apsemenu [accessed 1 May 2008].
2. T. Grønlie, 'Tiden etter 1945', in R. Danielsen et al., *Grunntrekk i norsk historie fra vikingtid til våre dager* (Oslo: Universitetsforlaget, 1991), p. 330.
3. On Norwegian minority policy, see K. E. Eriksen and E. Niemi, *Den finske fare. Sikkerhetsproblemer og minoritetspolitikk i nord 1860–1940* (Oslo: Universitetsforlaget, 1981); E. Niemi, 'Kategorienes etikk og minoritetene i nord. Et historisk perspektiv', in *Samisk forskning og forskningsetikk. Den nasjonale forskningsetiske komité for samfunnsvitenskap og humaniora* (Oslo: De nasjonale forskningsetiske komiteer, publikasjon 2, 2002), pp. 32–8; H. Minde, 'Assimilation of the Sami – Implementation and Consequences', *Acta Borealia*, 2 (2003), pp. 121–46.
4. B. Aarseth, *Norsk samepolitikk 1945–1990. Målsetting, virkemidler og resultater* (Oslo: Forlaget Vett og Viten/ Norsk Folkemuseums Samiske Samlinger, 2006), pp. 347–445.
5. See A. Andresen, 'In the Wake of the Kautokeino-Event: Changing Perception of Insanity and of the Sámi 1852–1965', *Acta Borealia*, 24:2 (2007), pp. 130–42; S. A. Skaalevaag, 'Medical Hermeneutics of Murder: Race, Medicine and Law in a Murder Case from Finnmark, 1911', *Acta Borealia*, 24:2 (2007), pp. 109–29.
6. F. Barth (ed.), *Ethnic Boundaries: The Social Organization of Culture Difference* (Bergen: Scandinavian University Books, 1969). See also L. I. Hansen and B. Olsen, *Samenes historie fram til 1750* (Oslo: Cappelen Akademisk Forlag, 2004), pp. 31–45.
7. V. Merton, 'Nå skal du høre ka æ mene med arv', *Samisk forståelse av arv som en utfordring i medisinsk genetikk*, ISM skriftserie nr. 90-2006 (Senter for samisk helseforskning/Institutt for samfunnsmedisin, Universitetet i Tromsø), pp. 177–9, 183–7.
8. A. B. Ross, Å. Johansson, M. Ingman and U. Gyllensten, 'Lifestyle, Genetics and Disease in Sami', *Croatian Medical Journal*, 47 (2006), p. 554.
9. For example, M. Ingman and U. Gyllensten, 'A Recent Genetic Link between Sami and the Volga-Ural Region of Russia', *European Journal of Human Genetics*, 15 (2007), pp. 115–20. This is one article in a long list of publications on genetic links. A similar interest in 'origins' has made an imprint upon genetic research in other parts of the world. See, for example, F. R. Santos, A. Pandya, C. Tyler-Smith, M. Schanfield, W. R. Osipova, M. H. Crawford and R. J. Mitchell, 'The Central Siberian Origin for Native American Y Chromosomes', *American Journal of Human Genetics*, 64:2 (1999), pp. 619–28.
10. Ross et al., 'Lifestyle, Genetics and Disease in Sami', pp. 553–65.
11. For example, L. Soininen and E. Pukkala, 'Mortality of the Sami in Northern Finland 1979–2005', *International Journal of Circumpolar Health*, 67:1 (2008), pp. 45.
12. Hansen and Olsen, *Samenes historie fram til 1750*, p. 44.
13. Ibid., pp. 44–5; A. Schanche, 'Rase, etnisitet og samisk forhistorie. Et forskningshistorisk tilbakeblikk', in J. E. Myhre, *Historie, etnisitet og politikk*, Stensilserie B, 59 (Institutt for historie, Universitetet i Tromsø, 2000), pp. 3–18.
14. N. Risch, E. Burchard, E. Ziv and H. Tang, 'Categorization of Humans in Biomedical Research: Genes, Race and Disease', at http://genomebiology.com/2003/3/7/comment/2007.1 [accessed 13 May 2008].
15. S. Kvernmo, 'Developing Sami Health Services – A Medical and Cultural Challenge', in H. Gaski (ed.), *Sami Culture in a New Era: The Norwegian Sami Experience* (Seattle, WA: University of Washington Press, 1998), p. 134; T. Ryymin, 'Opplysningens

former i et flerspråklig område. Opplysningsarbeid mot tuberkulose i Finnmark', in K. Malterud, K. T. Elvbakken and P. Solvang (eds), *Sunnhet og sykdom i kulturelt perspektiv* (Bergen: Rokkansenteret, Rapport 12, 2005), pp. 91–4.

16. Eriksen and Niemi, *Den finske fare*, pp. 298–9.
17. *Samordningsnemda for skoleverket oppnemd ved kongeleg resolusjon 7 mars 1947. Tilråding om Samiske skole- og opplysningsspørsmål* (Oslo: Brødrene Tengs, 1948); Aarseth, *Norsk samepolitikk*, pp. 33, 67–8; Minde, 'Assimilation of the Sami'.
18. Betenkning fra nomadskolinspektør, dr. israel Ruong og professor, dr. Knut Bergsland om felles skriftspråk for norske og svenske samer og bruken av det i folkeopplysningens tjeneste. Samordningsnemda for skoleverket 1948, p. 12.
19. Innstilling fra Komiteen til å utrede samespørsmål. Oppnevnt 3 august 1956 (Mysen: Indre Smaalenenes Trykkeri, 1959), pp. 3, 62.
20. J. Torgersen, 'Noen populasjonsgenetiske data fra samene', *Tidsskrift for den norske lægeforening* 75 (1956), pp. 809–10.
21. For the text of the 1950 document see, http://unesdoc.unesco.org/images/0012/001282/128291eo.pdf [accessed 12 May 2008].
22. See, for example, Ø. Jonassen, 'Sosiale og hygieniske forhold i flyttsamenes basisområde', *Tidsskrift for den norske lægeforening*, 79 (1959), pp. 113–8; Torgersen, 'Noen populasjonsgenetiske data fra samene', pp. 809–11; B. Getz, 'Medfødt hofteleddsluksasjon hos lapper', *Tidsskrift for den norske lægeforening* (1956), pp. 812–15.
23. For example, *Finnmark fylkestings forhandlinger* (hereafter *FF*) (Vadsø, 1961), pp. 253–5.
24. *Om kulturelle og økonomiske tiltak av særlig interesse for den samisktalende befolkning*, St. meld., nr. 21 (1962–63), p. 49.
25. *så lenge det fortsatt er en del nordmenn som bare nytter dette språk, eller har vansker med å forstå norsk*, St. meld., nr. 21 (1962–63), p. 49.
26. Statsarkivet i Tromsø. Fylkeslegen i Finnmark, pk. 60, 081.26. 'Behovet at gemensam nordisk satsning på forskning som berör Grönlands och Nordkalottens medicinska och sosiala problem'. Av Samarbetskommittén för Nordisk Arktisk Medicinsk forskning, januar 1971: 4. Also 60, 08. 'Letter from Kolbjørn Øygard to medical officials in Tana and Karasjok', 2 July 1974.
27. *Folketellingen i Norge 1 desember 1930*, 9:17 (Oslo: Det Statistiske Centralbyrå, 1933); *Folketellingen 1 desember 1950, åttende hefte*, 11:236 (Oslo: Statistisk Sentralbyrå, 1956), pp. 22–3.
28. 'For en lege med god medisinsk utdanning, allmennutdanning og menneskelig forståelse og innfølingsevne, bør imidlertid etter Sosialdepartementets oppfatning, ikke tilpasningsprosessen by på slike vansker at det gir seg utslag i kvaliteten av den medisinske ytelsen'. St. meld., nr. 21 (1962–63), p. 49.
29. R. Slagstad, *De nasjonale strateger* (Oslo: Pax Forlag A/S, 2001), p. 371.
30. Ibid., pp. 325–94.
31. St. meld., nr. 21 (1962–3), p. 49.
32. T. Bertelsen, *Kampen for et medisinsk fakultet i Tromsø* (Det medisinske fakultet, Bergen 1991), p. 38.
33. St. meld., nr. 196 (1962–3), p. 496.
34. *Plan for helse- og sosialtjenester til den samiske befolking i Norge. Avgitt til Sosial- og helsedepartementet 16. februar 1995*, Norges Offentlige Utredninger (NOU), 6 (1995), ch. 12.6.2.2. In 1995 the Sami quota at the school of nursing was 10 per cent.

35. 'Gjennomføring av offentlig helsesøstertjeneste i Finnmark. Innstilling fra A. Aune', *FF*, Sak 22 (22 May 1960).
36. *FF* (1963), p. 254.
37. Aarseth, *Norsk samepolitikk*, p. 77.
38. H. Minde, 'Samebevegelsen, det norske arbeiderparti og samiske rettigheter', in *Samene – urbefolkning og minoritet* (Oslo: Universitetsforlaget, 1980), pp. 101–9.
39. A. Schiøtz, *Doktoren. Distriktslegenes historie 1900–1984* (Oslo: Pax Forlag A/S, 2004) pp. 117–45.
40. Bertelsen, *Kampen for*, p. 77.
41. *FF* (1960), p. 65; *FF* (1962), p. 231.
42. Ibid., (1964), p. 258.
43. Schiøtz, *Doktoren*, p. 126.
44. N. Fulsås, *Universitetet i Tromsø 25 år* (Tromsø: Universitetet i Tromsø, 1993), p. 30.
45. Ibid., p. 36.
46. T. Bertelsen, 'Hvor kommer lægene fra og hvor blir de av?', *Tidsskrift for den norske læge-forening* (1963), pp. 861–70.
47. Bertelsen, 'Hvor kommer lægene fra', p. 866.
48. 'En landsdels lægestand må baseres på innfødte læger, og dette gjelder i særlig grad for landsdeler hvor klima og arbeidsforhold atskilelr seg fra resten av landet' (Bertelsen, 'Hvor kommer lægene fra', p. 869).
49. Bertelsen, *Kampen for et medisinsk fakultet*.
50. Ibid., p. 60.
51. Fulsås, *Universitetet*, pp. 61–3.
52. NOU, 6 (1995), ch. 12.3.2.1.
53. Ibid.
54. Fulsås, *Universitet*, p. 143.
55. O. H. Førde and D. S. Thelle, *The Tromsø Heart Study: Population Studies of Coronary Risk Factors with Special Emphasis on High Density Lipoprotein and the Family Occurrence of Myocardial Infarction*, ISM skriftserie, no. 4 (Tromsø: Institutt for samfunnsmedisin, Universitetet i Tromsø, 1979), p. 131.
56. Ibid., p. 11.
57. K. Westlund and A. J. Søgaard, *Helse, livsstil og levekår i Finnmark. Resultater fra Hjerte-karundersøkelsen i 1987–88. Finnmark III*, skriftserie no. 28 (Tromsø: ISM, 1993), pp. 100–3.
58. Schiøtz, *Doktoren*, pp. 170–6.
59. NOU, 6 (1995), chs. 12.2.6 & 12.2.7.
60. Lately, however, it has been asked: 'Where do the Sami physicians go?' The reason is that despite quotas to educate Sami-speaking physicians, recruitment of Sami-speaking physicians to positions in Finnmark is very difficult. On this issue see 'Hvor blir det av de samiske legene?', at http://www.forskning.no/artikler/2007/juni/1182507839.84/ print [accessed 19 May 2008].
61. NOU, 6 (1995), ch. 12.6.2.1. Per Omvik, 'Det medisinske fakultet i Bergen svarer', *Tidsskr Nor Lægefor* (2006), pp. 126–2144.
62. Bertelsen, *Kampen for*, p. 38.
63. The text of this document can be found at http://www.ilo.org/ilolex/cgi-lex/convde. pl?C169 [accessed 28 January 2010].
64. Ibid.
65. See Aarseth, *Norsk samepolitikk*.

66. NOU, 6 (6), ch. 1.1.1, pp. 6–7.
67. SANKS (Sami National Competence Centre for Mental Health) was established in 1997.
68. NOU, 6 (1995), ch. 11.
69. NOU, 6 (1995), ch. 3, pp. 63–128; ch. 12, pp. 382–418.
70. 'En satsing på lokal rekruttering vil være sammenfallende med de fleste samers ønske om en tilværelse som samer også etter fullført utdanning. Dette innebærer at de ønsker å bo og bruke sin utdanning i de samiske områder'. NOU, 6 (1995), ch. 12.7, p. 404.
71. J. B. Waldram, D. Ann Hering and T. Kue Young, *Aboriginal Health in Canada, Historical, Cultural and Epidemiological Perspectives*, 2nd edn (Toronto: University of Toronto Press, 2006), pp. 264–5.
72. In April 2008, a member of the Sami Parliament announced that 'Norske Samers Riksforbund' (a national Sami organization) wanted health services to the Sami to be organized in a 'Sami health enterprise' (*Samisk helseforetak*). This presumably would be similar to the four 'state regional health enterprises' that organize other hospitals and specialist health services. See the newspaper, *Nordlys* (24 April 2008). On the regional health enterprises see: T. Grønlie, 'Hospital Sector Structure and Organisation in Britain and Norway – Contributions Towards a Comparative Study', in A. Andresen, K. T. Elvbakken and T. Grønlie (eds), *Politics of Prevention, Health Propaganda, and the Organisation of Hospitals 1800–2000* (Bergen: Rokkansenteret, report 10-2005), pp. 157–8.
73. NOU, 6 (1995), ch. 1, pp. 11, 14.
74. Waldram et al., *Aboriginal Health*, p. 3.
75. Ibid., pp. 238–44.
76. 'Fornyet kjennskap til den empiriske bruk av folkemedisin bør være en del av en samisk kulturreisning'. NOU, 6 (1995), ch. 4.4, pp. 143–4.
77. See R. Solhaug, 'Alternativ behandling ved hvert fjerde sykehus'. Forskning. no., http://www.forskning.no.artikler/2004/januar/1073375146.21 [accessed 12 March 2008]. See also L. Johansdatter Salomonsen, S. Grimsgaard and V. Fønnebø, 'Bruk av alternativmedisinsk behandling ved norske sykehus', *Tidsskr Nor Lægeforen*, 5:123 (2003), pp. 631–3.
78. 'Med etnisk medisin menes kulturforståelse, kunnskap om flerkulturelle forhold, tospråklighet, forståelse av akkulturasjonsprosesser, samt konstruksjon og forvaltning av en etnisk minoritetsidentitet. En forståelse av etnisk medisin bør sette helse- og sosialpersonell i stand til å se utviklingen av sykdomstilstander og forekomsten av sosiale problemer i forhold til kulturelle og etniske aspekter. En slik forståelse bør ligge til grunn (for) teoriutvikling så vel som for utvikling av forskningsmetoder blant etniske minoriteter'. NOU, 6 (1995), ch. 12.6.1.3, p. 399.
79. *Utredning om etnisk medisin ved Universitetet i Tromsø. Et forslag om opprettelse av en avdeling for samisk helseforskning* (Tromsø: Senter for samiske studier, Universitetet i Tromsø, 1999), pp. 4–6.
80. Ibid., p. 13.
81. Ibid., pp. 15–16.
82. The Sami general practitioner and member of the Sami Medical Association, Ester Fjellheim: 'I forbindelse med utredningen av etnisk medisin lå det også et mandat til å utrede om vi ville være et nasjonalt senter for etnisk medisin. Og vi kunne blitt et slikt nasjonalt senter med vår erfaring. Men grunnen til at vi ikke ville fokusere på dette nå, var at vi ikke ville miste det samiske inn i innvandringsproblematikken'. See http://www.uib.no/isf/utposten/2003nr5/utp03502.htm [accessed 1 March 2007].

83. The Ministry of Health established the Norwegian Centre for Minority Health Research in Oslo in 2004.
84. 'Men vi må også ha for øye et en kanskje vel så interessant målgruppe er den delen av befolkningen med samisk bakgrunn som har skiftet identitet. For dette identitetsskiftet kan være ledsaget av lidelser som nettopp setter oss på sporet av hvordan majoritetsundertrykkelse kan avstedkomme bestemte helsemessige mønster'. *Utredning om etnisk medisin*, p. 28.
85. 'Etnisk identitet dreier seg i så måte om kjennetegn relatert til ulike tradisjoner, men den kan også være relatert til slektskap og gener. Men vi kan også studere etnisk identitet som noe som skapes og endres i møte mellom to folk, der de gjensidig påvirker hverandre. I den første sammenhengen er vi opptatt av etniske forskjeller som opprinnelige og varige forskjeller eller egenskaper. I den andre sammenhengen har vi oppmerksomheten rettet mot hva som foregår på grensen mellom de to folk eller kulturer'. *Utredning om etnisk medisin*, p. 13.
86. *Utredning om etnisk medisin*, p. 26.
87. A. Sajantila et al., 'Genes and Languages in Europe: An Analysis of Mithochondrial Lineages', *Genome Research*, 5 (1995), p. 49.
88. See Merton, '*Nå skal du høre*', pp. 177–9; E. Fjellheim, 'Jeg husker min første samiske pasient. Hun hadde et klart samisk utseende', at http://www.uib.no/isf/utposten/2003nr5/utp03502.htm [accessed 1 March 2007].

4 Dupree, 'Foreshadowing the Future'

1. J. Curnow, 'The Provision of Healthcare in Remote Communities', in C. Nottingham (ed.), *The NHS in Scotland: The Legacy of the Past and the Prospect of the Future* (Aldershot: Ashgate, 2000), pp. 124–37. Although this paper focuses on the 'internal periphery' of the Highlands and Islands, it should be seen in the context of Christopher Smout's point that there are hierarchies of centre (with a concentration of administrative, cultural or economic decision-making) and periphery, as in the relationship between Lerwick and the outer islands of Shetland, see C. Smout, 'Centre and Periphery in History; with some Thoughts on Scotland as a Case Study', *Journal of Common Market Studies*, 18 (1980), pp. 256–71, on pp. 263, 268.
2. D. Hamilton, 'The Highlands and Islands Medical Services', in G. McLachlan (ed.), *Improving the Common Weal: Aspects of Scottish Health Services 1900–1984* (Edinburgh: Edinburgh University Press, 1987), pp. 481–90, on p. 483; M. McCrae, *The National Health Service in Scotland: Origins and Ideals, 1900–1950* (East Linton: Tuckwell Press, 2003), p. 1; J. Jenkinson, 'Scottish Health Policy 1918–1948 – Paving the Way to a National Health Service?', in C. Nottingham (ed.), *The NHS in Scotland*, pp. 1–19, on pp. 8, 13, 15.
3. Scottish Home and Health Department, *General Medical Services in the Highlands and Islands* (Edinburgh: HMSO, 1967), [Cd 3257].
4. Ibid., p. 4. The Registrar General's tables are calculated to only one decimal place – hence this disconcerting figure.
5. See, for example, the chapter by Megan J. Davies on the Peace River region of British Columba, Canada.
6. Scottish Home and Health Department, *General Medical Services in the Highlands and Islands*, pp. 4–6; McCrae, *The National Health Service in Scotland*, p. 3.
7. *Report of the Highlands and Islands Medical Service Committee* (Dewar Report), (HMSO, 1912), [Cd 6559].

8.   Scottish Home and Health Department, *General Medical Services in the Highlands and Islands*, p. 3.
9.   Hamilton, 'The Highlands and Islands Medical Service', p. 486.
10. Dewar Committee Report, quoted in McCrae, *The National Health Service in Scotland*, p. 8.
11. Hamilton, 'The Highlands and Islands Medical Service', p. 486; McCrae, *The National Health Service in Scotland*, pp. 8–10.
12. Scottish Home and Health Department, *General Medical Services in the Highlands and Islands*, p. 9.
13. Ibid., p. 9. 'The groups comprised the "crofter and cottar" class and their families, the dependents of those insured under the National Health Insurance Act and what were rather vaguely known as "those of like economic class"'.
14. Ibid., pp. 9, 65.
15. Ibid., pp. 9–10.
16. Ibid., p. 10; R. Ferguson, 'Whose Nurse? The Doctor, the District and the NHS', in C. Nottingham (ed.), *The NHS in Scotland*, pp. 20–33; R. Dugald, 'Perceptions of Change: An Oral History of District Nursing in Scotland, 1940–1990' (PhD dissertation, Glasgow Caledonian University, 2002).
17. Scottish Home and Health Department, *General Medical Services in the Highlands and Islands*, p. 10; Hamilton, 'The Highlands and Islands Medical Service', p. 488.
18. Department of Health for Scotland, 'Committee on Scottish Health Services Report', (1935–6), pp. 220–33, [Cd 5204]. See also Dugald, 'Perceptions of Change', pp. 75–6.
19. Scottish Home and Health Department, *General Medical Services in the Highlands and Islands*, p. 11.
20. Ibid., pp. 10–11; Hamilton, 'The Highlands and Islands Medical Service', p. 488.
21. 'British Medical Association (Scottish Office): Conditions of Practice in Remote Areas (with special reference to the Highlands and Islands of Scotland): Appendix II. The Highlands and Islands Medical Service by Dr R. D. Martin' [1958]. HH102/1185/5, National Archives of Scotland, Home and Health Department, Edinburgh (hereafter NAS), f. 21.
22. Quoted in McCrae, *The National Health Service in Scotland*, p. 1. See also, C. Webster, *The Health Services Since the War, Vol.1: Problems of Health Care the National Health Service Before 1957*, 2 vols (London: HMSO, 1988), vol. 1, p. 104.
23. Scottish Home and Health Department, *General Medical Services in the Highlands and Islands*, p. 12.
24. Webster, *The National Health Services Since the War*, vols 1 & 2; C. Webster, *The National Health Service: A Political History* (Oxford: Oxford University Press, 1998).
25. In addition, the teaching hospitals were under the Regional Hospital Boards in Scotland while those in England were directly under the Minister, and there was a difference in responsibility for health centres.
26. 'What Everyone Should Know', *Shetland Times*, 16 July 1948, p. 8, quoted in Dugald, 'Perceptions of Change', p. 183.
27. L. Reid, *Scottish Midwives: Twentieth-Century Voices* (East Lindon: Tuckwell Press, 2000), p. 62.
28. Dugald, 'Perceptions of Change', pp. 181–7; Scottish Home and Health Department, *General Medical Services in the Highlands and Islands*, pp. 11, 53–4.

29. Scottish Home and Health Department, *General Medical Services in the Highlands and Islands*, p. 1.
30. 'British Medical Association (Scottish Office): Conditions of Practice in Remote Areas (with special reference to the Highlands and Islands of Scotland)' [*c.* 1961]. NAS, HH102/1185/5, ff. 1–26.
31. 'Lord Birsay', *The Times*, 1 December 1982, p. 14; Philip [Rt Hon. Lord Philip (Alexander Morrison Philip)], 'Sir Harald Robert Leslie (1905–1982)', *ODNB* (Oxford: Oxford University Press, 2004), at [http://www.oxforddnb.com/vies/article/39695, [accessed 9 May 2008]; 'Appendix' [*c.* 1965], NAS, HH102/1251/21. Lady Birsay also served with the British forces in Germany, and was among the first allied doctors to enter Belsen concentration camp.
32. 'Appendix' [*c.* 1965], NAS, HH102/1251/21.
33. Scottish Home and Health Department, *General Medical Services in the Highlands and Islands*, p. 2.
34. Ibid., p. 3.
35. Ibid., p. 17.
36. Ibid., p. 18.
37. Ibid., p. 30.
38. Ibid., p. 90.
39. Ibid., p. 81.
40. Ibid., p. 82.
41. Ibid., pp. 82–3.
42. Ibid., p. 83.
43. Ibid., p. 90.
44. Ibid., p. 83.
45. Ibid., pp. 83–4.
46. Ibid., p. 92.
47. Ibid., pp. 84–5.
48. Ibid., p. 84.
49. Ibid., pp. 2, 98.
50. Ibid., pp. 83, 92.
51. Webster, *The Health Services Since the War, Vol. 2: Government and Health Care: The National Health Service, 1958–1979*, 2 vols (London: Stationary Office, c.1996), vol. 2, pp. 331–51; Webster, *The National Health Service*, pp. 87–111.
52. C. Webster, *National Health Service Reorganisation: Learning from History?* (London: Office of Health Economics, 1998), pp. 13–18, 27.

5 Edvinsson, 'A Country Doctor'

1. The translation of *provinsialläkare* in several dictionaries is given as 'district medical officer'. This emphasizes their role as government civil servants responsible for public health care and less with their obligations as providers of personal health care. I have chosen to keep the translation 'district medical officer' with the reservation that it partly misrepresents their daily practice. This is something that will be discussed in more detail in this article.
2. Reports from district medical officers, RA, Medicinalstyrelsens arkiv, E5A, provinsialläkares årsberättelser (in the following these are referred to as Report, district and year). Many of these reports have been transcribed and are available at *Medicinalhis-*

torisk databas, Linköping Electronic Press. The transcriptions have facilitated the work
substantially. The difficult handwriting has, however, made it necessary to examine the
original sources. All reports for this period have been scanned and are available at the
website of SVAR (Swedish Archive Information), a unit within the Swedish National
Archives available at www.svar.ra.se. Some reports were also printed in the yearly relations of the National Board of Health (*Sundhets-Collegii underdåniga berättelser öfver
Sundhetstillståndet i Riket, 1851–1860*). On these medical reports, see S. Landahl
'Provinsialläkarnas årsberättelser i Medicinalstyrelsens arkiv', in I. Andersson (ed.),
Archivistica et Mediaevistica: Ernesto Nygren oblata (Stockholm: Norstedt, 1956), pp.
232–47.

3.   P. Baldwin, *Contagion and the State in Europe, 1830–1930* (Cambridge: Cambridge
University Press, 1999), pp. 2–10; E. H. Ackerknecht, 'Anti-Contagionism between
1821–1867', *Bulletin of the History of Medicine*, 22 (1948), pp. 117–55; C. Hannaway,
'Environment and Miasmata', in W. F. Bynum and R. Porter (eds), *Companion Encyclope-
dia of the History of Medicine* (London: Routledge, 1993), pp. 292–308.

4.   C. B. Valencius, 'Histories of Medical Geography', in N. A. Rupke (ed.), *Medical Geography in Historical Perspective: Medical History*, supplement no. 20, (2000), pp. 3–28.

5.   P. Sköld, *Kunskap och kontroll. Den svenska befolkningsstatistikens historia* (Umeå:
Demographic Data Base, 2001); K. Johannisson, *Det mätbara samhället: statistik och
samhällsdröm i 1700-talets Europa* (Stockholm: Norstedts, 1988).

6.   Kongl. Maj:ts Instruction för Provincial-Medici, dated 29 July 1774, Swedish Statute-
Book (SFS), (Stockholm, 1774).

7.   F. Berg, 'Some Extracts from Fredrik Theodor Berg's Autobiographical Memorandum',
Acta Paediatrica, 32 (1944), pp. 218–31.

8.   F. Th. Berg, 'Om Dödligheten i första lefnadsåret', *Statistisk tidskrift* (1869), pp. 435–93.

9.   Excerpts from some of them were sometimes included in the printed official reports of
the Swedish Medical Board. See *Sundhets-Collegii Underdåniga Berättelse om Medicinalverket i Riket 1851* (Stockholm, 1853).

10. *Sundhets-Collegii Underdåniga Berättelse om Medicinalverket i Riket 1851*, p. 9.

11. Kongl. Maj:ts Sundhets-Collegii Circulär till Läkarne i Riket om årliga berättelsers och
rapporters afgifwande, SFS [Swedish Statute Book], 1851:17.

12. Kongl. Maj:ts Instruction för Provincial-läkarne i Riket, dated 13 June 1822, SFS.

13. Kongl. Maj:ts Nådiga Förordning Angående Sockenstämmor och Kyrko-Råd, dated 26
February 1817, SFS.

14. On smallpox vaccination, see P. Sköld, *The Two Faces of Smallpox: A Disease and Its
Prevention in Eighteenth- and Nineteenth-Century Sweden* (Umeå: Demographic Data
Base, 1996), pp. 401–16.

15. G. Kearns, W. R. Lee and J. Rogers, 'The Interaction of Political and Economic Factors
in the Management of Urban Public Health', in M. C. Nelson and J. Rogers (eds), *Urban-
isation and the Epidemiologic Transition* (Uppsala: Reprocentralen, 1989), pp. 9–80.

16. C. Dahlborg, *Svenska Provinsialläkarföreningens historia 1881–1905* (Stockholm: s.n.,
1930), pp. 99–101.

17. Parliamentary Publications, *Presteståndets protokoll vid 1859 års riksdag* (Minutes from
the clergy estate, 1859), vol. 7, p. 219, statement of Dr Almqvist.

18. Kearns et al., 'The Interaction', p. 66.

19. Parliamentary Publications, Committee Report 1890, *Underdånigt betänkande afgifvet
den 5 april 1887, Förslag till instruktion för provinsialläkare med flere läkare*, 2 saml, 2
avd. 1 band p. 97.

20. Ibid.; *Sundhets-Collegii underdåniga berättelse om Medicinalverket i Riket* (Stockholm, 1851), pp. 3–6.

21. J. Hellstenius, 'Barnadödligheten inom första lefnadsåret i Vesternorrlands och Jemtlands län', *Statistisk tidskrift*, 73 (1887), pp. 153–68.

22. The reconstruction of the district medical officers comes mainly from J. Sacklén, J. Svensk Läkarehistoria, 1 (1822); J. Sacklén, Svensk Läkarehistoria, 2 (1823–24); J. Sacklén, Svensk Läkarehistoria, Supplement (1835); J. Sacklén, Svensk Läkarehistoria, New Supplement (1853); and from Reports, Härjedalen.

23. Minutes from National Board of Health, RA, Sundhetscollegii archive, A1A:38, 15 September 1850.

24. Sacklén, *Svensk Läkarehistoria*, Supplement (1835), p. 390 ff.; Sacklén, *Svensk Läkarehistoria*, New Supplement (1853), p. 152.

25. Parliamentary Publications, *Kongl. Maj:ts Nådiga Proposition till Riksens Ständer, angående anslag å Stat för en särskild Provincial-Läkare i Herjeådalen* Proposition 12, p 259 ff. (Government Bill on district medical officer in Härjedalen, 1823).

26. Parliamentary Publications, *Bihang till Samtlige Riks-Ståndens Protocoll* (1847/8), 4 saml, 1. avd, p. 27.

27. Minutes from National Board of Health, RA, Sundhetscollegii archive, A1A:38, 27 May 1850, 1 July 1850 and 8 July 1850.

28. Biographic data from C. Landelius, entry Johan Ellmin, in *Svenskt Biografiskt Lexikon*, 13 (Stockholm 1950), pp. 364–6.

29. Provinsialläkarens i Härjedalens arkiv, letter 5 December 1860, ÖLA (Regional archive in Östersund).

30. On the international arena this was expressed by Villermé in France and Virchow in Prussia at this time.

31. *Förhandlingar vid de skandinaviske naturforskarnes tredje möte i Stockholm den 13–19 juli 1842* (Stockholm, 1842), pp. 401 ff.

32. B. Olsson, *Att torgföra vetenskapen. Det vetenskapliga föredragets och populärvetenskapens teori, praktik och kultur* (Studentlitteratur, 2001), pp. 45 ff., online at http://www.studentlitteratur.se/files/sites/svensksakprosa/Olsson_rapp24.pdf [accessed 15 April 2007]. On his activities within Bildningscirkeln, see J. Ellmin, *Om Folkets Bildning och Bildningscirkelns i Stockholm första år* (1847; Stockholm, 1942) and C. Landelius, *1840–1850-talets Bildningscirklar och Arbetarföreningar i Sverige* (Stockholm 1936), parts 1 and 2.

33. Ellmin, *Om Folkets Bildning*, pp. 57 ff.

34. Landelius, *1840–1850-talets Bildningscirklar*, part 2, p. 191.

35. Ibid., part 1, pp. 27–34.

36. E. Gamby, *Pär Götrek och 1800-talets svenska arbetarrörelse* (Tidens förlag, Stockholm 1978), pp. 200 ff. Their differences with Marx and Engels appear in the role that the French utopian socialist, Etienne Cabet, played in the Scandinavian society. His goal was to create a Christian utopia in the United States of America called 'Icarie'.

37. On his activities during the last years in Stockholm, see Landelius, *1840–1850-talets Bildningscirklar*, part 1, pp. 136 ff, on 1836; and B. Anderson, 'Stockholms arbetareförening av 1850', in F. Lindberg (ed.), *Studier och handlingar rörande Stockholms stads historia* (Stockholm: Stadsarkivet, 1975).

38. 'Provinsialläkarens i Härjedalens arkiv', letter 5 December 1860, ÖLA.

39. Minutes from the National Board of Health, RA. Sundhetscollegii archive, A1A:38, 14 October, 2 December, 16 December and 19 December 1850.

40. Ellmin's reports from the 1850s have previously been described in F. Järnankar, 'Ett ohyfsat men fromsint folk', *Jämten* (1997), pp. 33–43.

41. Report, Härjedalen 1851.
42. Hellstenius, 'Barnadödligheten inom första lefnadsåret', pp. 157–163.
43. Report, Härjedalen 1851.
44. The role of odours in nineteenth-century medical thinking is described in A. Corbin, *The Foul and the Fragrant: Odor and the French Social Imagination* (Cambridge, MA: Harvard University Press, 1986).
45. Hannaway, 'Environment and Miasmata', p. 301.
46. Report, Härjedalen 1851.
47. M. Huss, *Alchoholismus Chronica* (Stockholm, 1851).
48. S. Willner, *Det svaga könet* (Linköping: Linköping Studies in Art and Science, Institutionen för Tema, 1999); S. Edvinsson, *Den osunda staden. Sociala skillnader i dödlighet i 1800-talets Sundsvall* (Umeå: Demographic Data Base, 1992), pp. 195–203.
49. Report, Härjedalen 1851.
50. Ibid., 1851.
51. Ibid., 1851, 1852.
52. Ibid., 1851.
53. Ibid., 1851.
54. Ibid., 1851.
55. Ibid., 1859.
56. Ibid., 1851, 1859.
57. Ibid., 1852.
58. Ibid., 1851.
59. Ibid., 1851. Conflicts of this sort have remained until modern times. There have been intense discussions and court cases concerning the rights for the Sami to practise their extensive herding in areas with a resident population and their more intensive agriculture.
60. Report, Härjedalen 1851.
61. Ibid., 1855.
62. Ibid., 1851.
63. Ibid., 1851.
64. Ibid., 1855, 1856.
65. Ibid., 1851, 1852, 1856.
66. Letter from Ellmin to Sundhetskollegium, RA, Sundhetscollegii arkiv, Inkomna handlingar, 1854, E2:147; Letter from Ellmin to Sundhetskollegium, RA, Sundhetscollegii arkiv, Inkomna handlingar, 1855, E2:151.
67. Report, Härjedalen 1851.
68. Å. Wahlqvist, *Anders Wallström: Soln-Anders. 1841–1921. Naturläkare* (Rönninge: printed for the author, 2003)
69. Report, Härjedalen 1856.

6 Larsen, 'Medical Reports from the 1800s'

1. See further discussion in Ø. Larsen, 'Health Care and Attitudes in Health Matters – Some Personal Reflections', in M. Dinges (ed.), *Health and Health Care between Self Help, Intermediary Organizations and Formal Poor Relief (1500–2005)* (Braga: Edições Colibri, 2007), pp. 93–106.

2.   See also Ø. Larsen, 'Diseases, Geography, and the Medical Profession', in Ø. Larsen (ed.), *The Shaping of a Profession: Physicians in Norway, Past and Present* (Canton, MA: Science History Publications, 1996), pp. 184–7.

3.   The history of the Norwegian medical reports has been covered in detail by H. P. Schjønsby, 'The Medical Reports from the District Physicians – An Indispensable Source to the Norwegian Past', *Michael*, 2 (2005), pp. 218–35.

4.   Comprehensive data on Norway are offered by Statistics Norway, at www.ssb.no. In addition, a 128-page article in the authoritative national encyclopaedia gives updated historical and contemporary information on Norway; see P. Henriksen (ed.), *Aschehougs og Gyldendals store norske leksikon*, 16 vols (Oslo: Kunnskapsforlaget, 2006), vol. 11, pp. 210–337.

5.   The function of the Sanitation Committees in a selection of municipalities in the lower Telemark region in the period 1860–1900 has been the focus of A. Storesund's dissertation, see A. Storesund, 'Akutt sykelighet og forebyggende helsearbeid i Telemark 1860–1900', *Michael*, 2 (2005), pp. 3–112.

6.   A. Schiøtz, *Doktoren: distriktslegenes historie 1900–1984* (Oslo: Pax, 2003); and A. Schiøtz, *Folkets helse – landets styrke 1850–2003. Det offentlige helsevesen i Norge 1603–2003 bind 2* (Oslo: Universitetsforlaget, 2003).

7.   Data for a selection of communicable diseases were excerpted from the medical records on county level for the period from 1868–1900 and used as basis for an atlas covering the geographical distribution of these diseases over time (Ø. Larsen, *Epidemic Diseases in Norway in a Period of Change: An Atlas of Some Selected Infectious Diseases and the Attitudes towards Them 1868–1900* (Oslo: Unipub forlag, 2000)). The *Atlas* also contains the basic tables and calculations. Tuberculosis was another large infectious disease problem in Norway in the period covered, but as this disease epidemiologically represented a special case, it was not included in the studies discussed here.

8.   Especially for these frequent but not so serious diseases, methodological questions may be posed as to, for example, the completeness in contemporary disease notification by the district physicians. Here, geographical differences are also probable. For obvious reasons, this factor can hardly be controlled for retrospectively. On the other hand, as the reports were compiled for reasons of comparison only, there are clues to indicate that this possible bias is not that important, at least when making comparisons over periods that are not too long.

9.   The correctness of this statement has been questioned, as doctors were engaged by kings in earlier historical periods, but it may be said that from this point onwards a new development came to sight, as the king seems to take on responsibility for the health of the population. On the other hand, for all practical purposes, the emergence of a public health service of some efficiency in Norway does not occur until the nineteenth century. However, the 400 years' celebration of state health care in 2003 included support for an extensive history of medicine research programme that included the creation of exhibitions and local projects all over the country, and a penetrating two-volume historical work: O. G. Moseng, *Ansvaret for undersåttenes helse 1603–1850. Det offentlige helsevesen i Norge 1603–2003 bind 1* (Oslo: Universitetsforlaget, 2003); and A. Schiøtz, *Folkets helse - landets styrke 1850-2003. Det offentlige helsevesen i Norge 1603-2003 bind 2* (Oslo: Universitetsforlaget, 2003). On public health services, see also H. P. Schjønsby, 'The Establishment of a Public Health System', in Larsen, *The Shaping of a Profession*, pp. 71–85.

10. The development of the medical profession in Norway has been described by a series of authors in Larsen, *The Shaping of a Profession*, published in the same year as a biographic encyclopaedia covering all known Norwegian physicians throughout the times

up to spring 1996; see Ø. Larsen (ed.), *Norges leger I–V* (Oslo: Den norske lægeforening, 1996). The development of the medical profession has also been discussed, with more emphasis on economic and organizational issues, in Ø. Larsen, O. Berg and F. Hodne, *Legene og samfunnet* (Oslo: Den norske lægeforening, 1986). Until 1946, when the new University of Bergen was opened, Christiania/Kristiania (renamed Oslo in 1924) was home to the only university in the country. The history of medical teaching in Christiania/Oslo is recounted in Ø. Larsen, *Mangfoldig medisin* (Oslo: Universitetet i Oslo, Det medisinske fakultet, 1989); and Ø. Larsen, *Legestudent i hovedstaden* (Oslo: Gyldendal Akademisk, 2002).

11. The title of the original thesis by Holst is 'Morbus, quem Radesyge vocant, quinam sit, quanamque ratione e Scandinavia tollendus?' A translated edition by A. K. Lie was published in 2005; see F. Holst, *Hva er sykdommen som kalles Radesyke, og på hvilken måte kan den utryddes fra Skandinavia?*, ed. A. K. Lie, trans. S. Oppedal, in *Michael*, 2, supplement 2 (2005). See also A. K. Lie, *Radesykens tilblivelse* (Oslo: Universitetet i Oslo, Det medisinske fakultet, 2008).

12. See M. Nylenna, 'Scientific Literature and the Shaping of a Medical Profession in Norway', in Larsen, *The Shaping of a Profession*, pp. 229–57.

13. Larsen et al., *Legene og samfunnet*.

14. See B. O. Olsen, 'Recreation or Professional Necessity – The Study Tours of Nineteenth Century Norwegian Physicians', in Larsen, *The Shaping of a Profession*, pp. 258–75; and H. W. Kvarenes, 'Travel Accounts in the "Norsk Magazin for Lægevidenskaben" 1840–1880', in Larsen, *The Shaping of a Profession*, pp. 276–82.

15. E. O. Rosvold and Ø. Larsen, 'Krankheiten im Arztberuf. Die Gesundheit norwegischer Ärzte und ihrer Angehörigen im ausgehenden 19. Jahrhundert', *Medizinhistorisches Journal*, 31 (1996), pp. 167–80.

16. See Ø. Larsen, *Legevakten* (Oslo: Oslo kommune, 2000).

17. See K. Kristiansen and Ø. Larsen (eds), *Ullevål sykehus i hundre år* (Oslo: Oslo kommune, 1987).

18. The method is described in detail in Ø. Larsen, H. Haugtomt and W. Platou, '*Sykdomsoppfatning og epidemiologi 1860–1900* (Oslo: Seksjon for medisinsk historie, Universitetet i Oslo, 1980).

19. The notion of an 'ecology of disease' in medical and social history is discussed in detail in A. E. Imhof and Ø. Larsen, *Sozialgeschichte und Medizin* (Oslo/Stuttgart: Universitetsforlaget/Fischer, 1975).

7 Connor, '"Medicine is Here to Stay"'

1. S. L. Barney, *Authorized to Heal: Gender, Class and the Transformation of Medicine in Appalachia, 1880–1930* (Chapel Hill, NC: University of North Carolina Press, 2000); G. G. Willumson, *W. Eugene Smith and the Photographic Essay* (Cambridge: Cambridge University Press, 1992), ch. 4; also A. Digby, *The Evolution of British General Practice, 1850–1948* (Oxford: Oxford University Press, 1999).

2. J. L. Barona and S. Cherry (eds), *Health and Medicine in Rural Europe* (Valcència: Seminari d'Estudis sobre la Ciencia, Universitat de València, 2005); J. Elliot, M. Stuart and C. Toman, eds., *Place and Practice in Canadian Nursing History* (Vancouver: UBC Press, 2008); M. J. Davies, 'Mapping "Region" in Canadian Medical History: The Case of British Columbia', *Canadian Bulletin of Medical History*, 17 (2000), pp. 73–92; and P. L.

Twohig, 'Written on the Landscape: Health and Region in Canada', *Journal of Canadian Studies*, 41 (2007), pp. 5–17.

3. W. Kamp (ed.), *Health in Rural Settings: Contexts for Action* (Lethbridge, AB: University of Lethbridge, 1999), see especially M. J. Troughton, 'Redefining "Rural" for the Twenty-First Century', pp. 21–38; G. W. N. Fitzgerald, 'The *Canadian Journal of Non-Urban Medicine?*', *Canadian Journal of Rural Medicine*, 11 (2006), pp. 183–4; A. E. Joseph and P. R. Bantock, 'Rural Accessibility of General Practitioners: The Case of Bruce and Grey Counties, Ontario, 1901–1981', *Canadian Geographer*, 28 (1984), pp. 226–39; R. W. Pong and R. J. Pitblado, 'Don't Take Geography for Granted! Some Methodological Issues in Measuring Geographic Distributions of Physicians', *Canadian Journal of Rural Medicine*, 6 (2001), pp. 103–12.

4. For an overview of the long and rich history of this region, see S. T. Cadigan, *Newfoundland and Labrador: A History* (Toronto: University of Toronto Press, 2009); Newfoundland Historical Society, *A Short History of Newfoundland and Labrador* (St John's: Boulder Publications, 2008); J. Hiller and P. Neary, *Twentieth-Century Newfoundland: Explorations* (St John's: Breakwater Books, 1994); and R. I. McAllister (ed.), *Newfoundland and Labrador: The First Fifteen Years after Confederation* (St John's: Dicks, [1965]). For an introduction to the political scene, see S. J. R. Noel, *Politics in Newfoundland* (Toronto: University of Toronto Press, 1971); P. Neary, *Newfoundland in the North Atlantic World, 1929–1949* (Montreal: McGill-Queen's University Press, 1998); and R. B. Blake, *Canadians at Last: Canada Integrates Newfoundland as a Province* (Toronto: University of Toronto Press, 2004).

5. R. Rompkey, *Grenfell of Labrador: A Biography* (Montreal: McGill-Queen's University Press, 2009) and R. Rompkey (ed.), *The Labrador Memoir of Dr. Harry Paddon, 1912–1938* (Montreal: McGill-Queen's University Press, 2003).

6. Memorial University of Newfoundland (hereafter cited as MUN), Centre for Newfoundland Studies (CNS), *Articles of Association, The Companies Act, The Notre Dame Bay Memorial Hospital Association*; annual reports for the Notre Dame Bay Memorial Hospital (NDBMH) for 1925–7, 1928, 1929; and broadsheet entitled *Appeal in Aid New Wing* (Twillingate: [*Twillingate Sun*], 1930); see also C. E. Parsons, 'The Notre Dame Bay Memorial Hospital', *Among the Deep-Sea Fishers*, 21 (1924), pp. 115–21. Popular histories of the hospital that contain other useful excerpted historical documents are *Notre Dame Bay Memorial Hospital, Twillingate, Newfoundland: 50 Years in the Life of Our Hospital, 1924–1974* (Twillingate: Triple Island Chapter, Association of Registered Nurses of Newfoundland, n.d.); J. C. Loveridge, *Brief History of Twillingate Marking 40th Year of Medical Service by John McKee Olds* (Twillingate: n.p., 1974); and G. L. Saunders, *Doctor Olds of Twillingate: Portrait of an American Surgeon in Newfoundland* (St John's: Breakwater Books, 1994); and J. T. H. Connor, 'Twillingate', *Newfoundland Quarterly*, 100:1 (2007), pp. 12–15, 30–3, which is a popular and abbreviated account of this chapter.

7. See annual reports of The Commonwealth Fund of New York for the years 1921 to 1933; I am grateful and indebted to Al Lyons for his generosity in sharing copies of this material. See also A. Lyons, 'Hospitals for Southern Rural Communities: The Commonwealth Fund and Experimental Origins of Community Organizing and the Hill-Burton Act', Conference paper presented at the 2006 Southern Association for the History of Medicine and Science, San Antonio, Texas, 2006. On the philanthropic role of the Commonwealth Fund, see A. McGehee Harvey and S. L. Abrams, 'For the Welfare of Mankind': The Commonwealth Fund and American Medi-

cine (Baltimore, MD: Johns Hopkins University Press, 1986), especially pp. 114–26; see also S. C. Wheatley, *The Politics of Philanthropy: Abraham Flexner and Medical Education* (Madison, WI: University of Wisconsin Press, 1988), pp. 115–16 to see how this agency differed from other medical philanthropies. On the supportive role of other philanthropic agencies in the region, but noting that the CF's contributions to Atlantic Canada appear to have gone unnoticed until now, see J. G. Reid, 'Health, Education, Economy: Philanthropic Foundations in the Atlantic Regions in the 1920s and 1930s', *Acadiensis*, 14 (1984–5), pp. 63–83. The Delano architectural firm had also previously designed another Grenfell building, the King George V Institute located in St John's; see P. Pennoyer and A. Walker, *The Architecture of Delano & Aldrich* (New York: Norton, 2003).

8.   W. Grenfell to C. Parsons, 7 August 1920, MUN, Archives and Manuscripts Division, Ecke Papers, coll. 355, file 6.03.005.

9.   In a letter from General Nieh's Headquarters, Wutaishan, Shansi and dated 19 July 1938, Bethune wrote to his New York friend, Elsie Siff: 'As you probably know, we, that is the nurse and I, arrived in Sian and later in Yenan, safely. Dr. Parsons fulfilled all of my forebodings, as he turned out a drunken bum. We were glad to get rid of him ...', quoted in R. Stewart, *The Mind of Norman Bethune* (Toronto: Fitzhenry & Whiteside, 1977), p. 101; see also p. 80 for a unique photograph of Bethune, Parsons and party en route to China. On Bethune, see also R. Stewart, *Bethune* (Markham: Paperjacks, 1973).

10.   Under the new Commission of Government health matters fared not too badly as the commissioner in charge of the newly restructured department of Public Health and Welfare, John C. Puddester, was a native Newfoundlander. Along with his departmental secretary, Dr H. M. Mosdell, Puddester managed to ensure that as much money as possible was made available for health and welfare purposes; see J. R. Martin, *Leonard A. Miller: Public Servant* (Toronto: Fitzhenry and Whiteside, 1998), esp. ch. 4.

11.   On Sir William Coaker and his Fishermen's Protective Union, see I. D. H. McDonald and J. K. Hiller, *'To Each His Own': William Coaker and the Fishermen's Protective Union in Newfoundland Politics, 1908–1925* (St John's: ISER, 1987); R. H. Cuff (ed.), *A Coaker Anthology* (St John's: Creative Publishers, 1986); and W. Coaker, *Past, Present and Future* (Port Union, NL: Fishermen's Advocate, 1932).

12.   'N.D.B.M. Hospital Contract', circular letter, MUN, Archives and Manuscripts Division, Ecke Papers, coll. 355, file 6.02.002.

13.   MUN, CNS, NDBMH annual report for 1939 (this report actually covers the years 1935 to 1939 inclusive). See also the typescript by J. M. Olds, *A Brief Account of Medical Services in Notre Dame Bay* (1966) located in MUN, Health Sciences Library, Historical Collections.

14.   See A. B. Mills, 'The Farmer Takes a Stand for Better Health and Medical Care', *Modern Hospital*, 64 (1945), pp. 74–5; F. D. Mott, 'Action Now Toward Better Rural Health', *Modern Hospital*, 66 (1946), pp. 88–90; and F. D. Mott and M. I. Roemer, *Rural Health and Medical Care* (New York: McGraw-Hill, 1948). The most comprehensive historical analysis to date is M. R. Grey, *New Deal Medicine: The Rural Health Programs of the Farm Security Administration* (Baltimore, MD: Johns Hopkins University Press, 1999).

15.   On Sigerist, see E. Fee and T. Brown (eds), *Making Medical History: The Life and Times of Henry E. Sigerist* (Baltimore, MD: Johns Hopkins University Press, 1997). Diary quotation is from N. Sigerist Beeson (ed.), *Henry E. Sigerist: Autobiographical Writings* (Montreal: McGill University Press, 1966), p. 94.

16. See Grey, *New Deal Medicine*, *passim*; D. S. Hirshfield, *The Lost Reform: The Campaign for Compulsory Health Insurance in the United States from 1932 to 1943* (Cambridge, MA: Commonwealth Fund-Harvard University Press, 1970); and M. I. Roemer, *Henry E. Sigerist on the Sociology of Medicine* (New York: MD Publications, 1960); M. M. Poen, *Harry S. Truman Versus the Medical Lobby: The Genesis of Medicare* (Columbia, MO: University of Missouri Press, 1979); and A. Derickson, *Health Security for All: Dreams of Universal Health Care in America* (Baltimore, MD: Johns Hopkins University Press, 2005).

17. William W. Lockwood to Robert Ecke, 3 March 1937, MUN, Archives and Manuscripts Division, Ecke Papers, coll. 355, file 3.37.004.

18. Mott and Roemer, *Rural Health and Medical Care*; also see M. I. Roemer, 'Historic Development of the Current Crisis of Rural Medicine in the United States', in S. R. Kagan (ed.), *Victor Robinson Memorial Volume: Essays on the History of Medicine* (New York: Froben Press, 1948), pp. 333–42. About the connections between health policy in Canada and the United States in the 1930s and 1940s, between Sigerist and Saskatchewan, see J. Duffin, 'The Guru and the Godfather: Henry Sigerist, Hugh MacLean, and the Politics of Health Care Reform in 1940s Canada', *Canadian Bulletin of Medical History/Bulletin canadien d'histoire de la médecine*, 9 (1992), pp. 191–218; and J. Duffin and L. A. Falk, 'Sigerist in Saskatchewan: The Quest for Balance in Social and Technical Medicine', *Bulletin of the History of Medicine*, 70 (1996), pp. 658–83.

19. Material for this biographical profile is from MUN, Archives and Manuscripts Division, Ecke Papers, coll. 355. This collection was transferred from the United States of America to Newfoundland under legal agreement by Ecke's executor in 2006; see B. Riggs, 'The Journey of the Ecke Papers', *Newfoundland Quarterly*, 100:1 (2007), p. 35.

20. Useful background on the Johns Hopkins medical school is available in T. B. Turner, *Heritage of Excellence: The Johns Hopkins Medical Institutions, 1914–1947* (Baltimore, MD: Johns Hopkins University Press, 1974); A. McGhee Harvey, G. Brieger, S. L. Abrams and V. A. McKusick, *A Model of Its Kind: A Centennial History of Medicine at Johns Hopkins*, 2 vols (Baltimore, MD: Johns Hopkins University Press, 1989); and A. McGhee Harvey, *Adventures in Medical Research: A Century of Discovery at Johns Hopkins* (Baltimore, MD: Johns Hopkins University Press, 1976), see esp. pp. 408–15 for a discussion of poliomyelitis research during Ecke's time at Hopkins. In addition to attracting the likes of Sigerist during the time Ecke was at Hopkins, the medical school also had the services of Dr George Canby Robinson who was instrumental in trying to 'humanize' medical practice and education by reintroducing a 'holistic' approach; see T. M. Brown, 'George Canby Robinson and "The Patient as a Person"', in C. Lawrence and G. Weisz (eds), *Greater Than the Parts: Holism in Biomedicine, 1920–1950* (New York: Oxford University Press, 1998), pp. 135–60; and G. C. Robinson, *The Patient as a Person: A Study of the Social Aspects of Illness* (New York: Commonwealth Fund, 1939).

21. The United States Typhus Commission was established by presidential order and functioned throughout the Second World War; it was involved in both research and applications related to louse-borne disease. For further details, see R. S. Ecke, A. G. Gilliam, J. C. Snyder, A. Yeomans, C. J. Zarafonetis and E. S. Murray, 'The Effect of Cox-Type Vaccine on Louse-Borne Typhus Fever', *American Journal of Tropical Medicine*, 25 (1945), pp. 447–62; H. T. Karsner, 'Pathology of Epidemic Typhus Fever', *Archives of Pathology*, 56 (1953), pp. 397–435; 512–53; and S. Bayne-Jones, 'Typhus Fevers', in J. B. Coates (ed.), *Medical Department, United States Army, Preventive Medicine in World*

War II – Communicable Diseases (Washington, DC: Office of the Surgeon General, Department of the Army, 1964), pp. 175–274.

22. The genre of doctors' memoirs is an overlooked historical source for collective biography. See J. T. H. Connor, 'Rural Medical Lives and Times', *Newfoundland and Labrador Studies*, 23 (2008), pp. 231–43; S. Mullally, 'History, Memory and Twentieth-Century Medical Life Writing: Unpacking a Cape Breton's Doctor's Black Bag', in E. A. Heaman, A. Li, and S. McKellar (eds), in *Essays in Honour of Michael Bliss* (Toronto: University of Toronto Press, 2008), pp. 435–69; and J. T. H. Connor, 'Putting the "Grenfell Effect" in its Place: Medical Tales and Autobiographical Narratives in Twentieth-Century Newfoundland and Labrador', *Papers of the Bibliographic Society of Canada/Cahiers de la Société bibliographique du Canada*, 48:1 (2010), pp. 77–118.

23. These generalizations of Ecke's practice are based on an overall reading of his published memoirs, R. S. Ecke, *Snowshoe & Lancet: Memoirs of a Frontier Newfoundland Doctor, 1937–1948* (Portsmouth, NH: Peter E. Randall, 2000).

24. Ecke, *Snowshoe & Lancet*. If a direct reference is made to this source in the body of the discussion, dates of diary entries are used rather than page numbers unless otherwise noted. If necessary to clarify any point, Ecke's 'original' typescript of his memoir has also been consulted; see MUN, Archives and Manuscripts Division, Ecke Papers, coll. 355, file 10.01.

25. MUN, CNS, NDBMH annual report for 1939 notes that on 1 August 1939 the hospital acquired an ECG machine and used it forty times during the rest of the year. That this equipment was not only purchased but actually used is doubly remarkable; this situation no doubt can be attributed to the leadership of Johns Hopkins medical school as a centre for the use of ECG technology. On the novelty of this technology in Newfoundland medical practice I am indebted to the insight of Dr Nigel Rusted who began his surgical career in 1933 (personal communication).

26. On cultural health attitudes of the 'old days', see R. R. Andersen, J. K. Crellin and B. O'Dwyer, *Healthways: Newfoundland Elders, Their Lifestyles and Values* (St John's: Creative Publishers, 1998), *passim*.

27. On the practice and demise of lay midwifery in Newfoundland, see C. M. Benoit, *Midwives in Passage: The Modernization of Maternity Care* (St John's: ISER, 1991); and L. Kealey, 'On the Edge of Empire: The Working Life of Myra (Grimsley) Bennett', in M. Rutherdale (ed.), *Caregiving on the Periphery: Historical Perspectives on Nursing and Midwifery in Canada* (Montreal: McGill-Queens University Press, 2010), pp. 84–105. By comparison, consider the thrust of a recent Newfoundland newspaper article exploring the merits of re-establishing licensed midwives in the province, M. Cook, 'When You're Pregnant, You're Not Sick', *Independent* (St John's), 25 April 2008, p. 7.

28. N. Murphy, *Cottage Hospital Doctor: The Medical Life of Dr. Noel Murphy, 1945–1954*, ed. M. Thackray (St John's: Creative Publishers, 2003), p. 245. The 'Cottage Hospital' network across the island was based on the experience of Scotland as outlined in the Dewar report; see *First Interim Report of the Royal Commission on Health and Public Charities, June 1930* (St John's: King's Printer, 1930). For development of this system, see Martin, *Leonard A. Miller*, esp. ch. 15; and J. K. Crellin, *The Life of a Cottage Hospital: The Bonne Bay Experience* (St John's: Flanker Press, 2007). For background of the Scottish model (the Highland and Islands Medical Service), see M. McCrae, *The National Health Service in Scotland: Origins and Ideals, 1900–1950* (East Linton, Scotland: Tuckwell Press, 2003); and the chapter by Marguerite Dupree in this volume. For comparison of

this system, see G. S. Lawson and A. F. Noseworthy, 'Newfoundland's Cottage Hospital System: 1920–1970', *Canadian Bulletin of Medical History*, 26 (2009), pp. 477–98.

29. Patient letters, MUN, Archives and Manuscripts Division, Ecke Papers, coll. 355, files 6.03.001 and 6.03.002.

30. For an 'introduction' to 'medical outportese' in which local dialect and folk aetiology of ailments figure prominently, see G. L. Saunders, *Doctor, When You're Sick You're Not Well: Forty Years of Outpatient Humour from Twillingate Hospital, Newfoundland* (St John's: Breakwater Books, 1998). More scholarly analyses of traditional healing practices and popular or vernacular medicine are available in J. K. Crellin, *Home Medicine: The Newfoundland Experience* (Montreal: McGill-Queen's University Press, 1994) and J. K. Crellin, *A Social History of Medicines in the Twentieth Century: To Be Taken Three Times a Day* (New York: Pharmaceutical Products Press, 2004). See also D. L. Davis, *Blood and Nerves: An Ethnographic Focus on Menopause* (St John's: ISER, 1983).

31. For a discussion of the 'frontier' thesis in North America other than in the United States of America, see F. Landon, *Western Ontario and the American Frontier* (Toronto: McClelland and Stewart, 1967); M. S. Cross, *The Frontier Thesis and the Canadas: The Debate on the Impact of the Canadian Environment* (Toronto: Copp Clark, 1970); and C. Berger, *The Writing of Canadian History: Aspects of English-Canadian Historical Writing Since 1900* (Toronto: University of Toronto Press, 1986).

32. Ecke, *Snowshoe & Lancet*, p. 125.

33. Ibid., pp. 212–25, *passim*.

34. On the general historical problem of alcoholism among doctors, see C. K. Warsh, *Moments of Unreason: The Practice of Canadian Psychiatry and the Homewood Retreat, 1883–1923* (Montreal: McGill-Queen's University Press, 1989), esp. ch. 10. For current analyses on this issue with an emphasis on the alcoholic 'country doctor' and the protective reaction of the community, see M. Winerip, 'Did You Hear About Doc Ogden', *New York Times*, 5 May 2002, pp. 42–7. For popular culture aspects, see the image of the drunken doctor in regional fiction as highlighted in the Newfoundland feature film *Young Triffie's Been Made Away With*, see http://www.telefilm.gc.ca/data/production/prod_4606.asp?lang=en& [accessed 28 April 2008]. This film was based on an earlier play by Newfoundland author Ray Guy. On Newfoundland and mummering, see E. Fowke, *Folklore of Canada* (Toronto: McClelland and Stewart, 1976); and http://www.batteryradio.com/Pages/mummers.html [accessed 1 February 2010].

35. Murphy, *Cottage Hospital Doctor*, pp. 128–31.

36. A totally rebuilt and enlarged Notre Dame Bay Memorial Hospital opened in 1976; see documents in MUN, CNS, *Notre Dame Bay Memorial Hospital, Twillingate, Official Opening, Friday, September 24, 1975* (n.p., n.d.) and *Welcome to the Official Opening*, (n.p., n.d).

8 Mullally, 'Policing Practitioners on the Periphery'

1. I would like to acknowledge support for this research from Associated Medical Services/ Hannah Institute (Toronto, Ontario), as well as the Canada Research Chair in Atlantic Canada Studies at the University of New Brunswick (Fredericton, New Brunswick). I am also indebted to the feedback and comments from participants of the Hannah Conference on Rural and Remote Medicine, held at the Memorial University of Newfoundland in May 2007. Finally, I would like to acknowledge the openness and generosity of the

New Brunswick College of Physicians and Surgeons, who allowed me to access this material in 1998 and copy these records.

2. Minutes of the Medical Council of the College of Physicians and Surgeons of New Brunswick, 13 March 1934, College of Physicians and Surgeons of New Brunswick Archives, Rothesay, New Brunswick, Canada (hereafter referred to as Council Minutes).

3. Although the College of Physicians and Surgeons of the Province of New Brunswick set no restrictions on my use of this material, at several points in this article I take care to protect the anonymity of physicians in cases where disciplinary actions, allegations of illegal activity or wrong-doing, as well as reports of unethical conduct, are related in the documents. Except in the case of Alfred Leger, where the prosecution is part of the public court records, I use initials to identify physicians and other practitioners named in the Minutes. Owing to the small sample size of physicians in the province (approximately 280 doctors) and the ready availability of physician names in medical directories, it may be possible for researchers to confirm the identities of physicians who were under investigation and prosecuted by the College/Medical Council through various cross-referencing strategies. Therefore, in all but a few cases, I also do not identify the communities where these physicians practised.

4. Council Minutes, 24 March 1931.

5. Ibid., 21 October 1931.

6. The Registrar read correspondence from the Massachusetts State Board of Registration and tabled letters exchanged between Dr Warwick, Chief Medical Officer for Massachusetts, and the New Brunswick Registrar Dr S. H. McDonald. Their meeting minutes cite a report from Mr E. P. Salt, Commissioner to the Royal Canadian Mounted Police (RCMP), as well as a letter from the local parish priest (Council Minutes, 18 July 1932).

7. Ibid.

8. P. Starr, *The Social Transformation of American Medicine* (New York: Basic Books, 1985).

9. S. E. D. Shortt, 'Before the Age of Miracles: The Rise, Fall and Rebirth of General Practice in Canada, 1900–1950', in *Health, Disease and Medicine: Essays in Canadian History*, ed. C. G. Roland (Toronto: Hannah Institute for the History of Medicine, 1982), pp. 123–52.

10. J. T. H. Connor, '"A Sort of *Felo-de-Se*": Eclecticism, Related Medical Sects, and their Decline in Victorian Ontario', *Bulletin of the History of Medicine*, 65:4 (1991), pp. 503–27; T. Romano, 'Professional Identity and the Nineteenth-Century Ontario Medical Profession', *Social History/Histoire sociale*, 28:55 (1995), pp. 77–98; P. O'Reilly, *Health Care Practitioners: An Ontario Case Study in Policy Making* (Toronto: University of Toronto Press, 2000). For a treatment of the professionalization as a broad process, see R. D. Gidney and W. P. J. Millar, *Professional Gentlemen: The Professions in Nineteenth-Century Ontario* (Toronto: Ontario Historical Studies Series/University of Toronto Press, 1994).

11. Region is a long-standing category of analysis in Canadian history; historians in Atlantic and western Canada have wrestled with the importance of region for several decades. See, for instance, the discussions *Acadiensis*: 'Forum: Roundtable on Re-Imagining Regions', *Acadiensis*, 25:2 (2006), pp. 127–68. Western Canadian scholar Gerald Friesen has argued convincingly that the idea of 'region' in Canada undergoes continual evolution in the social, political and historical discourse. In contemporary scholarship, he rightly acknowledges the growing importance of geography, culture and memory in defining the regions of Canada (p. 545). See G. Friesen, 'The Evolving Meanings of Region in Canada', *Canadian Historical Review*, 82:3 (2001), pp. 530–45.

12. M. Davies, 'Mapping "Region" in Canadian Medical History: The Case of British Columbia', *Canadian Bulletin for Medical History*, 17:1–2 (2000), pp. 73–92.

13. P. Twohig, *Labour in the Laboratory: Medical Laboratory Workers in the Maritimes, 1900–1950* (Montreal: McGill-Queen's University Press, 2005), pp. 13–15.

14. For a treatment of the recent literature on region and medicine in Canada, see C. Dooley, 'Reflections on "Region" in Recent Writings on the History of Health and Medicine in Canada', *Journal of Canadian Studies*, 41:3 (2007), pp. 166–84.

15. The Medical Act of 1920 also replaced and consolidated several medical statutes from 1903, 1911, 1913 and 1914. See *American Medical Directory 1921*, 7th edn (Chicago, IL: American Medical Association, 1921), pp. 1666–9. See *American Medical Directory 1921*, 7th edn (Chicago, IL: American Medical Association, 1921), pp. 1666–9. This Act, which replaced previous professional legislation from 1881, enabled the New Brunswick College of Physicians and Surgeons to take on an effective policing role. It accomplished this by vesting the management of licensure and registration with the Medical Council of the Provincial College of Physicians and Surgeons (after 1942, the Medical Licensing Board of New Brunswick) and set a clear set of penalties and fines for practising medicine without a licence. This legislation was further strengthened in 1928 and 1936 by raising these penalties to a fine of over 100 dollars and a possible jail sentence.

16. Legislative changes are captured in *American Medical Directory 1938*, 15th edn (Chicago, IL: American Medical Association, 1938), pp. 1870–3. Exceptions to these licensure laws were allowed for sectarians and midwives, but these must operate as 'drugless practitioners'. Ibid.

17. P. J. Mitham, 'For the Honour and Dignity of the Profession: Organized Medicine in Colonial New Brunswick', *Canadian Bulletin of Medical History*, 13:1 (1996), pp. 83–108. Mitham argues the medical profession looked for greater authority and protection under the law at this time following the advent of sectarian doctors in the province. Although personal tensions marked efforts to organize, the body did acquire 'a significant degree of authority' in the province following successful efforts to enlist legislative support.

18. Rural-urban political divides within the medical profession see occasional treatment in the historiography. See C. D. Naylor, 'Rural Protest and Medical Professionalism in Turn-of-the-Century Ontario', *Journal of Canadian Studies*, 21:1 (1986), pp. 5–20. Nonetheless, the ways in which physician organizations exercised and managed their growing professional power in rural Canada awaits systematic scholarly treatment.

19. The three 'Maritime Provinces' in Canada are New Brunswick, Nova Scotia and Prince Edward Island. The term 'Atlantic Provinces' has been in use since the 1950s and includes the Province of Newfoundland (now officially called Newfoundland and Labrador), which joined the Canada Confederation in 1949.

20. The province became officially bilingual in 1969, the same year as the Canadian nation-state. However, the French-speaking population growth approached one third of the provincial population by the Depression, and the growth of the rural Acadian populations was widely recognized in the province by that time. See M. Roy, 'Settlement and Population Growth in Acadia', *The Acadians of the Maritimes: Thematic Studies*, ed. J. Daigle (Moncton: Centre d'études acadiennes, 1982). For details of the 'Robichaud revolution' which took large strides in incorporating Francophone New Brunswickers into the leadership and apparatus of the province, see D. M. M. Stanley, *Louis Robichaud: A*

Decade of Power (Halifax: Nimbus Publishing, 1984). These strides were made possible, however, by the growth in the population of French-speaking communities of *Acadie*.

21. This precipitated a shift in the *alma maters* of registered physicians in the province: whereas the professional body was populated with many graduates of US diploma mills before the interwar period, after the Depression the *Medical Registry* sees many more graduates of Canadian schools such as McGill University (Montreal, Quebec), Dalhousie University (Halifax, Nova Scotia) and l'Université Laval (Quebec City, Quebec). American graduates on the roster get their training, increasingly, from elite schools like Harvard and the University of Pennsylvania. See the physician rosters in New Brunswick reported in *American Medical Directory 1921*, 7th edn, pp. 1669–71; and *American Medical Directory 1938*, 15th edn, pp. 1873–4.

22. In 1940, for instance, the Canadian Medical Association encouraged the New Brunswick Council to reinstate registration reciprocity with the British Medical Association, but the Council refused (Council Minutes, 28 March 1940).

23. See S. Mullally, 'Unpacking the Black Bag: Country Doctors and Rural Medicine in the Maritimes and New England, 1900–1950' (PhD dissertation, University of Toronto, 2005), pp. 166–7.

24. Ibid.

25. This average statistic for the nation is given by J. P. Willard, 'Has Canada Enough Doctors?' *Public Affairs* [Dalhousie], 11 (1947), pp. 22–8.

26. Council Minutes, 29 June 1939.

27. This mean rate for the province declined to just over 100 deaths per 1,000 live births over 1925–9, sinking once again to 85.3 deaths per 1,000 live births for the five years 1930–5. The rate in Madawaska declined as well, and the improvement between the first and second half of the 1920s was close to the provincial rate of decline. But this improvement stalled in later decades. This county reported a rate of 147.5 over 1925–9 and closed the period at 132.4 deaths per 1,000 live births between 1930–4. See New Brunswick Department of Health, *Annual Report of the Chief Medical Officer to the Minister of Health, 1926*, table 18; New Brunswick Department of Health, *Annual Report of the Chief Medical Officer to the Minister of Health, 1935*, table 18.

28. Charlotte County saw a very slight increase at this time as well, but only 1 per cent, from 62.2 in 1925–9 to 63.2 in 1930–4 (see ibid.).

29. Council Minutes, 8 July 1935.

30. Council Minutes, 21 October 1931. Some osteopaths entrenched in New Brunswick irritated the Medical Council, such as a Dr M based in Moncton, but legally the Council could only pursue prosecution if the individual charged for services not osteopathic in nature. Dr M is a problem mentioned in the Council Minutes of 20 March 1934 and 1 March 1935. In 1938 the provincial registrar suggested the Council engage in a legal lobbying effort to remove clauses from the Medical Act allowing osteopathic practitioners freedom as 'drugless practitioners', but his efforts were overruled by other members of the Council (Council Minutes, 15 October 1938).

31. In 1929 a new practitioner in Restigouche County wrote in to complain about midwives in his district who were making it difficult for him to break into practice. The correspondence was 'discussed and filed', a typical example of how these letters were treated. We do not hear from this physician again, although his name is still on the provincial registry a year later, suggesting he made a go of his practice (Council Minutes, 15 July 1929).

32. Ibid.

33. Council Minutes, 26 March 1929.

34. Council Minutes, 7 September 1936.
35. Ibid.
36. Council Minutes, 23 October 1935.
37. Council Minutes, 18 February 1936.
38. Council Minutes, 8 October 1930.
39. W. Mitchinson, *Giving Birth in Canada, 1900–1950* (Toronto: University of Toronto Press, 2002). See especially ch. 3, 'Midwives Did Not Disappear', pp. 69–103.
40. This is acknowledged in the introduction to I. Bourgeault, *Push!: The Struggle for Midwifery in Ontario* (Montreal and Kingston: McGill-Queen's University Press, 2006). Helene Laforce has argued that in Quebec the eclipse of midwifery was accomplished when medicine was effectively centralized in large hospitals and faculties of medicine; centralized medicine was easier to control via the mechanisms of the state. See H. Laforce, 'The Different Stages of the Elimination of Midwives in Quebec', in K. Arnup, A. Levesque and R. Pierson (eds), *Delivering Motherhood: Maternal Ideologies and Practices in the 19th and 20th Centuries* (London and New York, NY: Routledge, 1990), pp. 41–4.
41. Council Minutes, 24 March 1931.
42. Ibid.
43. Council Minutes, 15 July 1929.
44. Ibid.
45. Council Minutes, 15 March 1933.
46. Ibid.
47. Council Minutes, 20 March 1934.
48. Ibid.
49. Council Minutes, 24 October 1934.
50. Ibid.
51. Council Minutes, 7 September 1936.
52. Confirmation that Leger was 'back in the provincial hospital' was tabled in discussion at the meeting on 7 September 1936 (ibid.).
53. Council Minutes, 1 March 1935.
54. Ibid.
55. Council Minutes, 28 February 1935.
56. Ibid.
57. Council Minutes, 28 February 1935.
58. Council Minutes, 13 March 1934.
59. *American Medical Directory 1938*, pp. 1873–4.
60. Council Minutes, 13 March 1934.
61. Ibid.
62. Section 38.1 of the 1920 Medical Act reads, 'Forfeiture of right of Registration: (1) Any registered practitioner who shall have been convicted in any court of any crime punishable by imprisonment in a penitentiary, although a less penalty be imposed by the court or shall after due inquiry have been adjudged by the council to have been guilty of infamous conduct in any professional respect, shall thereby, subject to any appeal to a justice of the supreme court, forfeit his right to registration, and by direction of the council his name shall be erased from the register', *American Medical Directory 1921*, 7th edn, p. 1668. Perhaps because Dr C. was not in a 'penitentiary', this provided grounds for Council inaction.
63. Council Minutes, 8 July 1935.

64. Ibid.
65. Ibid. Other entries indicate the decision was difficult and some sympathy is expressed for the physician in discussions of the case on 23 October 1935. Letters from the local priest and several physicians from neighbouring communities accompanied his request for reinstatement, as did a member of the Canadian Senate. The physician also supplied a letter signed by all but one of the Northumberland County physicians advocating his re-registration.
66. Council Minutes, 7 September 1936.
67. Ibid.
68. C. Howell, 'Reform and the Monopolistic Impulse: The Professionalization of Medicine in the Maritimes', *Acadiensis*, 11 (1981), pp. 3–22.
69. This is another reason why 'place' is in many ways a better concept than 'region' to employ in this kind of analysis. As Erika Dyck has recently pointed out, the 'vocabulary of place' may be used to 'depoliticize' the analysis of region in Canada and move away from conceptualizations that always refer to federal-provincial or central-regional relationships. This paper has used the concept of place in this fashion to consider of heartland-hinterland relations even within jurisdictions, and within regions. E. Dyck, 'Land of the Living Sky with Diamonds?: A Place for Radical Psychiatry?', *Journal of Canadian Studies*, 41:3 (Fall 2007), pp. 42–66.
70. This is a trend observable in the history of medical institutions in the province. See W.G. Godfrey, *The Struggle to Serve: A History of the Moncton Hospital, 1895–1953* (Montreal and Kingston: McGill-Queen's University Press, 2004).
71. The records at this time show a shift in the activities of the Medical Council. They focused their war-time efforts dealing with the problem of licensing reciprocity within Canada, as well as international credential transfer.

9 Rønsager, 'The West Greenlandic Midwives'

1. O. Marquardt, 'Greenland's Demography, 1700–2000: The Interplay of Economic Activities and Religion', *Études/Inuit/Studies*, 26:2 (2002), pp. 47–69; M. Nuttall, 'Greenland: Emergence of an Inuit Homeland', in Minority Rights Group (ed.), *Polar Peoples: Self-Determination and Development* (London: Minority Rights Publications, 1994), pp. 1–28.
2. A. Bertelsen, 'Folkemedicin i Grønland i ældre og nyere Tid', *Det grønlandske Selskabs Aarsskrift* (1914), pp. 22–57; J. Robert-Lamblin, 'Life, Health and Therapy among the East Greenlanders: Tradition and Acculturation', presented at the Seventh Inuit Studies Conference, Inuit Studies Occasional Papers 4 Fairbanks, Alaska, 1990.
3. M. Rønsager, 'Grønlændernes sundheds- og sygdomsopfattelse 1800–1930. Statens Institut for Folkesundhed. Afdelingen for Grønlandsforskning', *SIFs Grønlandsskrifter*, 14 (2002), pp. 39, 77–81; P. P. Sveistrup and S. Dalgaard, 'Det Danske Styre af Grønland 1825–1850', *Meddelelser om Grønland*, 145 (1945), pp. 304–5, 312; A. K. Sørensen, *Danmark – Grønland i det 20. århundrede – en historisk oversigt* (København: Nyt Nordisk Forlag, Arnold Busck, 1983), pp. 14 ff.
4. J. C. Manniche, 'Sprogbeherskelse og Herskersprog – om sprog og kolonialisme i Grønland i 1800-tallet', Århus Universitet, Historisk Institut, *Arbejdspapirer*, 12 (2002).
5. In this chapter the term 'Danish' obstetrics and midwifery will be used. The Danish ways of obstetrics was rooted in European traditions, but the midwifery service differed from most of the European ones because of its high degree of control and effectiveness.

By 1810 the Danish midwives were regulated by a detailed statute with the purpose of reducing mortality among infants and mothers by ensuring that the best practices of birth attendance were applied to all births. By as early as around 1840 the public had completely adopted the Danish midwifery service and this made the Danish unique compared to the rest of Europe. Until the 1940s this birth attendance system was the most effective in the world measured by its ability to keep mortality at a very low level for both mothers and infants. For further information see A. Løkke, *Døden i barndommen. Spædbørnedødelighed og moderniseringsprocesser i Danmark 1800–1920* (København: Gyldendal, 1998).

6. A. Bertelsen, 'Ældre og nyere Tids Fødselshjælp i Grønland', *Tidsskrift for Jordemødre*, 9 (1911), pp. 105 ff., 117 ff.

7. In 1959 the ship *M/S Hans Hedtoft* was lost on her trip from Greenland to Denmark. Onboard the *Hans Hedtoft* was all the archival material from south Greenland, which was being sent to Rigsarkivet in Copenhagen. Today, therefore, it is only possible to reconstruct partially the archival material from the Southern Inspectorate. This goes for the health services as well. The archival material from the Northern Inspectorate is better preserved but with defects. For further information see K. Petersen, *Rapport om Rigsarkivets Grønlandssamlinger – med specielt henblik på KGH og Grønlands Styrelse* (København: Grønlands Arkiv, 1996).

8. H. Egede, *Relationer angaaende Den Grønlandske Mission 1738 samt Det gamle Grønlands nye Persulation eller Naturel – Historie 1741*, ed. Finn Gad. (1738; 1741; København: Rosenkilde and Bagger, 1971); H. J. F. Lerch, *Underretning for Jordemødre. unnersòutiksak ernisúksiortunnut kaládlit nunænnêtunnut* (København: Fabritius de Tengnagles Bogtrykkeri, 1829), p. 9.

9. 'Letter of the Inspector of North Greenland to Lerch', 2 March 1820; and 'Letter of the Inspector of North Greenland to Lerch', 2 April 1820, no. 158, Inspektøren for Nordgrønland, Inspektørens Arkiv, Kopibog for breve til Betjente 1819–21, Nunatta Katersugaasivia Allagaateqarfialu (NKA); Indretning til Det Kgl. Sundhedskollegium for Handelsaaret 1860 of Doctor Prosch in Julianehaab District, Sundhedskolliets Medicinalberetning Grønland 1820–1861, Rigsarkivet (RA); 'Letter of Rentekammeret to the Director of KGH', 7 February 1835, Styrelsen af Kolonierne i Grønland, Grønlands Handel og Styrelse. Korrespondancesager, RA.

10. It is impossible to know for certain the number of the Greenlandic midwives because of the loss of the *Hans Hedtoft* (see note 7 above). The names and other information concerning known midwives are given in M. Rønsager, 'Imellem læger og landsmænd. Den vestgrønlandske jordemoderinstitution 1820–1920' (PhD dissertation, Københavns Universitet, 2006).

11. Ibid.

12. P. P. Sveistrup, *Rigsdagen og Grønland. Den danske Rigsdag 1849–1949*, vol. 6, (København: J. H. Schultz Forlag 1953), pp. 208–11; F. Gad, *Grønland. Politikens Danmarkshistorie* (København: Politiken 1984), p. 220. Until 1910 the education of midwives took place in the Laying-in-Hospital and after 1910 in Rigshospitalet in Copenhagen. For further details, see J. Rødtness, 'Dagligt Liv paa Jordemoderskolen før og nu', in W. Nellemose (ed.), *Danmarks Jordemødre* (København: Den almindelige danske Jordemoderforening, 1935), pp. 149 ff.

13. See Rønsager, 'Imellem læger og landsmænd', pp. 105–6, 115–17.

14. A. Bertelsen, 'Grønlænderne i Danmark. Bidrag til Belysning af Grønlandsk Koloniarbejde fra 1605 til vor Tid', *Meddelelser om Grønland*, 145:2 (1945), pp. 1–211, on p. 109. Rønsager, 'Imellem læger og landsmænd.

15. C. E. Janssen, *En Grønlandspræsts Optegnelser 1844–49* (København: August Bangs Forlag, 1913), pp. 47, 72, 131–2.

16. In 1853, a part of Ilulissat church was converted into a room for patients. The first real hospital in Greenland was built in 1856 in Nuuk, with room for eight patients. In 1929 there were ten hospitals, with a total of 233 beds, in West Greenland. See A. Bertelsen, 'Sundhedsvæsnet i Grønland', *Ugeskrift for Læger*, 5:91, nos 48–50 (1929), pp. 1080–3, 1111–15, 1144–7.

17. C. van Haven, 'Om lægeforhold i Grønland', *Ugeskrift for Læger*, 4:5 (1882), pp. 159–62; M. Rønsager, *Grønlændernes sundheds- og sygdomsopfattelse 1800–1930*, pp. 63–77.

18. Bertelsen, 'Ældre og nyere Tids Fødselshjælp i Grønland', pp. 120–1; Rønsager, 'Imellem læger og landsmænd', pp. 141–2.

19. 'Medicinalberetning for Nordgrønland for 1900. Doctor Bentzen', Sundhedskollegiets Medicinalberetning, Grønland, 1889–1910, RA.

20. Styrelsen af Kolonierne i Grønland, Grønlands Handel og Styrelse, Lægevæsenet i alm. Forholdene v. Arsuk, Jordemodervæsenet, 1904–24, RA.

21. Rønsager, 'Imellem læger og landsmænd'.

22. H.-E. Rasmussen, 'Some Aspects of Reproduction of the West Greenlandic Upper Social Stratum, 1750–1959', *Arctic Anthropology*, 23:1–2 (1986), pp. 137–50.

23. Thirty-three Greenlandic women were educated in Denmark between 1820 and 1920: ten women were 'first generation mixed descent', twenty were of 'mixed descent related' and three were described by the doctors as 'pure Greenlanders'. For further details see Rønsager, 'Imellem læger og landsmænd', p. 111, supplement 9a.

24. Ibid., pp. 104–17.

25. R. Paine (ed.), *Patrons and Brokers in the East Arctic* ([St John's, NL]: Institute of Social and Economic Research, Memorial University of Newfoundland, 1971).

26. In the period 1820–1917 different Midwife Acts were used in Greenland depending on the midwife's place of education and her place of appointment. The Greenlandic midwives educated in Denmark followed the Midwife Acts applied to the Danish midwives, which were the ones that were also used by midwives in Denmark. On the other hand midwives educated in Greenland were subject to acts especially made for Greenlandic midwives. These acts varied with the place of appointment. In 1917 both the Greenlandic midwives educated in Denmark as well as those educated in Greenland were governed by the same Midwife Act. For further details see Rønsager, 'Imellem læger og landsmænd', pp. 137, 150 ff., 251–60.

27. Styrelsen af Kolonierne i Grønland, Grønlands Handel og Styrelse, Jordemødre 1847–1916, RA; Rønsager, 'Imellem læger og landsmænd', pp. 164–6, 183–93.

28. See for instance: 'Letter of Doctor Koppel to the Inspector of South Greenland', 29 June 1906; and 'Letter of Inspector O. Bendixen to the Director of RGTC', 14 February 1907, both Jordemodervæsenet i almindelighed 1887–1910, Jordemødrenes ansættelser og lønningsvæsen 1907–1908 m.m, NKA.; Bertelsen, 'Ældre og nyere Tids Fødselshjælp i Grønland', p. 121; Rønsager, 'Imellem læger og landsmænd', pp. 210 ff.

29. Rønsager, 'Imellem læger og landsmænd', pp. 212–22.

30. S. Thuesen, *Fremmed blandt Landsmænd. Grønlandske kateketer i kolonitiden* (Nuuk: Forlaget Atuagkat, 2007), pp. 312–14.

31. Ibid., pp. 315–23.

32. See for instance: 'Letter to Doctor Harald Larsen, Imalik, from Otto Larsen', dated 1910, Inspektøren for Nordgrønland. Jordemodervæsenet i almindelighed 1910–24, NKA.
33. Rønsager, 'Imellem læger og landsmænd', pp. 93–4.
34. Styrelsen af Kolonierne i Grønland, Grønlands Handel og Styrelse. Lægevæsenet i almindelighed. Forholdene ved Arsuk, Jordemodervæsenet 1904–24, RA, Rønsager, 'Imellem læger og landsmænd', pp. 171 ff.

10 Kealey, 'Delivering Health Care in Rural New Brunswick'

1. S. Buckley, 'Ladies or Midwives? Efforts to Reduce Infant and Maternal Mortality', in L. Kealey (ed.), *A Not Unreasonable Claim: Women and Reform in Canada, 1880s–1920s* (Toronto: Women's Press, 1979), pp. 131–49; Lady Harris, 'Outport Nursing', *The Newfoundland Quarterly*, 21:1 (July 1921), p. 1. See also H. Coombs-Thorne, 'Conflict and Resistance to Paternalism: Nursing with the Grenfell Mission Stations in Newfoundland and Labrador, 1939–81', and L. Kealey, 'On the Edge of Empire: The Working Life of Myra (Grimsley) Bennett', in M. Rutherdale (ed.), *Caregiving on the Periphery: Historical Perspectives on Nursing and Midwifery in Canada* (Montreal: McGill-Queen's University Press, 2010), chs. 8 and 3, respectively.
2. *A History of Red Cross Outposts in New Brunswick, 1922–1975* (n.p: N.B. Division, Canadian Red Cross Society, n.d.). Bronwyn McIntyre travelled the province interviewing former staff and volunteers as well as using the records of the Red Cross to write this short history. Staff at the Saint John, New Brunswick, headquarters of the Red Cross, could not locate the records she used. The Canadian Red Cross Society archives in Ottawa also did not have the files referred to in this short history. Many thanks to the staff in Saint John and Ottawa for their assistance.
3. 'Outpost Hospitals and Nursing Stations, 1958–1975 inclusive', chart, in 'Outpost Hospitals and Nursing Stations' (box), Canadian Red Cross Society Archives, Ottawa, Ontario (CRCS Archives). The last outpost hospital in New Brunswick was turned over to the community in 1958 leaving seven nursing stations in 1959 in the province.
4. See M. Stuart, 'Shifting Professional Boundaries: Gender Conflict in Public Health, 1920–1925', in D. Dodd and D. Gorham (eds), *Caring and Curing: Historical Perspectives on Women and Healing in Canada* (Ottawa: University of Ottawa Press, 1994), pp. 49–70.
5. J. Elliott, 'A Negotiated Process: Outpost Nursing under the Red Cross in Ontario, 1922–1984', in Rutherdale (ed.), *Caregiving on the Periphery*, ch. 10.
6. J. Elliott, 'Blurring the Boundaries of Space: Shaping Nursing Lives at the Red Cross Outposts in Ontario, 1922–1945', *Canadian Bulletin of Medical History*, 21:2 (2004), pp. 303–25, on p. 306.
7. M. I. Schonberg, 'Outpost Nursing – A Challenge to Canadian Nurses', *Canadian Nurse*, 43:8 (August 1947), pp. 615–18, on p. 615.
8. Ibid., p. 617.
9. Ibid., p. 618.
10. R. E. May, 'Outpost Nursing', *Canadian Nurse*, 63:3 (March 1967), pp. 34–5. See also Coombs-Thorne, 'Conflict and Resistance to Paternalism'. In the early days, New Brunswick's nursing stations differed, however, as they did not provide patient beds, only a clinic and the nurses' living quarters.
11. *Canadian Red Cross*, 1:1 (February 1922), p. 10; see also S. Myers, 'The Governance of Childhood: The Discourse of State Formation and the New Brunswick Child Welfare

Survey, 1927–1930' (PhD dissertation, University of New Brunswick, 2004), ch. 2. The Rockefeller Foundation also helped to fund public-health nursing. When, however, the Foundation offered in January 1925 to fund a dozen public-health nurses for two years as long as the municipalities agreed to pick up the costs thereafter, the municipalities declined. Myers provides the infant mortality rate per 1,000 live births (p. 114).

12. *Canadian Red Cross*, 2:6 (September 1923), p. 12. Ironically, New Brunswick had the first Department of Health in the British Empire, established in 1918.
13. 'In Campbellton', *Despatch*, 3:8 (October 1924), p. 13.
14. 'New Brunswick Division', *Despatch*, 4:2 (February 1925), p. 11.
15. Canadian Red Cross Society (CRCS), New Brunswick (NB) Division, *Annual Report for 1924*, pp. 36, 6; and *Annual Report for 1927*, p. 6. Infant mortality rates in New Brunswick had dropped to 102.4 in 1924, but 1926 and 1929 showed a jump to 105.9 and 106.5, respectively, with the highest rates in the francophone northern counties (Myers, 'The Governance of Childhood', p. 129, table 2.5, and p. 135, table 2.6).
16. Myers, 'The Governance of Childhood', p. 55. Correspondence in the Provincial Department of Health files, however, suggests resentment of the Red Cross for attempting to move locally raised funds to the provincial office of the Red Cross. Huilota Dykeman of the Public Health Nursing Service wrote to the chief medical officer on this item and also claimed that Red Cross supervision of public-health nurses was inappropriate. See H. Dykeman to G. G. Melvin, 23 October 1926, RS136.M2K, Department of Health records, Provincial Archives of New Brunswick.
17. CRCS, NB Division, *Annual Report for 1926*, pp. 26–7.
18. CRCS, NB Division, *Annual Report for 1927*, pp. 40–1; and CRCS, NB Division, *Annual Report for 1928*, p. 17.
19. CRCS, NB Division, *Annual Report for 1931*.
20. CRCS, NB Division, *Annual Report for 1935*, p. 11.
21. CRCS, NB Division, *Annual Report for 1942*, p. 2.
22. The others were located in Rexton, Stanley, Harvey, Fredericton Junction and Plaster Rock. See *A History of Red Cross Outposts*, pp. 11–18.
23. CRCS, NB Division, Annual Reports for 1944 and 1942.
24. *A History of Red Cross Outposts*, pp. 7–10; the Red Cross's mandate specified that hospitals should be turned over to the communities as soon as they were able to run the facilities successfully. CRCS, NB Division, *Annual Report for 1951*.
25. CRCS, NB Division, Annual Reports for 1951 and 1964.
26. 'Record of Outpost Hospitals & Nursing Stations 1958–1975 inclusive', chart, 'Outpost Hospitals and Nursing Stations' (box), CRCS Archives. By 1960 British Columbia/Yukon, Saskatchewan, Ontario, Quebec and New Brunswick maintained nursing stations, a policy continued into the 1970s; Ontario no longer staffed nursing stations after 1970 but continued to run outpost hospitals. The Hospital and Diagnostic Services Act (1957) provided federal, cost-shared funds to the provinces with their own hospital insurance plans.
27. 'Record of Outpost Hospitals and Nursing Stations 1958–1975 Inclusive', chart.
28. CRCS, NB Division, Annual Reports for 1951, 1952 and 1960.
29. CRCS, NB Division, *Annual Report for 1963*.
30. CRCS, NB Division, Annual Reports for 1967 and 1968. The latter indicated that only 35 per cent of patients paid the prescribed fee.

31. 'Programme Evaluation: Highway Safety Posts, First Aid, Outpost Hospitals and Nursing Stations', May 1968, A.D. Kelly, chairman, 'Outpost Hospitals and Nursing Station', (box), CRCS Archives; CRCS, NB Division, *Annual Report for 1969*.

32. The government of Louis Robichaud, 1960–70, initiated a modernization programme which included sweeping changes to social welfare, including health-care provision, reform of the higher education system and recognition of the rights of the francophone population under the concept of 'Equal Opportunity'. See D. Stanley, 'The 1960s: The Illusions and Realities of Progress', in E. R. Forbes and D. A. Muise (eds), *The Atlantic Provinces in Confederation* (Toronto: University of Toronto Press, 1993), pp. 421–59.

33. CRCS, NB Division, Annual Reports for 1970 and 1974; 'Record of Outpost Hospitals and Nursing Stations 1958–1975 Inclusive', CRCS Archives; *Annual Report for 1978*, CRCS, NB Division; all mentions of outpost nursing stations disappear from subsequent annual reports.

34. K. G. DeMarsh, 'Red Cross Outpost Nursing in New Brunswick', *Canadian Nurse*, 69 (June 1973), pp. 24–5; *Despatch*, 8:7 (November 1947), pp. 8–9.

35. *Despatch*, 8:14 (June 1947), p. 4.

36. *Despatch*, 8:13 (April–May 1947), p. 8.

37. DeMarsh, 'Red Cross Outpost Nursing', pp. 25, 26, 27.

38. *A History of Red Cross Outposts*, 'Outpost Nursing: Some Personal Memoirs'; *Despatch*, 12:4 (Fall 1951), p. 10.

39. DeMarsh, 'Red Cross Outpost Nursing', pp. 25–6.

40. Ibid., pp. 25, 27; CRCS, New Brunswick Division, *Annual Report for the Year 1944*. The CRCS, NB Division, *Annual Report for the Year 1950* noted other marriages and commented that most of the nursing personnel were now married.

41. CRCS, NB Division, *Annual Report for the Year 1948*.

42. Interview with Bessie Bass by Shirley Alcoe, 1996, vol. 54, Arlee H. McGee Collection, Nurses' Association of New Brunswick, New Brunswick Museum, Saint John, New Brunswick (hereafter McGee Collection).

43. Canadian Red Cross Society Correspondence, Mary Southern-Holt, Director, Maternal and Child Health, 'Paquetville', 30 January 1961, RS136 N2G4, Provincial Archives of New Brunswick; Elizabeth (Betty) Cripps, interview with author, 26 October 2006, Bathurst, NB, Labour History in New Brunswick (LHTNB) oral history collection [to be deposited at the Provincial Archives of New Brunswick].

44. CRCS, NB Division, Annual Reports for 1952, 1953 and 1954.

45. CRCS, NB Division, Annual Reports for 1955 and 1956.

46. CRCS, NB Division, Annual Reports for 1957, 1958 and 1965. Newspaper clipping files, August 1977, McGee Collection.

47. CRCS, NB Division, *Annual Report for 1978*; *A History of Red Cross Outposts*, p. 35.

48. *A History of Red Cross Outposts*, pp. 24–5; CRCS, NB Division, *Annual Report for 1961*.

49. Annual conferences of outpost nurses are mentioned in the annual reports for the years 1950–4, 1956 and 1960. In 1966 the conference was held in Fredericton to coincide with the annual meeting of the NANB. In addition to the annual conference in 1967, nurses from Canterbury, Paquetville and St Stephen visited the nursing station at Campobello Island and the nurse from Campobello visited Paquetville. The 1969 report mentions that instead of a provincial conference each nurse visited the provincial office of the Red Cross.

50. 'Helen McArthur Nursing Research Award', CRCS Archives. See also CRCS, NB Division, Annual Reports for 1948, 1951, 1952, 1953 and 1954.

51. M. Valverde, *The Age of Light, Soap and Water: Moral Reform in English Canada, 1885–1925* (Toronto: McClelland & Stewart, 1991).
52. See *A History of Red Cross Outposts*, p. 12, in which an interview with Lorna Russell Thompson completed in 1972 suggests that she married relatively late in her career is included in the footnotes.
53. D. Dodd, J. Elliott and N. Rousseau, 'Outpost Nursing in Canada', in C. Bates, D. Dodd and N. Rousseau (eds), *On All Frontiers: Four Centuries of Canadian Nursing* (Ottawa: University of Ottawa Press/Canadian Museum of Civilization, 2005), p. 152.

11 Davies, 'Mother's Medicine'

1. I would like to thank Wellcome Trust for funding this research, the University of Glasgow Centre for the History of Medicine for supporting my application for a Wellcome fellowship, and the wonderful women of the Peace who opened their doors to me in 2002 and 2005 and shared stories of their mothers. These tales were a profound revelation to a historian who had blindly been doing 'motherwork' for a decade without incorporating it into her analysis of health. My goal here is to balance an exploration of the social and political implications of the health work of Peace River women with a narrative which reclaims, honours and values their lives. Jon Swainger, a historian with a much more extensive knowledge of the Peace River region than I, has been generous with references, general knowledge and friendship. Bettina Bradbury, Colin Coates and Sasha Mullally have been tremendously helpful during the writing and editing stages of this paper. The opportunity to teach about health in the unique interdisciplinary milieu of the Department of Social Science at York University has served to foster my intellectual development in entirely new and positive directions. As always, Mab Coates-Davies, Bryn Coates-Davies and Colin Coates were ideal travelling companions for my 2002 road trip to the Peace.
2. I cobbled this story together from two slightly different accounts. Bear Flats (Taylor) native Blanche Dopp Hipkiss remembers the accident happening in the late 1920s or early 1930s, while Alice Summer believes it happened in 1924, when she was four years old. Alice pointed out that the moccasin needle would have been used because it has three sharp edges. The telegraphy had been extended from Edmonton to Hudson's Hope by this time, and Philip Tompkins had been able to get a little station at the farm. Alice's brother operated the telegraphy. Robinson had a long convalescence but had no permanent damage. 'Doc Buggins', an early dentist in Dawson Creek built him 'the most peculiar plate to fill in the teeth which he had knocked out', according to C. Ventress, M. Davies and E. Kyllo (authors-compilers), *The Peacemakers of North Peace* ([Fort St John, BC]: Davies, Ventress and Kyllo, 1973), p. 59; and Alice Summer, interview with the author, 26 July 2005, Hudson's Hope, BC.
3. Alice Summer, interview with the author.
4. Alice Summer stressed that her mother was midwife only to women in the immediate region of the family farm (Alice Summer, interview with the author). Emily Tompkins' midwifery work is noted in Ventress et al., *The Peacemakers of North Peace*, p. 68.
5. There is not a huge literature on the history of women's informal health work in Canada. See N. L. Lewis, 'Goose Grease and Turpentine: Mother Treats the Family', *Prairie Forum*, 15:1 (Spring 1990), pp. 67–84.
6. I take the phrase 'motherwork' from H. Rosenberg's 'The Home is the Workplace: Hazards, Stress and Pollutions in the Household', in S. Arat-Koc, M. Luxton and H.

Rosenberg (eds), *Through the Kitchen Window: The Politics of Home and Family* (Toronto: Garamond, 1990), pp. 57–80. Rosenberg defines 'motherwork' as the caregiving activities of women in the home and in the community, noting that it included a culturally organized set of tasks relating to children and other dependent family members. See also M. Luxton, *More Than a Labour of Love: Three Generations of Women's Work in the Home* (Toronto: Women's Press, 1980).

7.   My understanding of maternalism – as a social and political movement that posited 'motherwork' as a means by which women would reform modern society through their natural roles as women, mothers and citizens – is informed by S. Koven and S. Michel, 'Introduction: "Mother Worlds"', in S. Koven and S. Michel (eds), *Mothers of a New World: Maternalist Politics and the Origins of Welfare States* (New York, NY: Routledge, 1993), pp. 1–43. The key work regarding maternalism and construction of colonial power relations remains Anna Davin's early article on the subject. See A. Davin, 'Imperialism and Motherhood', *History Workshop Journal*, 5 (Spring 1978), pp. 9–66. Health and social welfare initiatives, such as mothers' pensions and well-baby clinics, put forward by government and women's groups such as the Women's Institutes, were part of this broad agenda in BC during the inter-war period. See M. J. Davies, 'Competent Professionals and Modern Methods: State Medicine in British Columbia during the 1930s', *Bulletin of the History of Medicine*, 76:1 (Spring, 2002), pp. 56–83; and M. J. Davies, '"Services Rendered, Rearing Children for the State": Mothers' Pensions in British Columbia', in B. K. Latham and R. J. Pazdro (eds), *Not Just Pin Money: Selected Essays on the History of Women's Work in British Columbia* (Victoria, BC: Camosun College Press, 1984), pp. 249–63.

8.   The important work on race and 'White' British Columbia is A. Perry's, *On the Edge of Empire: Gender, Race and the Making of British Columbia, 1849–1871* (Toronto: University of Toronto Press, 2001). Additional useful works also include A. Kobayashi and L. Peake, 'Racism out of Place: Thoughts on Whiteness and an Antiracist Geography in the New Millennium', *Annuals of the Association of American Geographers*, 90:2 (2000), pp. 392–403; L. Pulido, 'Reflections on a White Discipline', *The Professional Geographer*, 54:1 (2002), pp. 42–9; and H. Nast, 'Mapping the 'Unconscious': Racism and the Oedipal Family', *Annals of the Association of American Geographers*, 90:2 (2000), pp. 215–55.

9.   Historians of women in rural western Canada spotlight these aspects. See V. Strong-Boag, 'Pulling in Double Harness or Hauling a Double Load: Women, Work and Feminism on the Canadian Prairie', in R. D. Francis and H. Palmer (eds), *The Prairie West: Historical Readings* (Edmonton: Pica Pica Press, 1992), pp. 401–23; C. G. Bye, '"I Like to Hoe My Own Row": A Saskatchewan Farm Woman's Notions about Work and Womanhood', *Frontiers*, 26:3 (2005), pp. 135–67; C. A. Cavanaugh, '"No Place for a Woman": Engendering Western Canadian Settlement', in R. D. Francis and C. Kitzan (eds), *The Prairie West as Promised Land* (Calgary: University of Calgary, 2007), pp. 261–90.

10. See K. Pickles and M. Rutherdale, 'Introduction', in K. Pickles and M. Rutherdale (eds), *Contact Zones: Aboriginal and Settler Women in Canada's Colonial Past* (Vancouver: UBC Press, 2005), pp. 1–14; and K. Elswood-Holland, '"We Used to Scrump the Apples, We Used to Have Our Knickers Full of 'Em"', Growing up in the Countryside: Forging Feminities in Rural Somerset *c*: 1950–1970', in J. Little and C. Morris (eds), *Critical Studies in Rural Gender Issues* (Aldershot: Ashgate, 2005), pp. 123–40. Laurel Thatcher Ulrich is also inspirational for appreciating the importance of the material. L. Thatcher Ulrich, *The Age of the Homespun: Objects and Stories in the Creation of an*

American Myth (New York, NY: Vintage Books, 2001). The human body should be understood as both as a biological reality and a cultural and social construct – and the literature on the body and medicine is vast. For an overview see D. Lupton, *Medicine as Culture* (London: Sage Publications, 2003), pp. 22–53. For specific analysis of colonialism and the body, see M. Jolly, 'Colonizing Women: The Maternal Body and the Empire', in S. Gunew and A. Yeatman (eds), *Feminism and the Politics of Difference* (St Leonard's, Australia: Allen & Unwin, 1993), pp. 103–27.

11. On the first of my two field trips to the Peace (2002 and 2005) to do archival research and undertake oral histories, I was fortunate to obtain a comprehensive set of extensive local histories. Tales of birth, accidents and illness feature prominently in these valuable community narratives, which women played a significant role in compiling, making them excellent sources for this project.

12. I am not aware of recent surveys of local histories, but two older ones include: P. Voisey, 'Rural Local History and the Prairie West', in Francis and Palmer (eds), *The Prairie West: Historical Readings*, pp. 497–509; L. Hale and J. Barman, *British Columbia Local Histories: A Bibliography* (Victoria: British Columbia Heritage Trust, 1991).

13. The term 'belated frontier' is used by W. Stegner in *Wolf Willow: A History, a Story and a Memory of the Last Prairie Frontier* (Toronto: Macmillan, 1962), cited in P. Banting, 'Introduction', in P. Banting (ed.), *Fresh Tracks: Writing the Western Landscape* (Victoria, BC: Polestar Press, 1998), pp. 11–13.

14. Ibid., p. 13.

15. I am extrapolating these illustrations of biomedically managed births in inter-war Canada from W. Mitchinson, *Giving Birth in Canada, 1900–1950* (Toronto: University of Toronto Press, 2002), ch. 6.

16. My use of this concept was based in the first instance on the ideas of Mary Pratt, which apply to the dynamics between empire and colonies, the observers and the observed, how power and interpretation is negotiated by different parties. I thank Ruth Sandwell for pointing out the usefulness of interpretation as it applies to rural and urban contact. See M. L. Pratt, *Imperial Eyes: Travel Writing and Transculturation* (London: Routledge, 1992), introduction.

17. J. Crellin, *Home Medicine: The Newfoundland Experience* (Montreal: McGill-Queen's University Press, 1994), p. 5.

18. Here I am employing notions of medicine that 'travels', developed by Valentina Napolitano and Gerardo Mora Flores in their work on transcultural medicine in urban Mexico. For a closer study of this see V. Napolitano and G. Mora Flores, 'Complementary Medicine: Cosmopolitan and Popular Knowledge, and Transcultural Translations – Cases from Urban Mexico', *Theory, Culture and Society*, 20:4 (2003), pp. 79–95.

19. This means that BC's Peace River region is approximately the size of Great Britain.

20. B. McGillivray, *Geography of British Columbia: People and Landscapes in Transition* (Vancouver: UBC Press, 2000), pp. 17–18.

21. The history of the Peace River region has not yet been the subject of a sustained scholarly historical study. For works contemporary to the period, see F. H. Kitto, *The Peace River Country Canada: Its Resources and Opportunities* (Ottawa: National Development Bureau, 1930); C. A. Dawson and R. W. Murchie, *The Settlement of the Peace River Country – A Study of a Pioneer Region* (Toronto: The Macmillan Company of Canada Ltd, 1934); and 'The Peace River Country, Canada', in W. A. Mackintosh, *Prairie Settlement: The Geographical Setting* (Toronto: The Macmillan Company of Canada, Ltd, 1934), pp. 151–71. For recent historiography which considers crime and community in the Peace,

see J. Swainger, 'Breaking the Peace: Fictions of the Law-Abiding Peace River Country, 1940–1950', *BC Studies*, 119 (August 1998), pp. 5–25; J. Swainger, 'Police Culture in British Columbia and "Ordinary Duty" in the Peace River Country, 1910–1950', in J. Swainger and C. Backhouse (eds), *People and Place: Historical Influences on Legal Culture* (Vancouver: UBC Press, 2003), pp. 198–223; J. Swainger, 'Creating the Peace: Crime and Community Identity in North-Eastern British Columbia, 1930–1950', in L. Knafla (ed.), *Violent Crime in North America* (Westport, CT: Praeger, 2003), pp. 131–54. Work on First Nations in the region includes: A. Napoleon (ed.), *Bushland Spirit: Our Elders Speak* (Moberly Lake, BC: Twin Sisters Publishing Company, 1998); R. Ridlington, *Little Bit Know Something: Stories in a Language of Anthropology* (Vancouver: Douglas and McIntyre, 1990); H. Brody, *Maps and Dreams: Indians and the British Columbia Frontier* (Harmondsworth: Penguin Books Ltd, 1983); J. Goulet, *Ways of Knowing: Experience, Knowledge, and Power Among the Dene Tha* (Vancouver: UBC Press, 1998).

22. Kitto, *The Peace River Country Canada*, pp. 7, 26.

23. McGillivray, *Geography of British Columbia*, p. 7.

24. There is a limited historiography that considers health in rural BC. The most thought-provoking work is J. Norris, 'The Country Doctor in British Columbia: 1887–1975. An Historical Profile', *BC Studies*, 49 (Spring 1981), pp. 15–19. See also M. Andrews, 'Rural Medical Practice in the Smelter West, 1898–1923: A Case-Study Comparison', *Canadian Bulletin of Medical History*, 6:1 (1989) pp. 83–109; and M. Davies, 'Mapping "Region" in Canadian Medical History: The Case of British Columbia', *Canadian Bulletin of Medical History*, 17:1–2 (2000), pp. 73–92.

25. Winnie Williams told me that it would take about two days to get from Sunset Prairie to Pouce Coupe, where there was a doctor and a hospital, with a team and wagon or a sledge. Neighbours got a truck in 1933, but the roads were still difficult. Winnie Williams, interview with the author, 27 July 2005, Sunset Prairie, BC.

26. 'Dr. Brown: – Fort St. John's First Doctor', 984–116 Ms 40, Fort St John Archives, Fort St John, BC.

27. 'Dr. Hollies passes away', newsclipping, Calverley Collection, Dawson Creek Library, Dawson Creek, BC.

28. N. Dunn, 'Public Health Service South of the Peace River, B.C.', *Public Health Nurses' Bulletin* (hereafter *PHNB*), 1:9 (March, 1932), pp. 34–5.

29. I consider this and other inter-war public health initiatives in BC in M. J. Davies, 'Competent Professionals and Modern Methods: State Medicine in British Columbia during the 1930s', *Bulletin of the History of Medicine*, 76:1 (Spring 2002), pp. 56–83.

30. The link between female identity and the reproduction and rearing of children is an important aspect of the historiography of women on the frontier or in remote and rural areas. See, for example, E. L. Silverman, *The Last Best West: Women on the Alberta Frontier, 1880–1930* (Montreal: Eden Press, 1984), p. 59; and C. Benoit, 'Mothering in a Newfoundland Community: 1900–1940', in K. Arnup, A. Lévesque and R. Roach Pierson (eds), *Delivering Motherhood: Maternal Ideologies and Practices in the 19th and 20th Centuries* (London: Routledge, 1990), pp. 173–89. The capable woman was a strong theme in the oral histories which I collected in the Peace River.

31. I am borrowing the term 'fields of care' from work that has been done on therapeutic landscape. See K. Wilson, 'Therapeutic Landscapes and First Nations Peoples: An Exploration of Culture, Health and Place', *Health and Place*, 9 (2003), pp. 83–93.

32. Mitchinson makes some useful points in regard to the use of the term 'midwife', suggesting that the word has been used differently by different settings. I suggest that most

of the women who assisted in childbirth in the early years of white settlement in Peace River were local women who assisted neighbours in labour and thus gained a reputation as women who were capable in this regard. See Mitchinson, *Giving Birth in Canada*, pp. 70–1.

33. The concept of the 'neighbourhood midwife' is one developed by Jutta Mason and offered by her as a dominant motif in the history of Canadian midwifery, but Leslie Biggs argues that it is in fact best suited to specific settler situations – Biggs also discusses the 'myriad of cultural understandings of the figure of the midwife' which is shown in the different names used. See L. Biggs, 'Rethinking the History of Midwifery in Canada', in I. Bourgeault, C. Benoit and R. Davis-Floyd (eds), *Reconceiving Midwifery* (Montreal: McGill-Queen's University Press, 2004), pp. 17–45.

34. I encountered no sense of loss at the shift to physician-assisted hospital birth in the Peace River. Mitchinson deals with this question, stating that many women saw this shift as a sign of progress and modernization. See Mitchinson, *Giving Birth in Canada*, p. 92.

35. L. Ulrich, *A Midwife's Tale: The Life of Martha Ballard, Based on Her Diary, 1785–1812* (New York, NY: Vintage Books, 1991).

36. Ventress et al., *The Peacemakers of North Peace*, p. 19.

37. *Rolla Remembers, 1912–1952*, comp. Rolla History Book Committee (Rolla, BC: The Committee, 1991), p. 106. Mrs Miller was certainly used by the extended Coon family. See *Rolla Remembers*, pp. 110, 115.

38. *Rolla Remembers*, pp. 232, 235.

39. The story about Kate Edwards was written in 1934 by Clive Planta, MLA, and is quoted in *Rolla Remembers*, p. 121.

40. *Rolla Remembers*, pp. 112, 203; L. York (ed.), *Lure of the South Peace: Tales of the Early Pioneers to 1945* (Fort St John and Dawson Creek, BC: South Peace Historical Book Committee, 1981), p. 133.

41. Ventress et al., *The Peacemakers of North Peace*, pp. 55, 144.

42. Ibid., p. 149.

43. There is a parallel here, of course, with ties of family. To cite one example: Mabel Armitage's mother always went to help her sister-in-law give birth: 'She wasn't a midwife, but she'd always go help her sister-in-law of course'. Mabel Armitage, Belda Ireland and Martha Tower, collective interview with the author, Dawson Creek, BC, 29 July 2002. I am also not dealing here with instances, of which there were undoubtedly many, where the father assisted at a birth.

44. This took place between 1917 and 1923. Ventress et al., *The Peacemakers of North Peace*, p. 65.

45. Amy Smith, interview with the author, 29 July 2005, Fort St John, BC.

46. Ventress et al., *The Peacemakers of North Peace*, pp. 312–13.

47. Mabel Armitage, Belda Ireland and Martha Tower, collective interview with the author. The term 'chinooky day' refers to a chinook, a weather pattern common to western and southern Alberta as well as the Peace River, whereby a short spell of warm weather comes in the midst of winter. These weather conditions may well have made it impossible for Martha's mother to make it to the hospital.

48. Martha Tower told me that Mrs Trail was well into middle age with grown children when she helped birthing women. Mabel Armitage, Belda Ireland and Martha Tower, collective interview with the author. Mary Louis Miller (née Fey) was born in 1873 in Indiana and came to the Peace as a married woman with eight children. No mention is made of her midwifery in the local history, but she was clearly regarded as a healer in the

Rolla area: 'The nearest doctor and nurse were a hundred miles away at Grande Prairie. Mother was called on to ride many miles to take care of the sick'. *Rolla Remembers*, p. 164.

49. Alice Summer, interview with the author.

50. This birth, which was of the first white baby born at Cecil Lake, is recounted in several places. See Ventress et al., *The Peacemakers of North Peace*, p. 382; *A Community Tells Its Story: Cecil Lake, 1925–2000*, ed. Women's Institute History Book Committee (n.p., 2000), p.119; and Jean Mensink and Dorthea Smith, collective interview with the author, 30 July 2002, Cecil Lake, BC.

51. *A Community Tell Its Story*, p.119.

52. Jean Mensink and Dorthea Smith, collective interview with the author.

53. York (ed.), *Lure of the South Peace*, p. 196.

54. Holgates lived in the Rolla region between 1927 and 1942. She may have had nursing training in England. *Rolla Remembers*, p. 352.

55. Ventress et al., *The Peacemakers of North Peace*, p. H59.

56. Ibid., p. H59.

57. Amy Smith and Dorothy Campbell, interview with the author, 29 July 2005, Fort St John, BC. Both Smith (who commented, 'People in the community just have to admire her') and Campbell (who said, 'Her name will never die') paid tribute to Young's midwifery work. Amy and Dorothy told me that Young was paid by the Provincial Government for her midwifery work, but I have not been able to verify this using government sources. She was paid in the 1930s for working as a school nurse. Other references to Young's midwifery work include the 1947 birth of Kay Paris in Montney and her own settler biography. Ventress et al., *The Peacemakers of North Peace*, pp. 259, 293–5; and *Pioneers of Sunrise and Two Rivers* (Fort St John: Alaska Highway News, 1981), p. 114.

58. Alice Summer, interview with the author.

59. Ellen Dewetter, interview with the author, 28 July 2005, Pouce Coupe, BC.

60. Cecil Helman notes that the concept of clearing out 'blockage' is rooted in widespread British folk concepts that posit a 'good clear out' as necessary for good health. He is talking here about constipation, but I see a link here to spring tonics as well. C. Helman, *Culture, Health and Illness* (Oxford: Butterworth-Heinemann, 2000), p. 21. Crellin links the practice to 'autointoxication' and notes that there was widespread belief in and use of spring tonics in early-twentieth-century Newfoundland (*Home Medicine*, pp. 23, 227–30). Although Newfoundlanders used commercial tonics, I found no mention of these among my Peace River respondents.

61. Crellin makes this link between concepts of cleanliness and purges, but does not connect it with gender (*Home Medicine*, pp. 22–4).

62. Crellin identifies sulphur and molasses as a 'standard' springtime purgative in Newfoundland, noting that while sulphur was the medicinal element, molasses was also believed to have health-giving properties (*Home Medicine*, p. 224). Winnie Williams, interview with the author; Toulie Hamilton, interview with the author, 26 July 2005, Hudson's Hope, BC; Girlie Powell, interview with the author, 26 July 2005, Hudson's Hope, BC.

63. Girlie Powell, interview with the author.

64. Alice Summer, interview with the author. Like other interviewees, Alice noted that her mother was the person in the household who was in charge of the family diet.

65. For a reference to Aboriginal use of saskatoon berries, see A. MacKinnon, J. Pojar and R. Coupe (eds), *Plants of Northern British Columbia* (Vancouver: BC Ministry of Forests & Lone Pine Publishing, 1999), p. 46.

66. Jean Mensink and Dorthea Smith, collective interview with the author. The consumption of pigweed was recalled with some humour. Though not native to northern BC, pigweed grows in cultivated land. Its leaves can be eaten raw or boiled. See MacKinnon et al. (eds), *Plants of Northern British Columbia*, p. 199.

67. Crellin, *Home Medicine*, p. 228.

68. Jean Mensink told me this (Jean Mensink and Dorthea Smith, collective interview with the author). Elizabeth Gibbon made the point as well (Elizabeth M. Gibbon, interview with the author, 28 July 2005, Pouce Coupe, BC). But this is not to suggest that this was a universal pattern: Alice Summer does not remember a doctor's book in her parents' house at Halfway (Alice Summer, interview with the author). Toulie Hamilton's father had a little doctor's book, which she thinks came from his St John's Ambulance training in England, but her mother did not read it (Toulie Hamilton, interview with the author). For discussions of the history of popular health publications like doctors' books, see L. R. Murphy, *Enter the Physician: The Transformation of Domestic Medicine, 1760–1860* (Tuscaloosa, AL: University of Alabama Press, 1991), esp. chs. 4 and 5; J. B. Blake, 'From Buchan to Fishbein: The Literature of Domestic Medicine', in G. B. Risse, R. L. Numbers and J. W. Leavitt (eds), *Medicine Without Doctors: Home Health Care in American History* (New York: Neale Watson Academic Publications, 1977), pp. 11–30.

69. Ventress et al., *The Peacemakers of North Peace*, pp. 102–3.

70. The sterilized items were tools for delivering babies. Jean Mensink and Dorthea Smith, collective interview with the author.

71. Winnie Williams, interview with the author.

72. Elizabeth M. Gibbon, interview with the author.

73. Pointing out that her mother took care of humans, but also served as vet to the animals, Elizabeth reminded me that healthy livestock were very important (Elizabeth M. Gibbon, interview with the author).

74. Amy Smith and Dorothy Campbell, interview with the author, 29 July 2005, Fort St John, BC.

75. Winnie Williams, interview with the author.

76. Ventress et al., *The Peacemakers of North Peace*, p. 26.

77. Margaret Bidnlka, interview with the author, 30 July 2002, Fort St John, BC. Margaret, who called these 'barnagalias', believed that her mother Rose used remedies which she learnt from her own mother, a self-taught midwife who had been raised in a convent.

78. Bertha Lentendre, interview with the author, 27 July 2005, Moberly Lake, BC. Bertha told me if you had a bad cut you would get tobacco and a little white spruce tip and would chew it together and stick it on, and 'It would stop the blood dead'. Bertha's father Alexis Gauthier had knowledge of traditional healing, and her paternal grandfather, Tuskwala Gauthier, Dunneza who trapped near present-day Chetwynd, used traditional healing to cure damage to Bertha's brother Oliver's throat and vocal cords and spruce tips on a very bad cut Bertha got from a broad axe when she was four – both these incidents took place in the 1930s. Oliver Gauthier's story is in Napoleon (ed.), *Bushland Spirit*, p. 111.

79. Margaret Bidnlka, interview with the author.

80. The phrase 'country of home-mades' was used by Muriel Claxton. M. Claxton, 'North of the Peace River', *PHNB*, 2:2 (April 1935), p. 4.

81. *Peace River Block News (PRBN)*, 14 March 1933, p. 2.

82. Ibid., 20 June 1933, p. 3.

83. Ibid., 28 September 1934, p. 3.

84. Jean Mensink and Dorthea Smith, collective interview with the author.
85. Forbes is described by Winnie as part Indian and part Scottish, so this may be a Scottish remedy. Winnie Williams, interview with the author.
86. Ellen Dewetter (née McDonnell), interview with the author, 28 July 2005, Pouce Coupe. Ellen thought that the plant tincture was one that her mother got from *her* mother in Ontario, one of the old remedies. This may also have been related to commercial remedies for diarrhoea and stomach cramps which contained extract of wild strawberry. See Crellin, *Home Medicine*, p. 224.
87. For a discussion of humoral theory, see Helman, *Culture, Health and Illness*, pp. 18–20. Helman notes that humoral concepts persist in English folk beliefs concerning the environmental causes of colds and chills and the belief that they can be counteracted with heat in the form of warm drinks, warm foods and bed rest.
88. For a detailed discussion of remedies for pneumonia, see Crellin, *Home Medicine*, pp. 200–1. Prairie women used onion and mustard poultices for pneumonia. Silverman, *The Last Best West*, p. 130.
89. Winnie Williams, interview with the author. Mustard plasters, made from mixture of mustard, flour and water, were 'one of the best-known kitchen remedies from the early nineteenth century to the 1940s', and were used both for colds and for more 'serious' chest ailments. Crellin, *Home Medicine*, p. 188.
90. This took place in 1938 and what is interesting is that Dr Hollies of Pouce Coupe agreed that this was a good remedy for this situation and that Doonan had saved the baby from death by pneumonia. *Rolla Remembers*, p. 243.
91. Ventress et al., *The Peacemakers of North Peace*, pp. 102–3.
92. *Pioneers of Sunrise and Two Rivers*, pp. 45–52.
93. Crellin notes that mustard plasters were once recommended by physicians (*Home Medicine*, p. 188).
94. Ellen Dewetter (née McDonnell), interview with the author.
95. Jean Mensink and Dorthea Smith, collective interview with the author.
96. Toulie Hamilton, interview with the author; Girlie Powell, interview with the author.
97. Winnie Williams, interview with the author.
98. R. Blaustein, A. Cavender and J. Sluder, 'The Poor Man's Medicine Bag: The Empirical Folk Remedies of Tillman Waggoner', in E. Brady (ed.), *Healing Logics: Culture and Medicine in Modern Health Belief System* (Logan, UT: Utah State University, 2000), pp. 88–112. For the specific reference to kerosene, see pp. 97–8.
99. *PHNB*, 2: 4 (March 1937), p. 33.
100. Toulie Hamilton, interview with the author; Girlie Powell, interview with the author.
101. I am still trying to track down specific information about what would likely have been in 'stock dip' or 'sheep dip' in the 1920s and 1930s. Sheep dip, apparently invented in Coldstream, Scotland, in 1830, was based on arsenic power and exported from the nearby English port of Berwick-upon-Tweed. Sheep dip currently contains insecticides and fungicides.
102. Jean Mensink and Dorthea Smith, collective interview with the author.
103. Toulie Hamilton, interview with the author.
104. Mothers' medical 'kits' were mentioned in the Cecil Lake and Dawson Creek collective interviews. Mabel Armitage's mother had 'kits' already made up for dealing with injuries such as bad cuts. Mabel Armitage, Belda Ireland and Martha Tower, collective interview with the author; Jean Mensink and Dorthea Smith, collective interview with the author.

105. Amy Smith and Dorothy Campbell, interview with the author, 29 July 2005, Fort St John, BC.

106. Highlands and Islands Medical Service Committee, *Report to the Lords Commissioners of His Majesty's Treasury, Volume 1* (London: His Majesty's Stationery Office, 1912); Royal Commission on Health and Public Charities (St John's: King's Printer, 1930); John Crellin argues that this is debatable (*Home Medicine*, pp. 15–16).

107. Girlie Powell, interview with the author.

108. Amy Smith and Dorothy Campbell, interview with the author. These women told me that these men were common during the 1930s in Saskatchewan and probably all across Canada. Women sometimes did this work. It was customary for a customer to give them a free meal and they would sometimes stay over night.

109. Alice Summer, interview with the author.

110. Ellen Dewetter, interview with the author.

111. Girlie Powell, interview with the author. These themes of self-sufficiency and a 'hands off' attitude towards injuries is echoed in Toulie Hamilton's memory of an accident where a horse dragged her a distance and the hay 'rake' went over her, bruising her and marking her up. She does not remember her mother doing anything (Toulie Hamilton, interview with the author).

112. *PRBN*, 9 February 1939, p. 2.

113. *PHNB*, 2:3 (June 1936), pp. 53–4.

114. *Pioneers of Sunrise and Two Rivers*, pp. 24–8.

115. The concept of relational authority and its importance on understanding how authority works within folk medicine is explored by E. Brady, 'Introduction', in *Healing Logics*, pp. 3–12.

116. Fort St John Museum and Archives, Herbie Taylor Fonds, 984–130. Ventress et al., *The Peacemakers of North Peace*, pp. 30, 34. Also, Dorothy Campbell, interview with the author, 29 July 2005, Fort St John, BC. Charlotte Taylor's marriage to Herbie Taylor, one of the first white men in the region of Taylor Flats, was a common pattern in early years of white activity in a region, when white women were limited in number. However, oral and written evidence strongly indicated the high esteem with which Charlotte Taylor was held in her community, regardless of her ethnicity. For a discussion of Aboriginal wives and mothers in pioneer society, see J. Barman, 'Invisible Women: Aboriginal Mothers and Mixed Race Daughters in Rural Pioneer British Columbia', in R. W. Sandwell (ed.), *Beyond City Limits: Rural History in British Columbia* (Vancouver: UBC Press, 1999), pp. 159–79.

117. Amy Smith, interview with the author.

118. *Rolla Remembers*, p. 120.

119. Ibid.

120. L. York (ed.), *Petticoat Pioneers of the South Peace* (n.p.: Peace River Block News, 1979) p. 8.

121. Ventress et al., *The Peacemakers of North Peace*, p. 156.

122. Ibid., p. H56.

123. Girlie Powell, interview with the author.

124. Mabel Armitage, Belda Ireland and Martha Tower, collective interview with the author.

125. Jean Mensink and Dorthea Smith, collective interview with the author.

126. Amy Smith and Dorothy Campbell, interview with the author.

12 Junila, 'Call of the Wild'

1. M. Junila, 'Sairaanhoito sota-ajoilta nykypäiviin' in T. Manninen and M. Junila, *Lapin sairaanhoidon historia* (Rovaniemi: Lapin sairaanhoitopiirin kuntayhtymä, 2005); A. Yrjälä, *Public Health and Rockefeller Wealth. Alliance Strategies in the Early Formation of Finnish Public Health Nursing* (Åbo; Åbo Akademins University Press, 2005), pp. 86–87, 138–141; *Health Care Systems in Transition, Finland* (Copenhagen: World Health Organization Regional Office for Europe, 1996), pp. 12–13. See also Lääninterveyssisar Elli-Kaarina Oittisen esitelmä, 'Työntekijätarve Lapissa', *Terveyssisarten opinto- ja neuvottelupäivät Rovaniemellä*, 19 (22 September 1951), AMOPL, DVa, OMA.

2. The medical officer of the province (*lääninlääkäri*) was part of the state provincial administration as was the public health nurse of the province (*lääninterveyssisar*). Although public health nurses were employed by the municipalities rather than the state, these two officers supervised their work.

3. I will speak about 'the people of Lapland' or 'Lappish people' rather than 'the Lapps' because the latter term is sometimes used interchangeably with the Sami, the indigenous people who constitute only part of the Lappish population.

4. The collections used here are 'Hoitotyön muistot' (arranged by the Finnish Literature Society) and 'Lääkintää ja potilaita' (National Board of Antiquities). I have also made use of the contributions that were sent to a writing competition on 'Sairaana Lapissa' [Being ill in Lapland] which was organized for Lapin sairaanhoidon historia [The history of health care in Lapland].

5. Junila, 'Sairaanhoito sota-ajoilta nykypäiviin', p. 129; The Annual Report of the Public Health Nurse of the Province of Lapland for 1945, held at the Archives of the Medical Officer of the Province of Lapland (AMOPL), EIIe:1, at the Regional Archive of Oulu (hereafter OMA); The Report of the State Provincial Governor of Lapland for 1946, Documents of the Reconstruction Period, OMA; *Lapsi ja nuoriso*, 10 (1948), p. 203.

6. *Väestöpolitiikkamme taustaa ja tehtäviä, Väestöliiton vuosikirja 1* (Forssa, 1946), pp. 73–7; M. Mustonen, R. Suominen and K. Suonoja, *Imeväiskuolleisuuteen vaikuttavat sosiaaliset ja taloudelliset tekijät Suomessa 1910–1971*, Suomen Virallinen Tilasto [Statistics Finland] (SVT), 32:46 (Helsinki, 1976), p. 44; The Annual Report of the Public Health Nurse of the Province of Lapland for 1945, AMOPL, EIIe:1, OMA.

7. The Mannerheim League for Child Welfare also functioned as the department of child welfare of the Finnish Red Cross until 1950 when it became a fully independent organization. See A. Korppi-Tommola, *Terve lapsi – kansan huomen. Mannerheimin Lastensuojeliitto yhteiskunnan rakentajana 1920–1990* (Jyväskylä: Mannerheimin lastensuojeluliitto, 1990), p. 182; Sorvettula, *Johdatus suomalaiseen hoitotyön historiaan* (Jyväskylä: Gummerus, 1998), pp. 333–4; *Pohjois-Pohja* [newspaper], 12 April 1946; The Annual Report of the Public Health Nurse of the Province of Lapland for 1945 and 1946, AMOPL, EIIe:1, OMA.

8. *Pohjois-Pohja*, 12 April 1946; The Annual Report of the Public Health Nurse of the Province of Lapland for 1945 and 1946, AMOPL, EIIe:1, OMA.

9. Fabritius, 'Lapin piiriyhdistyksen toiminnasta', *Sairaanhoitajalehti* [Finnish Journal of Nursing], 11 (1948), p. 175.

10. Sorvettula, *Johdatus suomalaiseen hoitotyön historiaan*, pp. 220–1.

11. *Lapin Kansa* (newspaper), 24 November 1946; 'Lapin lapset – kovan työn kasvatit', *Vihuri*, 8 (1952), p. 7.

12. S. Wrede, 'Kenen neuvola? Kansanterveystyön "naisten huoneen" rakennuspuut', in I. Helén & M. Jauho, *Kansalaisuus ja kansanterveys* (Helsinki: Gaudemus, 2003), pp. 62, 78.

13. Fabritius, 'Lapin piiriyhdistyksen toiminnasta', pp. 172–5.
14. A. Bardy, 'Lapin synnytystupiin tutustumassa', *Kätilölehti* [Finnish Journal of Mid-wifery], 8 (1947), pp. 115–17, on p. 117.
15. 'Hoitotyön muistot', 3328–3333, held at the Suomalaisen Kirjallisuuden Seuran Kansanrunousarkisto (henceforth SKS/KRA) [The Folklore Archives of the Finnish Literature Society, Helsinki].
16. 'Hoitotyön muistot', 325–332, SKS/KRA.
17. 'Lääkintää ja potilaita', MV:K25/290, 52, 314, 61, 516, 721, 251, 198, 448; 784, 435; Story no. 8 in the collection 'Sairaana Lapissa'.
18. 'Hoitotyön muistot', 74.1998, Suomalaisen Kirjallisuuden Seuran Äänitearkisto (SKSÄ) [The recording archives of the Finnish Literature Society].
19. 'Hoitotyön muistot', 925–1081, SKS/KRA.
20. *Pohjois-Pohja*, 12 April 1946; Fabritius, 'Lapin piiriyhdistyksen toiminnasta', p. 177; The Annual Report of the Public Health Nurse of the Province of Lapland for 1945 and 1946, AMOPL, EIIe:1. OMA; *Suomen lääkärit 1946*, ed. G. Soininen and L. A. Kaprio (Helsinki: Suomen lääkäriliitto, 1947); *Suomen lääkärit 1952*, ed. P-E. Heikel (Helsinki: Suomen lääkäriliitto,1953); *Suomen lääkärit 1957*, ed. P-E. Heikel and A. Mikkola (Helsinki: Suomen lääkäriliitto, 1958); 'Hoitotyön muistot', 3328–3333, SKS/KRA.
21. H. Kamila, *Terveyssisar kinttupoluilla ja pitkospuilla* (Helsinki: Yliopistopaino, 2000), p. 32.
22. 'Kirje Ivalon aluesairaalan ylihoitajalle', 12 July 1949, Archives of the District Doctor of Inari and Utsjoki Ea:2, OMA; *Sairaanhoitajalehti*, 12 (1957), p. 418; 'Hoitotyön muistot', 74.1998, SKSÄ; Story no.12 in the collection 'Sairaana Lapissa'.
23. 'Hoitotyön muistot', 3328–3333, SKS/KRA.
24. 'Työntekijöiden luettelot Lapin läänin terveyssisarpiirissä 1942–1968', AMOPL, BIId:1, OMA; Story no. 8 in the collection 'Sairaana Lapissa'; Kamila, *Terveyssisar kinttupoluilla ja pitkospuilla*, p. 13.
25. 'Työntekijöiden luettelot Lapin läänin terveyssisarpiirissä 1942–1968', AMOPL, BIId:1, OMA.
26. See Suomen Matkailu, *Journal of the Finnish Tourist Association*, 1–3, 4 & 5 (1940), 3 (1941), 2 (1942), 1 and 2 (1943), 1 (1944), 2 (1946), 3 (1947), 2 & 4 (1948).
27. 'Lapin läänin neuvolat 1943, 1948–1970', Archives of the Medical Officer of the Province of Lapland BV:1; 'Lääninterveyssisar Elli-Kaarina Oittisen esitelmä "Työntekijätarve Lapissa"', Terveyssisarten opinto- ja neuvottelupäivät Rovaniemellä 19', 22 September 1951, AMOPL, DVa, OMA.
28. *Pohjois-Pohja*, 5 September 1946; SVT, XI:56, p. 48; SVT, XI:57, p. 24; SVT, XI:58, p. 20; SVT, XI:59, p. 35; SVT, XI:60, p. 5; SVT, XI:61, p. 41; SVT, 00:62, p. 91; The Annual Reports of the Public Health Nurse of the District of Kainuu in the Province of Oulu for 1950–9, held at the Archives of the Medical Officer of the Province of Oulu, Dc:9, OMA.
29. Junila, 'Sairaanhoito sota-ajoilta nykypäiviin', pp. 127–8.
30. 'Hoitotyön muistot', 370–414, SKS/KRA.
31. A. Punto, *Terveyssisarkoulutuksen ja terveyssisarten neuvontatoiminnan kehitys Suomessa 1912–1944* (Vaasa: Sairaanhoitajien koulutussäätiö, 1991), pp. 78–80, 95; Sorvettula, *Johdatus suomalaiseen hoitotyön historiaan*, pp. 334–6; Wrede, 'Kenen neuvola?', pp. 62–3.

32. Sorvettula, *Johdatus suomalaiseen hoitotyön historiaan*, pp. 220, 336; Wrede, 'Kenen neuvola?', p. 72.
33. The Annual Report of the Public Health Nurse of the Province of Lapland for 1945 and 1946, AMOPL, EIIe:1, OMA; Lapin läänin terveyshuollosta 1959, AMOPL, DV:b; Lääkintöhallituksen kirje, 17 May 1946, held at the Archives of the District Doctor of Inari and Utsjoki, Ea:2, OMA.
34. 'Hoitotyön muistot', 3328–3333, SKS/KRA.
35. 'Hoitotyön muistot', 325–32, SKS/KRA.
36. 'Taikauskoa ja uusia tapoja', *Terveydenhoitolehti* [The journal of health care], 6–7 (1953), p. 143; 'Neuvolaoloista', *Sairaanhoitajalehti*, 2 (1954), pp. 44–5; Apulaislääninlääkäri Aino Yliruokasen esitelmä 'Terveyssisaren osuus kotisairaanhoidossa Lapin läänissä' opintopäivillä, 12–13 September 1963, held at the Archives of the Medical Officer of the Province of Lapland, EIc:1, OMA.
37. 'Taikauskoa ja uusia tapoja', pp. 142–3.
38. Sorvettula, *Johdatus suomalaiseen hoitotyön historiaan*, pp. 340–1; The Annual Report of the Public Health Nurse of the Province of Lapland for 1964, 1967 and 1969, AMOPL, EIIe:1, OMA.
39. Wrede, 'Kenen neuvola?', pp. 72, 84; Junila, 'Sairaanhoito sota-ajoilta nykypäiviin', p. 179; 'Hoitotyön muistot', 74.1998, SKSÄ.
40. *Rovaniemi* (newspaper), 24 January 1947; M. Koskikallio, 'Välähdyksiä Lapin lasten oloista', *Lapsi ja nuoriso*, 9–10 (1948), pp. 203–4.
41. Pöytäkirja lääninterveyssisarien, -kätilöiden ja Mannerheimliiton terveyssisarien opinto- ja neuvottelupäiviltä Helsingissä, 21, 24 February 1949, AMOPL, EVe:1, OMA.
42. The Annual Report of the Public Health Nurse of the Province of Lapland for 1946, AMOPL, EIIe:1, OMA.
43. Lääninterveyssisar Elli-Kaarina Oittisen esitelmä 'Työntekijätarve Lapissa'. Terveyssisarten opinto- ja neuvottelupäivät Rovaniemellä, 19, 22 September 1951, AMOPL, DVa, OMA.
44. The Annual Report of the Public Health Nurse of the Province of Lapland for 1945 and 1946, AMOPL, EIIe:1, OMA.
45. 'Neuvolaoloista', p. 44; 'Hoitotyön muistot', 118 – 119.1999, SKSÄ.
46. *Rovaniemi*, 2 July 1952; 'Neuvolaoloista', p. 44; 'Muistio Lapin läänin kunnankätilöiden opinto- ja neuvottelupäiviltä', 23, 25 April 1957, AMOPL, EIc:1, OMA; Kamila, *Terveyssisar kinttupoluilla ja pitkospuilla*, pp. 21–2.
47. *Lapin Kansa* (newspaper), 13 August 1947, 28 September 1947; *Rovaniemi*, 20 March 1947; 'Neuvolaoloista', p. 43; 'Hoitotyön muistot', 2142–2233, SKS/KRA.
48. 'Hoitotyön muistot', 3328–3333, SKS/KRA.
49. 'Hoitotyön muistot', 326–332, SKS/KRA.
50. 'Pöytäkirja lääninterveyssisarien, -kätilöiden ja Mannerheimliiton terveyssisarien opinto- ja neuvottelupäivät Helsingissä', 21, 24 February 1949, AMOPL, EVe:1, OMA.
51. 'Hoitotyön muistot', 326–332, SKS/KRA.
52. 'Hoitotyön muistot', 118 –119.1999, SKSÄ; 2142–2233, SKS/KRA; Story no.12 in the collection 'Sairaana Lapissa'.
53. Story no. 12 in the collection 'Sairaana Lapissa'.
54. Story no. 6 in the collection 'Sairaana Lapissa'.
55. 'Hoitotyön muistot', 3328–3333, SKS/KRA.

56. Junila, 'Sairaanhoito sota-ajoilta nykypäiviin', p. 129; 'Apulaislääninlääkäri Aino Yliruokasen esitelmä "Terveyssisaren osuus kotisairaanhoidossa Lapin läänissä" opintopäivillä', 12, 13 September 1963, AMOPL, EIc:1, OMA.
57. 'Hoitotyön muistot', 3328–3333, SKS/KRA; The Annual Reports of the Public Health Nurse of the District of Kainuu in the Province of Oulu for1946, held at the Archives of the Medical Officer of the Province of Oulu, Dc:9, OMA.
58. 'Lapin läänin väestön yleinen terveydentila 1947', AMOPL, DV:b, OMA.
59. 'Lääkintää ja potilaita', MV:K29/208, 516; 'Apulaislääninlääkäri Aino Yliruokasen esitelmä "Terveyssisaren osuus kotisairaanhoidossa Lapin läänissä" opintopäivillä', 12–13 September 1963, AMOPL, EIc:1, OMA.
60. 'Hoitotyön muistot', 118–119.1999, SKSÄ.
61. Sorvettula, *Johdatus suomalaiseen hoitotyön historiaan*, pp. 336–7.
62. *Rovaniemi*, 24 January 1947; Koskikallio, 'Välähdyksiä Lapin lasten oloista', pp. 203–4.
63. 'Hoitotyön muistot', 118–119.1999, SKSÄ.
64. Kamila, *Terveyssisar kinttupoluilla ja pitkospuilla*, p. 27.
65. 'Taikauskoa ja uusia tapoja', p. 145; Kamila, *Terveyssisar kinttupoluilla ja pitkospuilla*, p. 27.
66. 'Hoitotyön muistot', 118.1999, SKSÄ.
67. Wrede, 'Kenen neuvola?', pp. 84–5.
68. Kamila, *Terveyssisar kinttupoluilla ja pitkospuilla*, p. 32.
69. 'Terveyssisartyöntutkimuksesta', *Sairaanhoitajalehti*, 3 (1954), p. 84; 'Hoitotyön muistot', 118–119.1999, SKSÄ.
70. A. Punto, *Terveyssisarkoulutuksen ja terveyssisarten neuvontatoiminnan kehitys Suomessa 1912–1944*, pp. 82–3.
71. 'Hoitotyön muistot', 326–332, SKS/KRA.
72. 'Lääkintää ja potilaita', MV:K25/251.
73. 'Taikauskoa ja uusia tapoja', pp. 142–3; SVT XI:56, pp. 52–3; Kamila, *Terveyssisar kinttupoluilla ja pitkospuilla*, p. 19; Junila, 'Sairaanhoito sota-ajoilta nykypäiviin', pp. 185–8; 'Lääkintää ja potilaita', MV:K25/448; 'Hoitotyön muistot', 925–1081, SKS/KRA; 118–19.1999, SKSÄ; The Annual Report of the Public Health Nurse of the Province of Lapland for 1945, AMOPL, EIIe:1, OMA; Apulaislääninlääkäri Aino Yliruokasen esitelmä 'Terveyssisaren osuus kotisairaanhoidossa Lapin läänissä' opintopäivillä, 12–13 September 1963, AMOPL, EIc:1, OMA.
74. 'Hoitotyön muistot', 908–924, SKS/KRA.
75. *Rovaniemi*, 24 January 1947; Bardy, 'Lapin synnytystupiin tutustumassa'; Koskikallio, 'Välähdyksiä Lapin lasten oloista', pp. 203 – 204; 'Arvio Lapin läänin tilasta vuonna 1961', AMOPL, DV:b. OMA; 'Hoitotytön muistot', 2142–2233, SKS/KRA.
76. 'Hoitotyön muistot', 118.1999, SKSÄ.
77. 'Hoitotyön muistot', 370–414, SKS/KRA.
78. 'Lääkintää ja potilaita', MV:K25/448.
79. Kamila, *Terveyssisar kinttupoluilla ja pitkospuilla*, p. 33.
80. Wrede, 'Kenen neuvola?', p. 73; 'Lääninlääkäri kirje Sodankylän kunnalle', 14 June 1947; 'Lääninlääkäri kirje lääkintöhallitukselle', 20 February 1948, AMOPL, DIV:1, OMA.
81. 'Arvio Lapin läänin tilasta vuonna 1961', AMOPL, DV:b, OMA.
82. Wrede, 'Kenen neuvola?', p. 66.
83. Sorvettula, *Johdatus suomalaiseen hoitotyön historiaan*, p. 220.
84. The Annual Report of the Public Health Nurse of the Province of Lapland for 1946, AMOPL, EIIe:1, OMA; 'Hoitotyön muistot', 118–119.1999, SKSÄ.

85. *Rovaniemi*, 15 January 1953; Laki 181/5.3.1948 kunnallisista terveyssisarista annetun lain muuttamisesta; The Annual Report of the Public Health Nurse of the Province of Lapland for 1946, AMOPL, EIIe:1, OMA; 'Hoitotyön muistot', 118.–199.1999, SKSÄ.
86. Sorvettula, *Johdatus suomalaiseen hoitotyön historiaan*, pp. 336–7.
87. 'Hoitotyön muistot', 370–414 ja 3328–3333, SKS/KRA; 118–119.1999, SKSÄ.
88. Wrede, 'Kenen neuvola?', pp. 85–6; SVT, XI, pp. 50–1, 56–7.
89. Junila, 'Sairaanhoito sota-ajoilta nykypäiviin', pp. 120–1.
90. *Rovaniemi*, 2 July 1952; 'Hoitotyön muistot', 370–414 ja 3328–3333, SKS/KRA.; 'Hoitotyön muistot', 118–119.1999, SKSÄ; The Annual Report of the Public Health Nurse of the Province of Lapland for 1968, AMOPL, EIIe:1, OMA.
91. 'Arvio Lapin läänin tilasta vuonna 1961', AMOPL, DV:b, OMA.
92. The Annual Report of the Public Health Nurse of the Province of Lapland for 1968, AMOPL, EIIe:1, OMA; 'Hoitotyön muistot', 370–414, SKS/KRA.
93. 'Lääkintöhallituksen kirje', 18 April 1947, Utsjoen kunnan kunnallislautakunnalle, Archives of the District Doctor of Inari and Utsjoki, OMA.
94. 'Lääninterveyssisari Elli-Kaarina Oittisen esitelmä terveyssisarten opinto- ja neuvottelupäivillä', 19–22 September 1951, Lapin lääninlääkärin arkisto DVa; The Annual Reports of the Public Health Nurses in Inari and Sevettijärvi for 1950 and 1951, Archives of the District Doctor of Inari and Utsjoki; Arvio Lapin läänin tilasta vuonna 1961, AMOPL, DV:b, OMA.
95. Terveyden- ja sairaanhoito Lapin läänissä 1953, 1959, 1961, AMOPL, DV:b; The Annual Report of the Public Health Nurse of the Province of Lapland for 1952, 1953, 1957, 1958, 1959, 1960 and 1962, AMOPL, EIIe:1, OMA.
96. Wrede, 'Kenen neuvola?' , pp. 76–7.
97. Fabritius, 'Lapin piiriyhdistyksen toiminnasta', p. 174.
98. The Annual Report of the Public Health Nurse of the Province of Lapland for 1946, AMOPL, EIIe:1, OMA.
99. 'Hoitotyön muistot', 3328–3333, SKS/KRA.
100. 'Lääkintää ja potilaita', MV:K25/16; The Annual Report of the Public Health Nurse of the Province of Lapland for 1946, AMOPL, EIIe:1, OMA; Lääninterveyssisari Elli-Kaarina Oittisen esitelmä 'Työntekijätarve Lapissa', Terveyssisarten opinto- ja neuvottelupäivät Rovaniemellä, 19–22 September 1951, AMOPL, DVa. OMA.
101. The Annual Report of the Public Health Nurse of the Province of Lapland for 1965, 1966 and 1967, AMOPL, EIIe:1, OMA.
102. See the discussion of D. Seers, 'What are We Trying to Measure', *Journal of Development Studies*, 8 (1972), pp. 21–36 in J. Othick, 'Development Indicators and the Historical Study of Human Welfare: Towards a New Perspective', *Journal of Economic History*, 43 (1983), pp. 63–4, 66–8.
103. Junila, 'Sairaanhoito sota-ajoilta nykypäiviin', pp. 133, 134–5, appendix 5.
104. 'Apulaislääninlääkäri Aino Yliruokasen esitelmä "Terveyssisaren osuus kotisairaanhoidossa Lapin läänissä" opintopäivillä', 12–13 September 1963, AMOPL, EIc:1, OMA.

INDEX

Milton Keynes UK
Ingram Content Group UK Ltd.
UKHW031144141024
449569UK00024B/1091